Statistics for
Epidemiology

CHAPMAN & HALL/CRC
Texts in Statistical Science Series

Series Editors
Chris Chatfield, *University of Bath, UK*
Martin Tanner, *Northwestern University, USA*
Jim Zidek, *University of British Columbia, Canada*

Analysis of Failure and Survival Data
Peter J. Smith

**The Analysis and Interpretation of
Multivariate Data for Social Scientists**
David J. Bartholomew, Fiona Steele,
Irini Moustaki, and Jane Galbraith

**The Analysis of Time Series —
An Introduction, Sixth Edition**
Chris Chatfield

**Applied Bayesian Forecasting and Time
Series Analysis**
A. Pole, M. West and J. Harrison

**Applied Nonparametric Statistical
Methods, Third Edition**
P. Sprent and N.C. Smeeton

**Applied Statistics — Handbook of
GENSTAT Analysis**
E.J. Snell and H. Simpson

**Applied Statistics — Principles and
Examples**
D.R. Cox and E.J. Snell

**Bayes and Empirical Bayes Methods for
Data Analysis, Second Edition**
Bradley P. Carlin and Thomas A. Louis

Bayesian Data Analysis, Second Edition
Andrew Gelman, John B. Carlin,
Hal S. Stern, and Donald B. Rubin

**Beyond ANOVA — Basics of Applied
Statistics**
R.G. Miller, Jr.

**Computer-Aided Multivariate Analysis,
Third Edition**
A.A. Afifi and V.A. Clark

A Course in Categorical Data Analysis
T. Leonard

A Course in Large Sample Theory
T.S. Ferguson

Data Driven Statistical Methods
P. Sprent

Decision Analysis — A Bayesian Approach
J.Q. Smith

**Elementary Applications of Probability
Theory, Second Edition**
H.C. Tuckwell

Elements of Simulation
B.J.T. Morgan

**Epidemiology — Study Design and
Data Analysis**
M. Woodward

Essential Statistics, Fourth Edition
D.A.G. Rees

A First Course in Linear Model Theory
Nalini Ravishanker and Dipak K. Dey

**Interpreting Data — A First Course
in Statistics**
A.J.B. Anderson

**An Introduction to Generalized
Linear Models, Second Edition**
A.J. Dobson

Introduction to Multivariate Analysis
C. Chatfield and A.J. Collins

**Introduction to Optimization Methods
and their Applications in Statistics**
B.S. Everitt

Large Sample Methods in Statistics
P.K. Sen and J. da Motta Singer

**Markov Chain Monte Carlo — Stochastic
Simulation for Bayesian Inference**
D. Gamerman

Mathematical Statistics
K. Knight

**Modeling and Analysis of Stochastic
Systems**
V. Kulkarni

Modelling Binary Data, Second Edition
D. Collett

Modelling Survival Data in Medical Research, Second Edition
D. Collett

Multivariate Analysis of Variance and Repeated Measures — A Practical Approach for Behavioural Scientists
D.J. Hand and C.C. Taylor

Multivariate Statistics — A Practical Approach
B. Flury and H. Riedwyl

Practical Data Analysis for Designed Experiments
B.S. Yandell

Practical Longitudinal Data Analysis
D.J. Hand and M. Crowder

Practical Statistics for Medical Research
D.G. Altman

Probability — Methods and Measurement
A. O'Hagan

Problem Solving — A Statistician's Guide, Second Edition
C. Chatfield

Randomization, Bootstrap and Monte Carlo Methods in Biology, Second Edition
B.F.J. Manly

Readings in Decision Analysis
S. French

Sampling Methodologies with Applications
Poduri S.R.S. Rao

Statistical Analysis of Reliability Data
M.J. Crowder, A.C. Kimber, T.J. Sweeting, and R.L. Smith

Statistical Methods for SPC and TQM
D. Bissell

Statistical Methods in Agriculture and Experimental Biology, Second Edition
R. Mead, R.N. Curnow, and A.M. Hasted

Statistical Process Control — Theory and Practice, Third Edition
G.B. Wetherill and D.W. Brown

Statistical Theory, Fourth Edition
B.W. Lindgren

Statistics for Accountants, Fourth Edition
S. Letchford

Statistics for Epidemiology
Nicholas P. Jewell

Statistics for Technology — A Course in Applied Statistics, Third Edition
C. Chatfield

Statistics in Engineering — A Practical Approach
A.V. Metcalfe

Statistics in Research and Development, Second Edition
R. Caulcutt

Survival Analysis Using S—Analysis of Time-to-Event Data
Mara Tableman and Jong Sung Kim

The Theory of Linear Models
B. Jørgensen

Statistics for Epidemiology

Nicholas P. Jewell

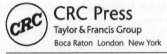

CRC Press
Taylor & Francis Group
Boca Raton London New York

CRC Press is an imprint of the
Taylor & Francis Group, an **informa** business
A CHAPMAN & HALL BOOK

Datasets and solutions to exercises can be downloaded at http://www.crcpress.com/e_products/downloads/.

Send correspondence to Nicholas P. Jewell, Division of Biostatistics, School of Public Health, 140 Warren Hall #7360, University of California, Berkeley, CA 94720, USA. Phone: 510-642-4627, Fax: 510-643-5163, e-mail: jewell@stat.berkeley.edu

Chapman & Hall/CRC
Taylor & Francis Group
6000 Broken Sound Parkway NW, Suite 300
Boca Raton, FL 33487-2742

© 2004 by Taylor and Francis Group, LLC
Chapman & Hall/CRC is an imprint of Taylor & Francis Group, an Informa business

No claim to original U.S. Government works

ISBN 13: 978-1-58488-433-0 (hbk)

**Visit the Taylor & Francis Web site at
http://www.taylorandfrancis.com**

**and the CRC Press Web site at
http://www.crcpress.com**

Library of Congress Cataloging-in-Publication Data

Statistics for epidemiology / by Nicholas P. Jewell.
    p. cm. — (Texts in statistical science series ; 58)
   Includes bibliographical references and index.
   ISBN 1-58488-433-9 (alk. paper)
    1. Epidemiology—Statistical methods. I. Jewell, Nicholas P., 1952- II. Texts in statistical science.

   RA652.2.M3S745 2003
   614.4′072′7—dc21   2003051458

Library of Congress Card Number 2003051458

To Debra and Britta, my very soul of life

Contents

1 Introduction   **1**
  1.1 Disease processes 1
  1.2 Statistical approaches to epidemiological data 2
      1.2.1 Study design 3
      1.2.2 Binary outcome data 4
  1.3 Causality 5
  1.4 Overview 5
      1.4.1 Caution: what is not covered 7
  1.5 Comments and further reading 7

2 Measures of Disease Occurrence   **9**
  2.1 Prevalence and incidence 9
  2.2 Disease rates 12
      2.2.1 The hazard function 13
  2.3 Comments and further reading 15
  2.4 Problems 16

3 The Role of Probability in Observational Studies   **19**
  3.1 Simple random samples 20
  3.2 Probability and the incidence proportion 21
  3.3 Inference based on an estimated probability 22
  3.4 Conditional probabilities 24
      3.4.1 Independence of two events 26
  3.5 Example of conditional probabilities—Berkson's bias 26
  3.6 Comments and further reading 28
  3.7 Problems 29

4 Measures of Disease–Exposure Association   **31**
  4.1 Relative risk 31
  4.2 Odds ratio 32
  4.3 The odds ratio as an approximation to the relative risk 33
  4.4 Symmetry of roles of disease and exposure in the odds ratio 34
  4.5 Relative hazard 35
  4.6 Excess risk 37
  4.7 Attributable risk 38

4.8   Comments and further reading   40
4.9   Problems   41

5 Study Designs   **43**
5.1   Population-based studies   45
      5.1.1   Example—mother's marital status and infant birthweight 46
5.2   Exposure-based sampling—cohort studies   47
5.3   Disease-based sampling—case-control studies   48
5.4   Key variants of the case-control design   50
      5.4.1   Risk-set sampling of controls   51
      5.4.2   Case-cohort studies   53
5.5   Comments and further reading   55
5.6   Problems   56

6 Assessing Significance in a 2 × 2 Table   **59**
6.1   Population-based designs   59
      6.1.1   Role of hypothesis tests and interpretation of p-values   61
6.2   Cohort designs   62
6.3   Case-control designs   64
      6.3.1   Comparison of the study designs   65
6.4   Comments and further reading   68
      6.4.1   Alternative formulations of the χ^2 test statistic   69
      6.4.2   When is the sample size too small to do a χ^2 test?   70
6.5   Problems   71

7 Estimation and Inference for Measures of Association   **73**
7.1   The odds ratio   73
      7.1.1   Sampling distribution of the odds ratio   74
      7.1.2   Confidence interval for the odds ratio   77
      7.1.3   Example—coffee drinking and pancreatic cancer   78
      7.1.4   Small sample adjustments for estimators of the odds ratio   79
7.2   The relative risk   81
      7.2.1   Example—coronary heart disease in the
              Western Collaborative Group Study   82
7.3   The excess risk   83
7.4   The attributable risk   84
7.5   Comments and further reading   85
      7.5.1   Measurement error or misclassification   86
7.6   Problems   90

**8 Causal Inference and Extraneous Factors: Confounding
    and Interaction**   **93**
8.1   Causal inference   94
      8.1.1   Counterfactuals   94
      8.1.2   Confounding variables   99

8.1.3   Control of confounding by stratification   100

8.2   Causal graphs   102

8.2.1   Assumptions in causal graphs   105

8.2.2   Causal graph associating childhood vaccination to
subsequent health condition   106

8.2.3   Using causal graphs to infer the presence of
confounding   107

8.3   Controlling confounding in causal graphs   109

8.3.1   Danger: controlling for colliders   109

8.3.2   Simple rules for using a causal graph to choose the
crucial confounders   111

8.4   Collapsibility over strata   112

8.5   Comments and further reading   116

8.6   Problems   119

9   Control of Extraneous Factors   **123**

9.1   Summary test of association in a series of 2×2 tables   123

9.1.1   The Cochran–Mantel–Haenszel test   125

9.1.2   Sample size issues and a historical note   128

9.2   Summary estimates and confidence intervals for the odds ratio,
adjusting for confounding factors   128

9.2.1   Woolf's method on the logarithm scale   129

9.2.2   The Mantel–Haenszel method   130

9.2.3   Example—the Western Collaborative Group Study: part 2 .   131

9.2.4   Example—coffee drinking and pancreatic cancer: part 2 . .   133

9.3   Summary estimates and confidence intervals for the relative risk,
adjusting for confounding factors   134

9.3.1   Example—the Western Collaborative Group Study: part 3 .   135

9.4   Summary estimates and confidence intervals for the excess risk,
adjusting for confounding factors   136

9.4.1   Example—the Western Collaborative Group Study: part 4 .   137

9.5   Further discussion of confounding   138

9.5.1   How do adjustments for confounding affect precision? . . .   138

9.5.2   An empirical approach to confounding   142

9.6   Comments and further reading   143

9.7   Problems   144

10 Interaction   **147**

10.1 Multiplicative and additive interaction   148

10.1.1 Multiplicative interaction   148

10.1.2 Additive interaction   149

10.2 Interaction and counterfactuals   150

10.3 Test of consistency of association across strata   152

10.3.1 The Woolf method   153

10.3.2 Alternative tests of homogeneity   155

10.3.3 Example—the Western Collaborative Group Study: part 5 .   156
10.3.4 The power of the test for homogeneity   158
10.4 Example of extreme interaction   160
10.5 Comments and further reading   161
10.6 Problems   162

11 Exposures at Several Discrete Levels   165
11.1 Overall test of association   165
11.2 Example—coffee drinking and pancreatic cancer: part 3   167
11.3 A test for trend in risk   167
    11.3.1 Qualitatively ordered exposure variables   169
    11.3.2 Goodness of fit and nonlinear trends in risk   170
11.4 Example—the Western Collaborative Group Study: part 6   171
11.5 Example—coffee drinking and pancreatic cancer: part 4   173
11.6 Adjustment for confounding, exact tests, and interaction   175
11.7 Comments and further reading   176
11.8 Problems   176

12 Regression Models Relating Exposure to Disease   179
12.1 Some introductory regression models   181
    12.1.1 The linear model   181
    12.1.2 Pros and cons of the linear model   183
12.2 The log linear model   183
12.3 The probit model   184
12.4 The simple logistic regression model   186
    12.4.1 Interpretation of logistic regression parameters   187
12.5 Simple examples of the models with a binary exposure   188
12.6 Multiple logistic regression model   190
    12.6.1 The use of indicator variables for discrete exposures   191
12.7 Comments and further reading   196
12.8 Problems   196

13 Estimation of Logistic Regression Model Parameters   199
13.1 The likelihood function   199
    13.1.1 The likelihood function based on a logistic regression model   201
    13.1.2 Properties of the log likelihood function and the maximum
           likelihood estimate   204
    13.1.3 Null hypotheses that specify more than one regression
           coefficient   206
13.2 Example—the Western Collaborative Group Study: part 7   207
13.3 Logistic regression with case-control data   212
13.4 Example—coffee drinking and pancreatic cancer: part 5   215
13.5 Comments and further reading   218
13.6 Problems   219

14 Confounding and Interaction within Logistic Regression Models   **221**

14.1 Assessment of confounding using logistic regression models . . . 221

    14.1.1 Example—the Western Collaborative Group Study: part 8 . 223

14.2 Introducing interaction into the multiple logistic regression
model 225

14.3 Example—coffee drinking and pancreatic cancer: part 6 227

14.4 Example—the Western Collaborative Group Study: part 9 230

14.5 Collinearity and centering variables 230

    14.5.1 Centering independent variables 233

    14.5.2 Fitting quadratic models 233

14.6 Restrictions on effective use of maximum likelihood techniques . . 235

14.7 Comments and further reading 236

    14.7.1 Measurement error 237

    14.7.2 Missing data 237

14.8 Problems 240

**15 Goodness of Fit Tests for Logistic Regression
Models and Model Building**   **243**

15.1 Choosing the scale of an exposure variable 243

    15.1.1 Using ordered categories to select exposure scale 244

    15.1.2 Alternative strategies 245

15.2 Model building 246

15.3 Goodness of fit 250

    15.3.1 The Hosmer–Lemeshow test 252

15.4 Comments and further reading 254

15.5 Problems 255

16 Matched Studies   **257**

16.1 Frequency matching 257

16.2 Pair matching 258

    16.2.1 Mantel–Haenszel techniques applied to
pair-matched data 262

    16.2.2 Small sample adjustment for odds ratio estimator 264

16.3 Example—pregnancy and spontaneous abortion in relation to
coronary heart disease in women 264

16.4 Confounding and interaction effects 265

    16.4.1 Assessing interaction effects of matching variables 265

    16.4.2 Possible confounding and interactive effects due to
nonmatching variables 266

16.5 The logistic regression model for matched data 269

    16.5.1 Example—pregnancy and spontaneous abortion in
relation to coronary heart disease in women: part 2 271

16.6 Example—the effect of birth order on respiratory distress
syndrome in twins 274

16.7 Comments and further reading 276

      16.7.1 When can we break the match? 277
      16.7.2 Final thoughts on matching 278
  16.8 Problems 279

17 Alternatives and Extensions to the Logistic Regression Model   **285**
  17.1 Flexible regression model 285
  17.2 Beyond binary outcomes and independent observations 289
  17.3 Introducing general risk factors into formulation of the relative
      hazard—the Cox model 290
  17.4 Fitting the Cox regression model 293
  17.5 When does time at risk confound an exposure–disease relationship? 295
      17.5.1 Time-dependent exposures 296
      17.5.2 Differential loss to follow-up 296
  17.6 Comments and further reading 297
  17.7 Problems 298

18 Epilogue: The Examples   **301**

References   **303**

Glossary of Common Terms and Abbreviations   **311**

Index   **319**

Acknowledgments

The material in this book has grown out of a graduate course in statistical methods for epidemiology that I have taught for more than 20 years in the School of Public Health at Berkeley. I wish to express my appreciation for the extraordinary students that I have met through these classes, with whom I have had the privilege of sharing and learning simultaneously. My thanks also go to Richard Brand, who first suggested my teaching this material, and to Steve Selvin, a lifelong friend and colleague, who has contributed enormously both through countless discussions and as my local S-Plus expert. The material on causal inference depended heavily on many helpful conversations with Mark van der Laan. Several colleagues, especially Alan Hubbard, Madukhar Pai, and Myfanwy Callahan, have selflessly assisted by reading parts or all of the material, diligently pointing out many errors in style or substance. I am forever grateful to Bonnie Hutchings, who prepared the earliest versions of handouts of some of this material long before a book was ever conceived of, and who has been a constant source of support throughout. I also owe a debt of gratitude to Kate Robertus for her incisive advice on writing issues throughout the text.

Finally, my enjoyment of this project was immeasurably enhanced by the love and support of my wife, Debra, and our daughter, Britta. Their presence is hidden in every page of this work, representing the true gift of life.

CHAPTER 1

Introduction

In this book we describe the collection and analysis of data that speak to relationships between the occurrence of diseases and various descriptive characteristics of individuals in a population. Specifically, we want to understand whether and how differences in individuals might explain patterns of disease distribution across a population. For most of the material, I focus on chronic diseases, the etiologic processes of which are only partially understood compared with those of many infectious diseases. Characteristics related to an individual's risk of disease will include (1) basic measures (such as age and sex), (2) specific risk exposures (such as smoking and alcohol consumption), and (3) behavioral descriptors (including educational or socioeconomic status, behavior indicators, and the like). Superficially, we want to shed light on the "black box" that takes "inputs"—risk factors such as exposures, behaviors, genetic descriptors—and turns them into the "output," some aspect of disease occurrence.

1.1 Disease processes

Let us begin by briefly describing a general schematic for a disease process that provides a context for many statistical issues we will cover. Figure 1.1, an adapted version of Figure 2.1 in Kleinbaum et al. (1982), illustrates a very simplistic view of the evolution of a disease in an individual.

Note the three distinct stages of the disease process: *induction, promotion*, and *expression*. The etiologic process essentially begins with the onset of the first cause of the resulting disease; for many chronic diseases, this may occur at birth or during fetal development. The end of the promotion period is often associated with a clinical diagnosis. Since we rarely observe the exact moment when a disease "begins," induction and promotion are often considered as a single phase. This period, from the start of the etiologic process until the appearance of clinical symptoms, is often called the *latency period* of the disease. Using AIDS as an example, we can define the start of the process as exposure to the infectious agent, HIV. Disease begins with the event of an individual's infection; clinical symptoms appear around the onset and diagnosis of AIDS, with the expression of the disease being represented by progression toward the outcome, often death. In this case, the induction period is thought to be extremely short in time and is essentially undetectable; promotion and expression can both take a considerable length of time.

Epidemiological study of this disease process focuses on the following questions:

- Which factors are associated with the induction, promotion, and expression of a disease? These *risk factors* are also known as *explanatory variables, predictors,*

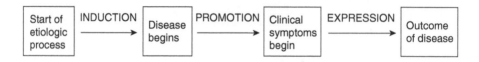

Figure 1.1 *Schematic of disease evolution.*

covariates, independent variables, and *exposure variables*. We will use such terms interchangeably as the context of our discussion changes.

- In addition, are certain factors (not necessarily the same ones) associated with the duration of the induction, promotion, and expression periods?

For example, exposure to the tubercule bacillus is known to be necessary (but not sufficient) for the induction of tuberculosis. Less is known about factors affecting promotion and expression of the disease. However, malnutrition is a risk factor associated with both these stages. As another example, consider coronary heart disease. Here, we can postulate risk factors for each of the three stages; for instance, dietary factors may be associated with induction, high blood pressure with promotion, and age and sex with expression. This example illustrates how simplistic Figure 1.1 is in that the development of coronary heart disease is a continuous process, with no obvious distinct stages. Note that factors may be associated with the outcome of a stage without affecting the duration of the stage. On the other hand, medical treatments often lengthen the duration of the expression of a chronic disease without necessarily altering the eventual outcome.

Disease intervention is, of course, an important mechanism to prevent the onset and development of diseases in populations. Note that intervention strategies may be extremely different depending on whether they are targeted to prevent induction, promotion, or expression. Most public health interventions focus on induction and promotion, whereas clinical treatment is designed to alter the expression or final stage of a disease.

1.2 Statistical approaches to epidemiological data

Rarely is individual information on disease status and possible risk factors available for an entire population. We must be content with only having such data for some fraction of our population of interest, and with using statistical tools both to elucidate the selection of individuals to study in detail (sampling) and to analyze data collected through a particular study. Issues of study design and analysis are crucial because we wish to use sample data to most effectively make applicable statements about the larger population from which a sample is drawn. Second, since accurate data collection is often expensive and time-consuming, we want to ensure that we make the best use of available resources. Analysis of sample data from epidemiological studies presents many statistical challenges since the outcome of interest—disease status—is usually binary. This book is intended to extend familiar statistical approaches for continuous outcome data—for example, population mean comparisons and regression—to the binary outcome context.

1.2.1 Study design

A wide variety of techniques can be used to generate data on the relationship between explanatory factors and a putative outcome variable. I mention briefly only three broad classes of study designs used to investigate these questions, namely, (1) *experimental studies*, (2) *quasi-experimental studies*, and (3) *observational studies*. The crucial feature of an experimental study is the investigator's ability to manipulate the factor of interest while maintaining control of other extraneous factors. Even if the latter is not possible, control of the primary risk factor allows its randomization across individual units of observation, thereby limiting the impact of uncontrolled influences on the outcome. Randomized clinical trials are a type of experimental study in which the main factor of interest, treatment type, is under the control of the investigator and is randomly assigned to patients suffering from a specific disease; other influencing factors, such as disease severity, age, and sex of the patient, are not directly controlled.

Quasi-experimental studies share some features of an experimental study but differ on the key point of randomization. Although groups may appear to differ only in their level of the risk factor of interest, these groups are not formed by random assignment of this factor. For example, comparison of accident fatality rates in states before and after the enactment of seat-belt laws provides a quasi-experimental look at related safety effects. However, the interpretation of the data is compromised to some extent by other changes that may have occurred in similar time periods (did drivers increase their highway speeds once seat belts were required?). A more subtle example involved an Austrian study of the efficacy of the PSA (prostate specific antigen) test in reducing mortality from prostate cancer; investigators determined that, within 5 years, the death rate from prostate cancer declined 42% below expected levels in the Austrian state, Tirol, the only state in the country that offered free PSA screening. Again, comparisons with other areas in the country are compromised by the possibility there are other health-related differences between different states other than the one of interest. Many *ecologic* studies share similar vulnerabilities. The absence of randomization, together with the inability to control the exposure of interest and related factors, make this kind of study less desirable for establishing a causal relationship between a risk factor and an outcome.

Finally, observational studies are fundamentally based on sampling populations with subsequent measurement of the various factors of interest. In these cases, there is not even the advantage of a naturally occurring experiment that changed risk factors in a convenient manner. Later in the book we will focus on several examples including studies of the risk of coronary heart disease where primary risk factors, including smoking, cholesterol levels, blood pressure, and pregnancy history, are neither under the control of the investigator nor usually subject to any form of quasi-experiment. Another example considers the role of coffee consumption on the incidence of pancreatic cancer, again a situation where study participants self-select their exposure categories.

In this book, we focus on the design and analysis of observational epidemiological studies. This is because, at least in human populations, it is simply not ethical to randomly assign risk factors to individuals. Although many of the analytic techniques are immediately applicable and useful in randomized studies, we spend a considerable amount of effort dealing with additional complications that arise because of the absence of randomization.

1.2.2 Binary outcome data

In studying the relationship between two variables, it is most effective to have refined measures of both the explanatory and the outcome variables. Happily, substantial progress is now being made on more refined assessment of the "quantity" of disease present for many major diseases, allowing a sophisticated statistical examination of the role of an exposure in producing given levels of disease. On the other hand, with many diseases, we are still unable to accurately quantify the amount of disease beyond its presence or absence. That is, we are limited to a simple binary indicator of whether an individual is diseased or not.

Similarly, in mortality studies, while death is a measurable event, the level and quality of health of surviving individuals are notoriously elusive, thus limiting an investigator use of the binary outcome, alive or not. For this reason, we focus on statistical techniques designed for a binary outcome variable. On the other hand, we allow the possibility that risk factors come in all possible forms, varying from binary (e.g., sex), to unordered discrete (e.g., ethnicity), to ordered discrete (e.g., coffee consumption in cups per day), to continuous (e.g., infant birthweight). However, we assume that risk factors or exposures have a fixed value and therefore do not vary over time (although composite values of time-varying measurements, such as cumulative number of cigarette pack-years smoked, are acceptable). Methods to accommodate exposures that change over time, in the context of longitudinal data, provide attractive extensions to the ideas of this book and, in particular, permit a more effective examination of the causal effects of a risk factor. We briefly touch on this again in Chapter 17, and also refer to Jewell and Hubbard (to appear) for an extensive discussion of this topic.

Statistical methodology for binary outcome data is applicable to a wide variety of other kinds of data. Some examples from economics, demography, and other social sciences and public health fields are listed in Table 1.1. In these examples, the nature of a risk factor may also be quite different from traditional disease risk factors.

Table 1.1 *Examples of binary outcomes and associated risk factors*

Binary Outcome	Possible Risk Factors
Use/no use of mental health services in calendar year 2003	Cost of mental health visit, sex
Moved/did not move in calendar year 2003	Family size, family income
Low/normal birthweight of newborn	Health insurance status of mother
Vote Democrat/Republican in 2004 election	Parental past voting pattern
Correct/incorrect diagnosis of patient	Place and type of medical training
Covered/not covered by health insurance	Place of birth, marital status

1.3 Causality

As noted in Section 1.2.1, observational studies preclude, by definition, the randomization of key factors that influence the outcome of interest. This may severely limit our ability to attribute a *causal* pathway between a risk factor and an outcome variable. In fact, selecting from among the three design strategies discussed in Section 1.2.1 hinges on their ability to support a causal interpretation of the relationship of a risk factor or intervention with a disease outcome. This said, most statistical methods are not based, *a priori*, on a causal frame of thinking but are designed for studying associations between factors not necessarily distinguished as input "risk factors" or outcome; for example, the association between eye color and hair color. In short, observational data alone can rarely be used to separate a causal from a noncausal explanation. Nevertheless, we are keenly interested in establishing causal relationships from observational studies; fortunately, even without randomization, there are simple assumptions, together with statistical aspects of the data, that shed light on a putative causal association. In Chapter 8, we introduce much recent work in this regard, including the use of counterfactuals and causal graphs. As noted above, longitudinal observational studies provide greater possibilities for examining causal relationships.

1.4 Overview

Our goal is to introduce current statistical techniques used to collect and analyze binary outcome data (sometimes referred to as *categorical data*) taken from epidemiological studies. The first 11 chapters set the context of these ideas and cover simple methods for preliminary data analysis. Further chapters cover regression models that can be used for the same data. Chapter 16 discusses the special design technique known as *matching* and describes the particular analytic methods appropriate for matched data.

I assume that readers are familiar with basic ideas from a first course in statistics including random variables and their properties (in particular, expectation and variance), sampling, population parameters, and estimation of a population mean and proportion. Of particular importance is the concept of the sampling distribution of a sample estimator that underpins the ideas of interval estimation (confidence intervals) and hypothesis testing (including Type I and Type II errors, p-values, and power). I further anticipate that readers have previously encountered hypothesis tests to compare population means and proportions (for example, the various t-tests and, at least, the one degree of freedom χ^2 test). Familiarity with the binomial, normal, and χ^2 distributions is expected, and experience with the techniques associated with multiple linear regression, while not essential, will make Chapters 12 to 15 much easier to follow. Moore and McCabe (1998) provides an excellent source to review these topics. While mathematical proofs are eschewed throughout, some algebra is used where it can bolster insight and intuition. Fear not, however. Readers are not assumed to have knowledge of techniques that use calculus. The overall goal here is to give some basic driving lessons, not to get under the hood and tinker with the mechanics of the internal combustion engine!

Regression models, found in the second half of the book, can be used to incorporate the simpler analyses from earlier chapters. Some readers may be tempted to jump directly to these methods, arguing that the earlier stratification methods are really only of historical interest. My view is that basic tabulations with related analyses are important not only to develop a general basis for understanding more complex regression models, but also for gaining a sense of what a particular data set is "saying" before launching a full-scale regression analysis.

I want to say a few words here about developing a personal philosophy about data analysis. Although statistical methodology has an inevitable feel of mathematics, it is more than simply the application of a set of mathematical rules and recipes. In fact, having the perfect recipe is a wonderful advantage, but it does not guarantee a perfect meal. It is crucial that each data analyst construct his own "artistic" principles that can be applied when unraveling the meaning of data. Asking the right questions and having a deep understanding of the context in which a study is designed and implemented are, of course, terrific help as you begin a data analysis. But some general feel for numbers and how to manipulate and illustrate them will also bear considerable fruit. For instance, a sense for the appropriate level in precision in numerical quantities is a valuable tool. As a rough rule of thumb, I do not pay attention to discrepancies between two quantities that are less than 10% of their size. This is not useful in some contexts—knowing a telephone number to within 10% does not get you too far—but in epidemiological studies, this level of difference is often much less than the size of random, let alone other systematic, error. Focusing on such comparisons in the presence of substantial imprecision is putting the priority in the wrong place; it is my statistical version of "don't sweat the small stuff!" Each reader needs a personal style in deciding how best to approach and report a data analysis project. Many other statistical rules of thumb can be found in van Belle (2002), which includes an entire section on epidemiology.

As a brief add-on to the last paragraph, results of data analyses in this book are frequently given as numerical quantities to the second or third decimal place. This is to allow the reader to reconstruct numerical computations and is not meant to reflect how these quantities should be reported in publications or other forms of dissemination.

This book uses a case study approach to illustrate the statistical ideas in ever-expanding generality. Three primary examples are used: the Western Collaborative Group Study of risk factors for coronary heart disease in men (Rosenman et al., 1975), a case-control study of coffee drinking and pancreatic cancer (MacMahon et al., 1981), and a matched pair case-control study of pregnancy and spontaneous abortion in relation to coronary heart disease in women (Winkelstein et al., 1958). There is nothing particular to these choices; most similar examples would be equally effective pedagogically. Because of the use of case studies, the book is intended to be read through chapter by chapter. While much can be gleaned by a quick glance at an isolated chapter, the material is deliberately constructed so that each chapter builds on the previous material.

Analyzing the same examples repeatedly allows us to see the impact of increasingly complex statistical models on our interpretation and understanding of a single data set. The disadvantage is that readers may not be interested in the specific topics covered in these examples and prefer to see the generality of the methods in the context of a wide range of health issues. Therefore, as you follow the ideas, I encourage you to bring an epidemiological "sketchbook" in which you can apply the ideas to studies of immediate interest, and in which you can note down questions—and perhaps some answers—that arise from your reading of the epidemiological literature. How did an investigator sample a population? How did they measure exposure? How did they deal with other relevant factors? Was matching involved? How were the risk factors coded in a regression model? What assumptions did these choices involve? How is uncertainty reported? What other issues might affect the accuracy of the results? Has causality been addressed effectively?

This is an appropriate time to emphasize that, like most skills, statistical under-standing is gained by "doing" rather than "talking." At the end of each chapter, a set of questions is posed to provide readers an opportunity to apply some of the ideas conveyed during the chapter. To return to the analogy above, these assignments give us a chance to take the car out for a spin after each lesson! They should help you dif-ferentiate which points you understand from those you might like to review or explore further. They also give illustrative examples that expand on ideas from the chapter.

1.4.1 Caution: what is not covered

The material in this book is loosely based on a one-semester class of interest to be-ginning graduate students in epidemiology and related fields. As such, the choice of topics is personal and limited. Inevitably, there is much more to implementing, ana-lyzing, and interpreting observational studies than covered here. We spend little or no time on the conceptual underpinnings of epidemiological thinking or on crucial com-ponents of many field investigations, including disease registries, public databases, questionnaire design, data collection, and design techniques. Rothman and Greenland (1998) provides a superb introduction to many of these topics.

There are also many additional statistical topics that are not explored in this book. We will not spend time on the appropriate interpretation of p-values, confidence in-tervals, and power. The Bayesian approach to statistical inference, though particularly appealing with regard to interpretation of parameter uncertainty, is not discussed here. Nor will we delve much into such issues as the impact of measurement error and miss-ing data, standardization, sample size planning, selection bias, repeated observations, survival analysis, spatial or genetic epidemiology, meta-analysis, or longitudinal stud-ies. At the end of each chapter, we include a section on further reading that provides extensions to the basic ideas.

1.5 Comments and further reading

The material in this book has been influenced by three excellent books on the analysis of epidemiological data: Fleiss (1981), Breslow and Day (1980), and Rothman and Greenland (1998). Fleiss (1981) covers the material through Chapter 9, but does not include any discussion of regression models. Breslow and Day (1980) is a beautifully written account of all the methods we discuss, albeit targeted at the analysis of case-control studies. The statistical level is higher and assumes a familiarity with likelihood methods and the theory thereof. Rothman and Greenland (1998) provides an overview of epidemiological methods extending far beyond the territory visited here, but spends less time on the development and underpinnings of the statistical side of the subject.

Hosmer and Lemeshow (2000) discusses in detail the logistic regression model, but does not include simpler stratification analysis techniques. Collett (2002) is at a similarly high level, and both books approach the material for a general rather than epidemiological application. Schlesselman (1982) has considerably more material on other aspects of epidemiological studies, but a slimmer account of the analysis techniques that are the primary focus here. Kleinbaum et al. (1982) covers all the topics we consider and more, and is encyclopedic in its treatment of some of these ideas. In addition to the above books, more advanced topics can be found in Selvin (1996) and Breslow and Day (1987). Two recent books on similar topics are Woodward (1999) and Newman (2001).

A plethora of statistical packages exist that analyze epidemiological data using methods described in this book. Some of these, including SAS®, SPSS®, GLIM®, and BMDP®, are well known and contain many statistical techniques not covered here; other programs, such as EGRET®, are more tailored to epidemiological data. Collett (2002) contains a brief comparison of most of these packages. A free software package, Epi Info 2000, is currently available online from the Centers for Disease Control. In this book, all data analyses were performed using STATA® or S-Plus®. All data sets used in the text and in chapter questions are available online at http://www.crcpress.com/e_products/downloads/.

I love teaching this material, and whenever I do, I take some quiet time at the beginning of the term to remind myself about what lies beneath the numbers and the formulae. Many of the studies I use as examples, and many of the epidemiological studies I have had the privilege of being a part of, investigate diseases that are truly devastating. Making a contribution, however small, to understanding these human conditions is at the core of every epidemiological investigation. As a statistician, it is easy to be immersed in the numbers churned up by data and the tantalizing implications from their interpetation. But behind every data point there is a human story, there is a family, and there is suffering. To remind myself of this, I try to tap into this human aspect of our endeavor each time I teach. One ritual I have followed in recent years is to either read or watch the Pulitzer prize-winning play, *Wit* by Margaret Edson (or *W;t: a Play*, the punctuation being key to the subject matter). A video/DVD version of the film starring Emma Thompson is widely available. The play gives forceful insight to a cancer patient enrolled in a clinical trial, with the bonus of touching on the exquisite poetry of John Donne.

CHAPTER 2

Measures of Disease Occurrence

A prerequisite in studying the relationship between a risk factor and disease outcome is the ability to produce quantitative measures of both input and output factors. That is, we need to quantify both an individual's exposure to a variety of factors and his level of disease.

Exposure measurement depends substantially on the nature of the exposure and its role in the disease in question. For the purposes of this book, we assume that accurate exposure or risk factor measurements are available for all study individuals. See Section 2.3 for literature on exposure assessment. On the other hand, though fine levels of an outcome variable enhance the understanding of disease and exposure associations, most disease outcomes—and all here—are represented as binary; quantifying a continuous level of disease can involve invasive methods and therefore might be impractical or unethical in human studies. As a consequence, epidemiologists are often reduced to assessing an outcome as disease present or absent. As with risk factors, we assume that accurate binary measurements are available for the disease of interest. Underlying this approach is the simplistic assumption that a disease occurs at a single point of time, so that before this time the disease is not present, and subsequently it is. Disease in exposed and unexposed subgroups of a population is usually measured over an interval of time so that disease occurrences can be observed. This allows for a variety of definitions of the amount of disease in subgroups.

In light of these introductory comments, it is important to note that error in measurement of either exposure or disease or both will compromise the statistical techniques we develop. If such errors are present, this effect must be addressed for us to retain a valid assessment of the disease–exposure relationship. Fortunately, substantial advances have been made in this area and, although beyond the scope of this book, we point out available literature when possible.

2.1 Prevalence and incidence

Disease prevalence and incidence both represent proportions of a population determined to be diseased at certain times. Before we give informal definitions, note that the time scale used in either measurement must be defined carefully before calculation of either quantity. Time could be defined as (1) the age of an individual, (2) the time from exposure to a specific risk factor, (3) calendar time, or (4) time from diagnosis. In some applications, a different kind of time scale might be preferred to chronological time; for example, in infectious disease studies, a useful "time" scale is often defined in terms of the number of discrete contacts with an infectious agent or person.

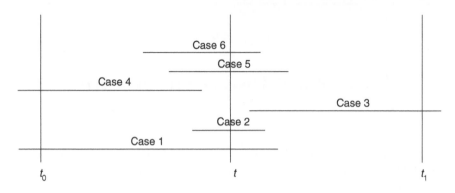

Figure 2.1 *Schematic illustrating calculation of an incidence proportion and point prevalence. Six cases of disease in a population of, say, 100 individuals are represented. Lines represent the duration of disease.*

The *point prevalence* of a disease is the proportion of a defined population at risk for the disease that is affected by it at a specified *point* on the time scale. *Interval prevalence*, or *period prevalence*, is the proportion of the population at risk affected at any point in an interval of time.

The *incidence proportion* is the proportion of a defined population, all of whom are at risk for the disease at the beginning of a specified time interval, who become new cases of the disease before the end of the interval. Since this quantity includes all individuals who become cases over the entire interval, it is sometimes referred to as the *cumulative incidence proportion*. To be "at risk" can mean that an individual has previously been unaffected by the disease, or that susceptibility has been regained after previously contracting the disease and recovering (e.g., as with the common cold to which no sufferer becomes fully immune). There are situations where certain individuals cannot be affected by a disease, e.g., women cannot develop prostate cancer, and so are never at risk.

Figure 2.1 demonstrates schematically the calculation of the incidence proportion and point prevalence in a contrived example of a population of 100 individuals, 6 of whom become cases of a disease during the time period from t_0 to t_1. Using data from the figure, the point prevalence at time t is either 4/100 or 4/99, depending on whether case 4 is considered to be at risk of the disease at t or not, respectively. The incidence proportion in the interval $[t_0, t_1]$ is 4/98, since cases 1 and 4 are not at risk for the disease at the beginning of the interval. This simple scenario reflects that calculations of disease occurrence vary according to definitions of who is "at risk"; take care to compute these quantities according to the appropriate definition!

Neither prevalence (or interval prevalence) nor an incidence proportion carries any units—they are all proportions, sometimes expressed as percentages, that must lie between 0 and 1. The simplest use of these measures of disease occurrence is their comparison across subgroups that have experienced different levels of exposure. For example, one might compare the prevalence of lung cancer among adult males who have smoked at any point in their lives against adult males who have never smoked.

Table 2.1 *Prevalence and incidence data (proportions) on CHD in males*

	Incidence (10 year)		Prevalence	
Cholesterol	CHD	No CHD	CHD	No CHD
High	85 (75%)	462 (47%)	38 (54%)	371 (52%)
Low	28 (25%)	516 (53%)	33 (46%)	347 (48%)

Source: Friedman et al. (1966).

The principal disadvantage with the use of prevalence measures to investigate the etiology of a disease is that they depend not only on initiation, but also on the duration of disease. That is, a population might have a low disease prevalence when (1) the disease rarely occurs or (2) it occurs with higher frequency, but affected individuals stay diseased for only a short period of time (either because of recovery or death). This complicates the role of risk factors, because duration may be influenced by many factors (such as medical treatment) that are unrelated to those that cause the disease in the first place. In addition, risk factors may change during the risk interval and so may assume different values at various times. Thus, prevalence difference across subgroups of a population is often difficult to interpret.

These points are well illustrated by coronary heart disease (CHD), from which a significant proportion of cases has high early mortality. Data (from the Framingham Heart Study, Friedman et al., 1966) relating levels of cholesterol and CHD for men aged 30 to 59 years are shown in Table 2.1. Here, incidence data refer to a group of men, initially free of CHD, whose cholesterol was measured at the beginning of a 10-year follow-up period, during which incident cases of CHD were counted. Cholesterol levels were categorized into four quartiles ("high" and "low" in the table refer to the highest and lowest quartiles). Soon we will discuss methods of analyzing such data with regard to the issue of whether, and by how much, the higher cholesterol group suffers from an elevated risk for CHD. Yet even without analysis, it is immediately clear from the incidence data that there is a substantially larger fraction of CHD cases in the high cholesterol group as compared with the low cholesterol group. This is not apparent in the prevalence data, where cholesterol and CHD measurements were taken at the *end* of the 10-year monitoring period. This discrepancy in the two results might then arise if high cholesterol is associated only with those CHD cases who suffered rapid mortality (dying before the end of the interval) and thus were not included in the prevalence analysis. An alternative explanation is that surviving CHD patients modified their cholesterol levels after becoming incident cases so that their levels at the end of the follow-up period became more similar to the levels of the CHD-free men. (The latter possibility is supported by a more detailed analysis of the Framingham data [Friedman et al., 1966].) This example illustrates the dangers of using prevalence data in attempts to establish a causal association between an exposure and initiation of a disease.

While the statistical methods introduced apply equally to prevalence and incidence data, for most of the discussion and examples we focus on incidence proportions. Why? Because if causality is of prime concern, it is almost always necessary to use incidence, rather than prevalence, as a measure of disease occurrence.

2.2 Disease rates

Before leaving this brief introduction to disease occurrence measures, it is worth broadening the discussion to introduce the concept of a *rate*. If the time interval underlying the definition of an incidence proportion is long, an incidence proportion may be less useful if, for some groups, cases tend to occur much earlier in the interval than for other groups. First, this suggests the need for a careful choice of an appropriate interval when incidence proportions will be calculated. It does not make sense to use an age interval from 0 to 100 years if we want to compare mortality patterns. In the other direction, a study of food-related infections showed much higher mortality effects when individuals were followed for a full year after the time of infection, rather than considering only acute effects (Helms et al., 2003; see Question 5.5). Second, with long risk intervals, there may be substantial variation in risk over the entire period; for example, a person over 65 is at a far higher risk of mortality than an 8 year old. Third, when time periods are long, not all individuals may be at risk over the entire interval; when studying breast cancer incidence, for example, it may make little sense to include premenarcheal childhood years as time at risk. To address the latter point, rates that adjust for the amount of time at risk during the interval are often used.

Specifically, the (average) *incidence rate* of a disease over a specified time interval is given by the number of new cases during the interval divided by the total amount of time at risk for the disease accumulated by the entire population over the same interval. The units of a rate are thus $(\text{time})^{-1}$.

Figure 2.2 is a schematic that allows comparison of the computation of a point prevalence, incidence proportion, and incidence rate. If we assume that the disease under study is chronic in the sense that there is no recovery, then

- The point prevalence at $t = 0$ is $0/5 = 0$; at $t = 5$ it is $1/2 = 0.5$.
- The incidence proportion from $t = 0$ to $t = 5$ is $3/5 = 0.6$.
- The incidence rate from $t = 0$ to $t = 5$ is $3/(5 + 1 + 4 + 3 + 1) = 3/14 = 0.21$ cases per year.

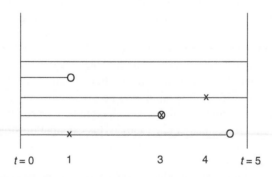

Figure 2.2 *Schematic illustrating calculation of an incidence proportion, point prevalence, and incidence rate. Population of 5; the symbols represent:* O, *death;* x, *incident case of disease. Here, lines represent time alive.*

If population size and follow-up periods are unknown or unclear, or if multiple events per person are possible, the above incidence rate is often referred to by 0.21 cases per person-year, or 0.21 cases per person per year. Note that if the disease is acute, with the property that individuals who recover immediately return to being at risk, then the incidence rate would be $3/(5 + 1 + 5 + 3 + 4.5) = 0.16$ cases per year.

2.2.1 The hazard function

Returning to the second point of the first paragraph of Section 2.2, if either the population at risk or the incidence rate changes substantially over the relevant time interval, it will be necessary to consider shorter subintervals in order to capture such phenomena. That is, both an incidence proportion—a cumulative measure—and an incidence rate—an average rate over the risk interval—are summary measures for the entire interval and, as such, conceal within-interval dynamics. Unfortunately, limited population size often means that there will be very few incident events in short intervals of time. Nevertheless, in sufficiently large populations it may be possible to measure the incidence rate over smaller and smaller intervals. Such calculations yield a plot of incidence rate against, say, the midpoint of the associated interval on which the incidence rate was based. This kind of graph displays the changes in the incidence rate over time, much as a plot of speed against time might track the progress of an automobile during a journey. This process, in the hypothetical limit of ever smaller intervals, yields the *hazard function, h(t)*, which is thus seen as an instantaneous incidence rate.

Figure 2.3 shows a schematic of the hazard function for human mortality among males, where the time variable is age. Looking at mortality hazard curves may feel morbid, particularly for those who find themselves on the right-hand incline of Figure 2.3. However, it is worth remembering that, as Kafka said, the point of life is that it ends. (I have always thought that one of the fundamental points of *The Odyssey* is also that the finiteness of life is what imbues it with meaning.) In Figure 2.3, the hazard function, plotted on the Y-axis, yields the mortality rate (per year) associated with a given age. In a population of size N, a simple interpretation of the hazard function at time t is that the number of cases expected in a *small and unit* increment of time is $Nh(t)$. For example, if $N = 1000$ and the hazard function at time t is 0.005/year, then we roughly anticipate five cases in a year including the time t somewhere near the middle.

If we write the time interval of interest as $[0, T]$, there is a direct link between the hazard function, $h(t)$, for $0 \le t \le T$, and the incidence proportion over the interval $[0, t]$, which we denote by $I(t)$. (We assume here that an incident case is no longer at risk after contracting the disease, and that this is the only way in which an individual ceases to be at risk.) The plot of $I(t)$ against t is necessarily increasing—as $I(t)$ measures the cumulative incidence proportion up to time t—and therefore has a positive slope at any time t. It can be shown that

$$h(t) = \frac{dI(t)}{dt} \Big/ (1 - I(t)), \qquad (2.1)$$

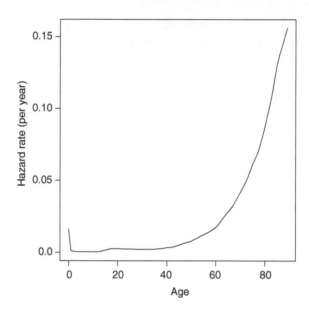

Figure 2.3 *Schematic of the hazard function based on mortality data for Caucasian males in California in 1980.*

where $dI(t)/dt$ represents the slope of $I(t)$ at time t. Note that the term in the denominator accounts for the proportion of the population still at risk at time t. This relationship provides a way of uniquely linking any cumulative incidence proportion, $I(t)$, to a specific hazard function $h(t)$, and vice versa. Oops—I promised no calculus, but this correspondence between incidence and hazard is worth an exception.

When the outcome of interest is disease mortality rather than incidence, we often look at the function $S(t)$, simply defined by $S(t) = 1 - I(t)$. Known as the *survival function*, $S(t)$ measures the proportion of the population that remains alive at age t. Figure 2.4 shows the survival function corresponding to the hazard function of Figure 2.3.

One of the appeals of hazard functions is the ease with which we can extract dynamic information from a plot of the hazard function, as compared with corresponding plots of the incidence proportion or survival function, against time. Even though Figures 2.3 and 2.4 contain exactly the same information, the hazard curve is considerably easier to interpret. For example, to quantify mortality risk for males in the first year of life, observe in Figure 2.3 that this level is roughly the same (yearly) mortality risk faced by 60-year-old males. This comparison is extremely difficult to extract from Figure 2.4. Note the steep increase in mortality risk after age 65 that restricts the chance of extremely long lives. While this phenomenon can be inferred from the graph of the survival function, where a drop occurs at later ages, specific comparative information regarding mortality risks is harder to interpret from the survival function than the hazard function.

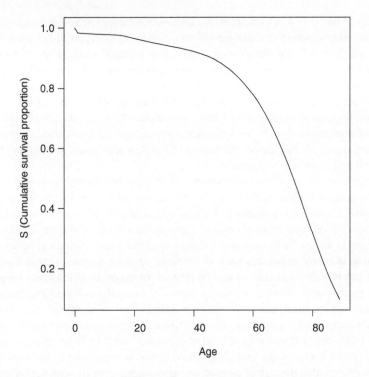

Figure 2.4 *Schematic of the survival function (for mortality) among Caucasian males in California in 1980.*

2.3 Comments and further reading

While we do not consider this matter further here, we cannot understate the value of effective assessment of exposures. With common exposures—tobacco and alcohol consumption, for example—there is substantial literature from previous studies that provides detailed methodology and examples. As a general guide, we refer to the book by Armstrong et al. (1994). In the context of a specific example, there is an excellent discussion of many relevant issues regarding the measurement of exposure to environmental tobacco smoke in the National Academy report on this topic (National Research Council, 1986). For nutritional exposures, the book by Willett (1998) is very useful. Some exposures can only be exactly measured by complex and perhaps invasive procedures so that accurate proxies must often be sought. There is considerable expertise available in questionnaire design and interview procedures to assess exposures determined from a survey instrument.

The definition of an incidence proportion assumes a closed population; that is, no new individuals at risk are allowed to enter after the beginning of the risk period. That this restriction is relaxed when using an incidence rate is one of its principal advantages. That said, it is still possible to estimate an incidence proportion when some individuals enter the population during the risk period. This is sometimes referred to as delayed entry, or left truncation. An important example arises in studying risks during pregnancy, where the risk period commences at conception but most study participants do not begin observation until a first prenatal visit, or at least until a pregnancy has been detected. The issue of closed vs. open populations will be echoed in our description of study designs in Chapter 5. Variations in incidence rate by exposure are not studied further here, but such data are widely available. The use of Poisson regression models is an attractive approach to rate data, corresponding to the use of regression models for incidence proportions that are studied extensively in Chapters 12 to 15. For further discussion of Poisson regression, see Selvin (1996) and Jewell and Hubbard (to appear).

Comments about exposure assessment are extremely cursory here, and fail to demonstrate many of the complex issues in classifying individuals into differing levels of exposure. Exposure information is often only available in proxy form including self-reports, job records, biomarkers, and ecologic data. To some degree, all exposure measurements are likely to only approximate levels of a true biological agent, even when using standard exposures such as smoking or alcohol consumption histories. Often, it may be valuable to obtain several proxies for exposure, at least on a subgroup of study participants. Validation information—for example, using an expensive but highly accurate exposure measurement on a subset of sampled individuals—is often a crucial component for estimating the properties of exposure measurement error.

In the following chapters, a fixed level of exposure over time is generally assumed. However, chronic exposures, including smoking and occupational conditions, accumulate, implying that the risk of disease will also change over the risk period for this if for no other reason. Composite summary measure of exposure, like pack-years of smoking, should be used with extreme care, since they only capture average exposure information. For example, in studies of fetal alcohol syndrome, episodes of binge drinking may be a better measure of alcohol exposure than average consumption measures. Exposures that vary over time are often best handled with hazard models, which are examined in Chapter 17, where regression methods for incidence proportions are briefly compared with those commonly used for hazard functions. Further details on estimation and inference for hazard functions, and related topics in survival analysis, can be found in Kalbfleisch and Prentice (2002), Hosmer and Lemeshow (1999), and Collett (1994).

2.4 Problems

Question 2.1

Figure 2.5 illustrates observations on 20 individuals in a study of a disease D. The time (i.e., horizontal) axis represents age. The lines, one per individual, represent the evolution of follow-up: the left endpoint signifies the start of follow-up, while the right endpoint indicates the age at onset of D, except in cases of withdrawal for a variety of reasons, marked with a W. For example, the first subject (the lowest line above the axis) started follow-up before his 50th birthday and developed the disease early in his 67th year, i.e., just after turning 66. Calculate for this small population:

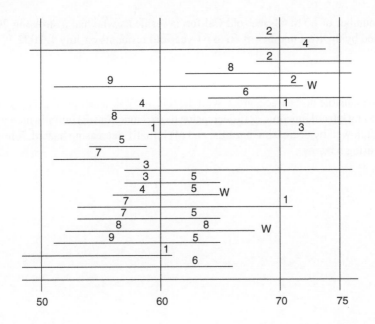

Figure 2.5 *Schematic showing onset of disease at different ages in population of 20 individuals.*

1. The incidence proportion for the disease between the ages 50 and 60 (assume that the disease is chronic so that those with the disease are no longer at risk).

2. The incidence proportion between (a) ages 60 and 70, and (b) ages 70 and 75.

3. The incidence rate for the intervals (a) ages 50 to 60, (b) ages 60 to 70, and (c) ages 70 to 75.

Comment on your findings.

Question 2.2

Indicate whether each of the following computed indices should be considered a point prevalence, incidence proportion, or an incidence rate:

1. The number of children born with congenital heart defects in California in 2002, divided by the number of live births in California in 2002.

2. The number of persons who resided in California on January 1, 2002, and who developed colon cancer during 2002, divided by the total number of disease-free persons who were California residents on January 1, 2002.

3. The number of myopic children under the age of 13 in California on July 1, 2002, divided by the total number of children under the age of 13 in California on July 1, 2002.

4. The number of 60 to 64-year-old California residents who had a stroke in 2002, divided by the total number of 60 to 64-year-old residents on July 1, 2002.

Question 2.3

Describe plausible disease scenarios, with the relevant risk intervals, that suggest (1) an increasing hazard function; (2) a decreasing hazard function; (3) initially increasing hazard, followed by decreasing hazards; and (4) initially decreasing hazard, followed by increasing hazards.

CHAPTER 3

The Role of Probability in Observational Studies

As indicated in the introduction, it is assumed that the reader is familiar with the basic concepts and manipulation of probability and random variables. In this chapter the use of probabilistic terms in epidemiological studies is discussed and some of the simplest ideas are reviewed. One goal of this chapter is to understand what we mean by the risk or probability of a disease. Does it mean that there is some random mechanism inside our bodies that decides our fate? While rejecting that notion, the source of randomness in epidemiological investigations, a key step in quantifying the uncertainty inherent in such studies, is also described. First, some basic understanding of the language and meaning surrounding a probability statement is needed.

Two fundamental components necessary to describe the probability of an occurrence are (1) a *random experiment* and (2) an *event*. A random experiment is a process that produces an identifiable *outcome* not predetermined by the investigator. An event is a collection of one or more distinct possible outcomes. An event occurs if the observed outcome of the experiment is contained in the collection of outcomes defining the event. For example, in tossing a coin one usually thinks of only two possible outcomes—"heads" and "tails." Here, the experiment is the toss of a coin, and an event might be that the coin comes up heads. A qualitatively similar situation occurs with the administration of a specific therapy to a patient with a certain disease. Here, the random experiment is application of treatment, with possible events being "patient cured" or "patient not cured"; note that "not cured" may be defined in terms of combinations of simple outcomes such as blood pressure reading or amount of inflammation.

What is the probability that a tossed coin comes up heads? More generally, in any random experiment, what is the probability of a particular event? Denote the probability of an event A by the term $P(A)$. A heuristic definition of probability is as follows:

> In a random experiment, $P(A)$ is the fraction of times the event A occurs when the experiment is repeated many times, independently and under the exact same conditions.

To express this formally, suppose that a random experiment is conducted K times and the event A occurs in K_A of the total K experiments. As K grows larger and larger, the fraction of times the event A occurs, K_A/K, approaches a constant value. This value is $P(A)$, the probability of A occurring in a single experiment.

3.1 Simple random samples

A special type of random experiment is illustrated by the sampling of individuals from a population that contains N distinct members; suppose you wish to select a sample of n of these members for study. If the members are selected "at random," then the sample is called a *random sample*. As in a random experiment, "at random" implies that although the investigator sets the sample size n, she does not predetermine which n individuals will be selected. An important kind of random sample is the *simple random sample*, with the defining property that every possible sample of size n is equally likely to occur, or is chosen with equal probability. Consider the special case $n = 1$; since there are N members in the population, there are exactly N samples of size $n = 1$, each distinct sample containing one particular member of the population. Since the N samples are equally likely to occur, each sample occurs with probability $1/N$. We refer to this below as random selection of a population member.

To fix the ideas, consider a simple example. Imagine drawing a single card at random from a deck of 52 playing cards. We wish to take a simple random sample of size $n = 1$ (one card) from a population of $N = 52$ cards. Now we wish to calculate the probability of a particular event associated with our sample of one card. For example, suppose we wish to compute the probability that the selected card is from the clubs suit—we will call this event A. Using the "long run" definition of probability above, we must ask what fraction of K independent simple random samples of size $n = 1$ will produce the outcome of a club card. Since each possible sample (i.e., each of 52 distinct playing cards) is equally likely, on each repetition we would expect each distinct playing card to appear $1/52$ times in the long run, and thus $K/52$ times in K draws. Thirteen of the cards are clubs; therefore, in the long run, the fraction of K draws that produces a club will be $((K/52) \times 13)/K = 1/4$. This is thus the probability of drawing a club on a single draw.

It is useful to draw a general conclusion from this example. When randomly selecting a single object from a group of N objects, the probability that the selected object has a specific attribute (event A) is just the fraction of the N objects that possess this attribute. We illustrate this by referring to Table 3.1, which lists the vital status of all births in the United States in 1991, 1 year after date of birth, and categorized by the marital status of the mother at the birth and the birthweight of the infant. By convention, low birthweight is defined as a birth where the newborn's weight is less than 2500 g. Suppose our "experiment" is now the random selection of one of these 4,111,059 births. If the event A refers to the death of this randomly chosen infant within 1 year of its birth, then $P(A)$ is the probability of an infant death in 1991 and is the fraction of the entire population of infants who died in their first year. The population information derived from the table shows this probability to be $35,496/4,111,059 = 0.0086$, or 8.6 deaths per 1000 births. Similarly, if event B refers to a randomly chosen infant with normal birthweight, then $P(B)$ is the probability of a normal birthweight infant, given by the fraction of all births that have a normal birthweight, that is, $3,818,736/4,111,059 = 0.93$.

Table 3.1 *1991 U.S. infant mortality by mother's marital status and by birthweight*

	Mother's Marital Status		
Infant Mortality	Unmarried	Married	Total
Death	16,712	18,784	35,496
Live at 1 year	1,197,142	2,878,421	4,075,563
Total	1,213,854	2,897,205	4,111,059

	Birthweight		
Infant Mortality	Low Birthweight	Normal Birthweight	Total
Death	21,054	14,442	35,496
Live at 1 year	271,269	3,804,294	4,075,563
Total	292,323	3,818,736	4,111,059

Source: National Center for Health Statistics.

3.2 Probability and the incidence proportion

These simple probability ideas can now be related to the measures of disease occurrence introduced in Chapter 2. As a general example, consider the incidence proportion for a disease. Each member of the relevant population at risk can be assigned the characteristic of being an incident case in the specified time interval—underlying the definition of the incidence proportion—or not. For convenience, label this characteristic D. By definition, the incidence proportion is just the fraction of the population that possesses characteristic D. As discussed in the last section, if an individual is drawn at random from the population, the probability that he will have characteristic D is $P(D)$, that is, the incidence proportion. Thus the incidence proportion can either be interpreted as the proportion of a population who are incident cases in a given interval, or, equivalently, as the probability that a randomly chosen member of the population is an incident case.

Similar statements can, of course, be made if the characteristic D is defined in terms of a point or interval prevalence. However, for reasons discussed in Section 2.1, we assume that D refers to incident cases so that $P(D)$ is interpreted as an incidence proportion. Further, we also use the terminology $P(E)$ to reflect the probability that a randomly selected individual from a population has an exposure characteristic labeled by E; E might be a qualitative or quantitative measure of exposure or risk. For convenience, with any event A, we sometimes use $\bar{A}$ to refer to the event "not A."

In the following, we often use the terms $P(D)$ and $P(E)$ to refer explicitly or implicitly to the "probability of being diseased" or the "probability of being exposed." This language may mislead us into thinking that a disease or exposure characteristic is random in some sense. In fact, as seen above, the randomness referred to in these statements arises entirely from random sampling from a population. Although it is possible that some disease outcomes or exposures might have a purely random component (for example, a disease dependent on the occurrence of a specific random mutation, or exposure to certain kinds of infectious agents), this issue is not germane to our treatment that is based solely on the randomness introduced by taking a random sample from a population. Specifically, in the following chapters, techniques are introduced that use sample quantities to convey information on population characteristics of interest such as $P(D)$ and $P(E)$, the incidence proportion and population exposure frequency, respectively. Understanding random sampling allows quantification of the uncertainty inherent in using samples to infer properties of a larger population from which the sample is drawn. The next section briefly reviews estimation of the probability of a single characteristic based on a simple random sample and the uncertainty that is inherent to this sample estimator.

3.3 Inference based on an estimated probability

We rarely observe an entire population with appropriate risk factor information as was possible for the infant mortality data reported in Table 3.1. Our strategy will instead be to draw a (simple) random sample that will provide us with appropriate data we can use to estimate a population probability or proportion. We now briefly review methods to compute confidence intervals, one approach to describing the uncertainty associated with a sample estimator of a population proportion.

Suppose we are interested in estimating $P(A)$, the probability of a characteristic A in a given population. We draw a simple random sample of size n from the population and let n_A denote the number in the sample with characteristic A. For simplicity, write $p = P(A)$. An obvious estimate of p is $\hat{p} = n_A/n$, the proportion of the sample that shares characteristic A. From sample to sample, the random number n_A follows a binomial sampling distribution with expectation (or mean) given by np and variance by $np(1 - p)$. This is just the sampling distribution of n_A. (In fact, this statement assumes we sample with replacement or that the population is infinitely large; this is only an issue when n represents a substantial fraction of the population.) For a sufficiently large n, this sampling distribution is close to a Normal distribution with the same expectation and variance. Thus, $\hat{p}$ has an approximate Normal sampling distribution with expectation p and variance $p(1 - p)/n$. The variance can be estimated from our sample data by plugging in $\hat{p}$ for p, yielding an approximate Normal sampling distribution with expectation p and variance $\hat{p}(1 - \hat{p})/n$.

We now have a simple method to construct a confidence interval for the unknown proportion p using our sample. Using the approximate sampling distribution,

$$P\left(\frac{|\hat{p} - p|}{\sqrt{\frac{\hat{p}(1-\hat{p})}{n}}} \leq z_{1-\frac{\alpha}{2}} \right) = P\left(-z_{1-\frac{\alpha}{2}} \leq \frac{\hat{p} - p}{\sqrt{\frac{\hat{p}(1-\hat{p})}{n}}} \leq z_{1-\frac{\alpha}{2}} \right) = 1 - \alpha, \quad (3.1)$$

where $z_{1-\frac{\alpha}{2}}$ is the $[1 - (\alpha/2)]$th percentile of a standard Normal distribution. Note that the probability in this statement refers to the experiment of repeatedly drawing simple random samples of size n from the population.

Equation 3.1 tells us, probabilistically, how close the sample estimate $\hat{p}$ is to the unknown p. But knowing this is the same as knowing how close p is to $\hat{p}$. That is,

$$\frac{|\hat{p} - p|}{\sqrt{\frac{\hat{p}(1-\hat{p})}{n}}} \leq z_{1-\frac{\alpha}{2}} \quad \text{if and only if} \quad \hat{p} - z_{1-\frac{\alpha}{2}}\sqrt{\frac{\hat{p}(1-\hat{p})}{n}} \leq p \leq \hat{p} + z_{1-\frac{\alpha}{2}}\sqrt{\frac{\hat{p}(1-\hat{p})}{n}}.$$

(3.2)

The right-hand part of Equation 3.2 then defines a $100(1 - \alpha)\%$ confidence interval for p.

For example, suppose that a random sample of 100 births were drawn from infants born in the U.S. in 1991 (see the data in Table 3.1) and that in this sample 35 births were associated with unmarried mothers. The estimate of the population proportion of unmarried mothers is then $35/100 = 0.35$, and a simple 95% confidence interval is

$$0.35 \pm \left(1.96\sqrt{\frac{0.35 \times 0.65}{100}}\right) = 0.35 \pm (1.96\sqrt{0.002275}) = (0.257, 0.443).$$

We might report this 95% confidence interval as (0.26, 0.44); it clearly makes no sense to report results to the third decimal place here, given the size of the margin of error ± 0.093. (The true population probability from Table 3.1 is 0.295.) Recall that the correct interpretation of this (random) confidence interval is that it includes the true value, 0.295, with probability 0.95.

A popular interpretation of a confidence interval is that it provides values for the unknown population proportion that are "compatible" with the observed data. But we must be careful not to fall into the trap of assuming that each value in the interval is equally compatible. In the example of the above paragraph, the value $p = 0.35$ is much more plausible than the value $p = 0.44$, although the data do not allow us to definitively rule out that possibility. Computing (and reporting) two confidence intervals with differing confidence coefficients reinforces this point. Using the data above, the 90% confidence interval for the population proportion of unmarried mothers is

$$0.35 \pm \left(1.644\sqrt{\frac{0.35 \times 0.65}{100}}\right) = (0.272, 0.428).$$

We have been using an approximate sampling distribution for $\hat{p}$ that is effective when the sample size n is "large." Most investigators agree that the question of whether n is large enough can be checked by ensuring that $n\hat{p}$ and $n(1 - \hat{p})$ are both greater than 5. In cases with sample sizes that fail to meet this criterion, the estimate $\hat{p}$ is very close to either 0 or 1, and the confidence interval described in Equation 3.2 should not be used. The simple technique for small or large $\hat{p}$ is not useful, particularly since it introduces the possibility that the confidence interval will stretch beyond the allowable interval (from 0 to 1) for a probability or proportion. Never fear—there exists a more complex method for calculating the interval that avoids this concern. Return for a moment to the approximate sampling distribution for $\hat{p}$ given by the Normal distribution with expectation p and variance $p(1 - p)/n$. Without trying to estimate the variance, this approximation tells us that

$$P\left(\frac{|\hat{p} - p|}{\sqrt{\frac{p(1-p)}{n}}} \leq z_{1-\frac{\alpha}{2}}\right) = 1 - \alpha.$$

Now

$$\frac{|\hat{p} - p|}{\sqrt{\frac{p(1-p)}{n}}} \leq z_{1-\frac{\alpha}{2}} \quad \text{if and only if} \quad (\hat{p} - p)^2 \leq z_{1-\frac{\alpha}{2}}^2 \times \frac{p(1 - p)}{n}.$$

The second inequality of this statement is quadratic in p and can be solved to yield

$$\frac{2n\hat{p} + z_{1-\frac{\alpha}{2}}^2 - z_{1-\frac{\alpha}{2}}\sqrt{z_{1-\frac{\alpha}{2}}^2 + 4n\hat{p}(1 - \hat{p})}}{2\left(n + z_{1-\frac{\alpha}{2}}^2\right)} \leq p$$

$$\leq \frac{2n\hat{p} + z_{1-\frac{\alpha}{2}}^2 + z_{1-\frac{\alpha}{2}}\sqrt{z_{1-\frac{\alpha}{2}}^2 + 4n\hat{p}(1 - \hat{p})}}{2\left(n + z_{1-\frac{\alpha}{2}}^2\right)}.$$

This provides a more accurate confidence interval for p that can never give values outside of the range [0, 1]. For the example used above to illustrate the simple method, with $\hat{p} = 35/100$ and $n = 100$, we have 95% confidence limits given by

$$\frac{(2 \times 100 \times 0.35) + 1.96^2 \pm 1.96\sqrt{1.96^2 + (4 \times 100 \times 0.35 \times 0.65)}}{2(100 + 1.96^2)}$$

$$= (0.264, 0.447),$$

or, more appropriately, (0.26, 0.45) to two decimal places. In this calculation, since n is reasonably large and $\hat{p}$ is well away from zero, the complex method gives almost exactly the same result as the simpler technique.

Both methods have the advantage that they can be computed without specialized software. Many computing packages now offer the possibility of an exact confidence interval for p, that is, one that uses the exact sampling distribution of $\hat{p}$, based on the binomial distribution. STATA® calculates for our example an exact 95% confidence interval corresponding to the estimate $\hat{p} = 35/100$ as (0.257, 0.452), or (0.26, 0.45) to two decimal places. The exact interval is always more effective than the simple method when p is close to 0 or 1, or when the sample size, n, is small, and precludes the need for a continuity correction that improves the Normal approximation to the binomial (see Moore and McCabe, 2002, Chapter 5.1).

3.4 Conditional probabilities

In Section 3.1, we discussed the probability that a randomly selected infant dies within 1 year of birth for the population summarized in Table 3.1. But what if we want to know this probability for important subgroups of the population? For example, we may be interested in the probability of death within a year of birth for a birth associated with an unmarried mother or for a normal birthweight infant. In either case we are looking for the *conditional probability* of the outcome. The conditional probability of event A given that event B occurs, notated as $P(A|B)$, is the "long run" fraction of times that event A occurs, the fraction being restricted to *only those events for which B occurs*. For example, if A represents the event that a randomly chosen infant dies within a year from birth, and B is the event that a randomly chosen birth is associated with an unmarried mother, then $P(A|B)$ is the probability that a randomly chosen infant dies within a year of birth, given that this infant has an unmarried mother.

To further understand a conditional probability, let us look at the heuristic definition of probability given earlier in this chapter. To compute the conditional probability $P(A|B)$, we have to calculate the long run fraction of times the event A occurs among events where B occurs. In a series of K independent equivalent experiments, let $K_{A\&B}$ denote the number of those experiments where both events A and B occur. Then the fraction of times that event A occurs amongst those experiments where event B occurs is just $K_{A\&B}/K_B$. Thus, the conditional probability $P(A|B)$ is the "long run" value of $K_{A\&B}/K_B$. But, by dividing both the numerator and denominator of this expression by K, we see that this conditional probability is given by the "long run" value of $K_{A\&B}/K$ divided by the "long run" value of K_B/K. More simply,

$$P(A|B) = \frac{P(A\&B)}{P(B)}. \tag{3.3}$$

An immediate consequence of this expression is a formulation for the probability of the composite event, A and B:

$$P(A\&B) = P(A|B) \times P(B). \tag{3.4}$$

By reversing the roles of the events A and B, it follows that $P(B|A) = P(A\&B)/P(A)$ so that

$$P(A\&B) = P(B|A) \times P(A).$$

For conditional probabilities, there is an analog to the statement in Section 3.1 that when we select a random member of a population, the probability that the selected individual has a specific characteristic is just the population proportion of individuals with this attribute. That is, for a randomly selected individual, the conditional probability that an individual has characteristic A, given that they possess characteristic B, namely, $P(A|B)$, is the population proportion of individuals with characteristic A amongst the subpopulation who have characteristic B. Thus, referring to Table 3.1, if A denotes death in the first year and B denotes having an unmarried mother, then $P(A|B)$, the conditional probability of death within a year of birth, given the infant has an unmarried mother, is $16,712/(1,197,142 + 16,712) = 16,712/1,213,854 = 0.014$, or 14 per 1,000 births. This conditional probability can also be calculated using Equation 3.3: since $P(A\&B) = 16,712/4,111,059 = 0.0041$, and $P(B) = 1,213,854/4,111,059 = 0.295$, we derive $P(A|B) = 0.0041/0.295 = 0.014$.

It is important to note that the conditional probability of $A|B$ is quite different from that of $B|A$. If A is infant death within the first year and now B is a normal birthweight infant, then the conditional probability $P(A|B)$ is the probability of an infant death, given that the child has normal birthweight. From Table 3.1, this conditional probability is given by $14,442/3,818,736 = 0.0038$, or 3.8 deaths per 1,000 births. On the other hand, the conditional probability $P(B|A)$ is the probability that an infant had normal birthweight, given that the infant died within 1 year from birth. Again, the data in Table 3.1 show that this conditional probability is $14{,}442/35{,}496 = 0.41$. These two conditional probabilities are quite different.

3.4.1 Independence of two events

A natural consequence of looking at the conditional probability of an infant death within a year of birth, given that the mother is unmarried, is to examine the same conditional probability for married mothers. Many questions then follow: Are these two conditional probabilities the same in this population? If not, how different are they? The two conditional probabilities $P(A|B)$ and $P(A|\bar{B})$ being identical reflects that the frequency of event A is not affected by whether B occurs or not. When A and B are defined in terms of the presence of certain characteristics, this can be interpreted as the two characteristics being unrelated. Formally, an event A is said to occur independently of an event B if the conditional probability $P(A|B)$ is equal to the (unconditional) probability of the event A, $P(A)$. That is, event A is independent of event B if and only if $P(A|B) = P(A|\bar{B}) = P(A)$. In other words, an infant's 1-year mortality is independent of its mother's marital status if the probability of an infant's death in the first year of life is not influenced by the marital status of the mother.

From Equation 3.4, it follows that if the event A is independent of event B, then $P(A\&B) = P(A) \times P(B)$. On the other hand, if $P(A\&B) = P(A) \times P(B)$, then, from the expression for the conditional probability $P(A|B)$, we have $P(A|B) = P(A\&B)/P(B) = [P(A) \times P(B)]/P(B) = P(A)$, so that the event A is independent of event B. Also, by reversing the roles of the events A and B, we can see that the event B is independent of event A if and only if the event A is independent of event B. Hence, events A and B are independent if and only if $P(A\&B) = P(A) \times P(B)$. For infant mortality and a mother's mortality status, recall that $P(\text{infant death}) = 0.0086$ and $P(\text{unmarried mother}) = 0.295$. If these two characteristics were independent, then $P(\text{unmarried mother and infant death}) = 0.0086 \times 0.295 = 0.0025$. In fact, Table 3.1 yields $P(\text{unmarried mother and infant death}) = 16{,}712/4{,}111{,}059 = 0.0041$. In this population, therefore, the two characteristics are clearly not independent. Here, the two characteristics, unmarried mother and infant death, occur together much more frequently than would be predicted if they were independent.

Finally, we note some other useful identities. First, if the events A and B are independent, $P(A \text{ or } B) = P(A) + P(B) - (P(A) \times P(B))$. Second, for any two events A and B, $P(A) = P(A|B)P(B) + P(A|\bar{B})P(\bar{B})$. Third, again for any two events A and B, $P(A|B) = P(B|A)P(A)/P(B)$; this relationship is known as *Bayes' formula* and allows us to link the probabilities of the two distinct events $A|B$ and $B|A$. These identities follow directly from the definitions of probability and conditional probability.

3.5 Example of conditional probabilities—Berkson's bias

In the earlier part of the last century it was believed that a possible cause or promoter of diabetes was a condition known as cholecystitis, or inflammation of the gall bladder. At one point, some physicians were removing the gall bladder as a treatment for diabetes. Berkson (1946) considered whether hospital or clinic records

Table 3.2 *Cholecystitis and diabetes in hypothetical hospital records using refractive error as reference group*

		Diabetes	Refractive Error	
Cholecystitis	C	626	9,504	10,130
	not C	6,693	192,060	198,753
	Total	7,319	201,564	208,833

Source: Berkson (1946).

Table 3.3 *Cholecystitis and diabetes in hypothetical population using refractive error as reference group*

		Diabetes	Refractive Error	
Cholecystitis	C	3,000	29,700	32,700
	not C	97,000	960,300	1,057,300
	Total	100,000	990,000	1,090,000

Source: Berkson (1946).

could be used to investigate the association between the presence of cholecystitis and diabetes. In particular, it seemed useful to look at the occurrence of cholecystitis amongst diabetic patients as compared to those without diabetes. Recognizing that cholecystitis might be associated with other diseases that lead to clinic use, he suggested that a condition known to be unrelated to cholecystitis be the reference group, and so he used individuals who came to the clinic with various refractive errors in an eye.

Berkson constructed some hypothetical data to illustrate possible findings. Table 3.2 shows information on the prevalence of cholecystitis amongst diabetic patients and in individuals with refractive error. For convenience we have labeled the three conditions, cholecystitis, diabetes, and refractive error, as C, D, and RE, respectively. If our population of interest is individuals with hospital records, then $P(C|RE) = 9,504/201,564 = 0.0472$, and $P(C|D) = 626/7,319 = 0.0855$. If we assume that $P(C|RE)$ is a reasonable proxy for the population value of $P(C)$, these two probabilities suggest that diabetes and cholecystitis are not independent, with cholecystitis occurring much more frequently in individuals with diabetes than in nondiabetic patients.

However, Table 3.3 expands Berkson's hypothetical data to the entire population. Note that the data of Table 3.2 are contained in Table 3.3. In the general population, we now see that $P(C|D) = 3,000/100,000 = 0.0300$, and $P(C|RE) = 29,700/990,000 = 0.0300$, also. So, here we see no evidence of association between cholecystitis and diabetes. This apparent contradiction has arisen because of variation in clinic/hospitalization use depending on the various factors affecting an individual.

Table 3.4 *Hypothetical data on cholecystitis, diabetes, and refractive error in both a hospitalized and general population*

	C and D	C and RE	Not C and D	Not C and RE
H	626	9,504	6,693	192,060
Not H	2,374	20,196	90,307	768,240
Total	3,000	29,700	97,000	960,300

Source: Berkson (1946).

Note: H refers to the existence of hospitalization records; C, D, and RE to the presence of cholecystitis, diabetes, and refractive error, respectively.

For each of four combinations of conditions (cholecystitis or not by diabetes and refractive error), Table 3.4 restates the information in Tables 3.2 and 3.3 in terms of the frequency of hospitalization or clinic use, labeled by H. Note that the hospitalization probabilities are quite different: $P(H|C\&D) = 626/3,000 = 0.21$, $P(H|C\&RE) = 9,504/29,700 = 0.32$, $P(H|\text{not } C\&D) = 6,693/97,000 = 0.07$, and $P(H|\text{not } C\&RE) = 192,060/960,300 = 0.20$.

This example illustrates the danger of using hospital or clinic users as a population to study the association of characteristics. It is interesting to note that the varied hospitalization rates represented in Table 3.4 were generated using different hospitalization frequencies separately for each of the three conditions—cholecystitis, diabetes, and refractive error—and then combining such probabilities with the assumption that hospitalization for any condition is independent of hospitalization from another. That is, no additional likelihood of hospitalization was assumed to arise for a subject suffering from more than one condition than expected from having each condition separately. Additional distortion inevitably arises when hospitalization rates for individuals with multiple conditions are greater than predicted from looking at each condition separately. Roberts et al. (1978) give an example of Berkson's fallacy with real data arising from household surveys of health care utilization.

3.6 Comments and further reading

The discussion in this and subsequent chapters is based on the assumption that data arise from a *simple* random sample of the population. There are other, often more effective sampling techniques, including stratified and cluster sampling, that are used to obtain estimates of a population proportion or probability. In more complex sampling schemes, the basic philosophy for constructing interval estimates remains the same, but expressions for both proportion estimators and their associated sampling variability must be modified to incorporate relevant sampling properties. We refer to Levy and Lemeshow (1999) for an extensive discussion of the advantages and disadvantages of various sampling schemes, with thorough descriptions of the appropriate estimation and confidence interval methods for a specific sampling design. A particular kind of stratified sampling forms the basis of matched studies (as covered in Chapter 16).

In many nonexperimental studies, participants are often not selected by any form of random sampling. Nevertheless, confidence intervals are usually calculated using the exact same techniques, with the tacit assumption that the data are being treated *as if they arose from a simple random sample*. This is a risky assumption to rely on consistently, since factors influencing a participant's selection are often unknown and could be related to the variables of interest. Such studies are thus subject to substantial bias in estimating probabilities and proportions. Of special concern is when study subjects are self-selected, as in volunteer projects. In restricted populations, sometimes all available population members are selected for study, with the same confidence interval procedures used. Here, confidence intervals are used to apply findings to a conceptually larger population, not to describe characteristics of a highly specified population. In fact, when the entire population is sampled, there is no sampling error, but the data may not be of broad interest. We return to this issue again when we discuss study designs in Chapter 5.

3.7 Problems

Question 3.1

The original data from the Chicago Western Electric Study (Shekelle et al., 1981) gave information on deaths from coronary heart disease (CHD) among middle-aged men who were free from CHD at entry into the study and who were followed for 25 years. There were 205 men who reported eating no fish at entry. Of these individuals, 42 subsequently died from CHD. Compute the 95% confidence interval for the unknown CHD mortality proportion for this group using both methods described in Section 3.3.

Repeat the calculations for the group of 261 men who reported consuming more than 35 g of fish per day at entry. Of these, 34 died from CHD during the study.

Question 3.2

Weitoft et al. (2003) investigated the impact of children growing up with a single parent in terms of the children's mental health morbidity and mortality, both total and cause-specific. Data were taken from Swedish national registries, covering almost the entire national population. Children were identified as living with (i) the same single adult or (ii) with two adults if their living situation remained the same in 1985 and 1990, with no requirement that the adults be biological parents. All such children were then tracked from 1991 until the end of 1999, at which point the youngest child was 14 years old and the oldest 26. Table 3.5 describes a very small amount of their data and ignores key variables including the sex of the child, socioeconomic factors, and other demographic factors.

Suppose a child is randomly selected from this population; based on Table 3.5, compute the probability that this child (1) was raised by a single parent; (2) died during the follow-up period; and (3) committed suicide during the same period. Compute the mortality and suicide probabilities conditional on whether the child lived with one or two parents. Comment on the possibility of association between their living arrangement and both mortality and suicide risk.

Table 3.5 *Mortality in children living with one or two parents in Sweden*

| | Total Mortality | | |
Child's Living Arrangement	Death	Survival	Total
With single parent	56	65,029	65,085
With two parents	608	920,649	921,257
Total	664	985,678	986,342

| | Suicide | | |
Child's Living Arrangement	Suicide	No Suicide	Total
With single parent	19	65,066	65,085
With two parents	96	921,161	921,257
Total	115	986,227	986,342

Source: Weitoft et al. (2003).

Question 3.3

Section 3.3 indicates that, in large samples, the standard deviation of a proportion estimate $\hat{p}$ of a population probability or proportion p is given by the square root of $p(1 - p)/n$, where n is the sample size. Compute this standard deviation for $n = 16$, 25, 100, 1000, 1500, and 2000 when $p = 0.5, 0.3, 0.1$, and 0.01. At a fixed sample size, for which values of p does the estimate have the highest standard deviation? If $p = 0.5$, how large a sample size is needed to guarantee that the *width* of a 95% confidence interval is no larger (i) than 0.05 and (ii) than 0.02?

CHAPTER 4

Measures of Disease–Exposure Association

Good old elementary fractions sit at the core of our discussion in this chapter. Just as they did in school, fractions can seem innocuous at first, only to cause you unbelievable confusion as soon as you take your eyes off them for a second. A classic puzzle, resurrected in one of National Public Radio's *Car Talk* books (Magliozzi et al., 1999), asks the following teaser: you have a 100-lb bag of potatoes in your car and your prize vegetables comprise 99% water and 1% solid potato, where solid material and water content are assumed to weigh the same. You are worried that your buyers will find the potatoes too mushy and so you set out to extract some of the water. But it is difficult and, after much huffing and puffing, you can only reduce the water content to 98%. After you throw away the extracted water, how much does your bag of potatoes weigh? The answer is not 99 lb, not 98 lb, but just 50 lb! The moral of the story is that doubling a small proportion can have a much bigger impact even when portrayed as reducing a fraction from 99 to 98%.

Enough teasers—what about linking risk factors to disease outcomes? Does a mother's marital status affect the risk of a baby's death its first year? By how much? What about birthweight? Which of these two risks has a stronger effect? With such questions ringing in our ears, we return to studying the association between a risk factor or exposure and the occurrence of a disease. For simplicity, we first look at the simplest type of risk factor, namely, one that can take only two values, e.g., "exposed" or "not exposed." As before, we label the (binary) incident disease outcome by D and the risk factor by E. There are therefore only four kinds of individuals in our population of interest, those with both factors (D & E), those with just one factor, and those with neither. Using the tools of conditional probabilities and the idea of independence, it makes sense to compare the incidence proportions $P(D|E)$ and $P(D|\bar{E})$. The following sections illustrate several alternative ways of quantifying this comparison.

4.1 Relative risk

The *Relative Risk* for an outcome D associated with a binary risk factor E, denoted by RR, is defined as follows:

$$RR = \frac{P(D|E)}{P(D|\bar{E})} = \frac{P(D|E)}{P(D|\text{not } E)}. \tag{4.1}$$

Some simple implications immediately follow from this definition. First, the RR must be a nonnegative number; the value $RR = 1$ is a *null* value since it is equivalent to saying that $P(D|E) = P(D|\bar{E})$ or that D and E are independent. If $RR > 1$, then there is a greater risk or probability of D when exposed (E) than when unexposed $(\bar{E})$; the reverse is true when $RR < 1$.

The Relative Risk is the basis of a multiplicative model for risk in the sense that, to obtain the risk of disease for an exposed individual, you take the baseline— unexposed—risk and *multiply* it by RR. It is easy to interpret: for example, if you smoke cigarettes, your lifetime risk of lung cancer increases tenfold, i.e., the Relative Risk for lung cancer associated with cigarette smoking is 10. One disadvantage is the restricted lower limit of RR, in that it cannot be negative, and an implicit upper bound whereby, for a given measure of baseline risk, $P(D|\bar{E})$, the RR must be less than or equal to $1/P(D|\bar{E})$. For instance, if $P(D|\bar{E}) = 1/3$, then $RR \leq 3$ since $P(D|E)$ can be no larger than 1. This restriction on the range of RR only becomes an issue with common disease outcomes.

A final important comment on the Relative Risk is that it is not symmetric in the role of the two factors D and E. The Relative Risk for E associated with D is a different measure of association; that is,

$$\frac{P(D|E)}{P(D|\text{not } E)} \neq \frac{P(E|D)}{P(E|\text{not } D)}.$$

The data given in Table 3.1 is used to illustrate the computation of Relative Risks in a population. From the definition, the Relative Risk for infant mortality in the U.S. in 1991, associated with a mother being unmarried at the time of birth, is $(16,712/1,213,854)/(18,784/2,897,205) = 2.12$, showing that the risk of an infant death with an unmarried mother is a little more than double the risk when the mother is married. The Relative Risk for infant mortality in the U.S. in 1991, associated with a low-birthweight infant, is $(21,054/292,323)/(14,442/3,818,736) = 19.0$, indicating the much greater effect of birthweight on infant mortality than we saw for a mother's marital status.

4.2 Odds ratio

We have been measuring the risk of the outcome D through the risk or probability $P(D)$; an alternative quantity is the *odds* of D as given by $P(D)/P(\text{not } D)$. The odds provide exactly the same information as $P(D)$ in that each of these quantities immediately determines the other. Gamblers are fond of the odds since it gives the likelihood of D occurring relative to it not occurring—"how likely am I to win?" as compared to "how likely am I to lose?" For example, an even odds event D (odds of D are 1) is equivalent to $P(D) = 1/2$, that is, the same chance of winning as losing.

Just as the Relative Risk measures association by comparing $P(D|E)$ to $P(D|\bar{E})$, the *Odds Ratio* measures association by comparing the odds of D in the exposed and unexposed subgroups. The Odds Ratio for D associated with E is defined by:

$$OR = \frac{P(D|E)}{P(\text{not } D|E)} \Big/ \frac{P(D|\text{not } E)}{P(\text{not } D|\text{not } E)}. \tag{4.2}$$

As with the Relative Risk, the null value of the Odds Ratio is $OR = 1$, again equivalent to independence of D and E; in addition, $OR > 1$ when there is a greater risk of D with E present, and $OR < 1$ when there is a lower risk of D if E is present.

The Odds Ratio is also the basis of a multiplicative model for the risk of D. Like RR, OR must be nonnegative, but unlike RR, OR has no upper limit whatever the baseline risk $P(D|\bar{E})$ for the unexposed. Thus, the Odds Ratio can be effectively used as a scale for association even when $P(D|\bar{E})$ is large.

Using the data from Table 3.1, the Odds Ratio for infant mortality associated with an unmarried mother is $[(16,712/1,213,854)/(1,197,142/1,213,854)]/[(18,784/2,897,205)/(2,878,421/2,897,205)] = (16,712 \times 2,878,421)/(18,784 \times 1,197,142) = 2.14$. Associated with low birthweight, the Odds Ratio is $[(21,054/292,323)/(271,269/292,323)/(14,442/3,818,736)/(3,804,294/3,818,736)] = (21,054 \times 3,804,294)/(14,442 \times 271,269) = 20.4$.

Comparing these Odds Ratios with the analogous Relative Risks computed in Section 4.1, we observe that the two measures are very similar, with the Odds Ratio just a little bigger in each case. We now investigate the generality of these comparisons between the measures.

4.3 The odds ratio as an approximation to the relative risk

From the definition of the Odds Ratio, we see immediately that

$$OR = \frac{P(D|E)}{P(D|\text{not } E)} \times \frac{P(\text{not } D|\text{not } E)}{P(\text{not } D|E)}$$

$$= RR \times \frac{P(\text{not } D|\text{not } E)}{P(\text{not } D|E)}. \tag{4.3}$$

Now, if $RR > 1$, then

$$P(D|E) > P(D|\text{not } E)$$

$$\Rightarrow 1 - P(D|E) < 1 - P(D|\text{not } E)$$

$$\Rightarrow P(\text{not } D|E) < P(\text{not } D|\text{not } E)$$

$$\Rightarrow \qquad OR > RR, \text{ using (4.3).}$$

Similarly, if $RR < 1$, then $OR < RR$. Thus, the Odds Ratio is always farther away from the null value, 1, than the Relative Risk, except when both measures equal 1.

But how much farther away from 1 is the Odds Ratio compared with the Relative Risk? This depends on the two conditional probabilities $P(D|E)$ and $P(D|\text{not } E)$, which are the ingredients of both measures of association. If the risk of disease is low—that is, the disease is rare—in *both* exposed (E) and unexposed (not E) subgroups, then this implies that $P(\text{not } D|E)$ and $P(\text{not } D|\text{not } E)$ are both close to 1, so that $OR \approx P(D|E)/P(D|\text{not } E) = RR$ (see Equation 4.3); that is, the Odds Ratio and the Relative Risk are approximately equal.

For a more detailed look at the difference between the Odds Ratio and the Relative Risk, Table 4.1 compares the values of the two measures given different conditional

Table 4.1 *Comparison of relative risk and odds ratio at various risk levels*

Risk in Unexposed $P(D\vert \text{not } E)$	Risk in Exposed $P(D\vert E)$	Relative Risk (RR)	Odds Ratio (OR)	Relative Difference $\frac{OR-RR}{RR} \times 100$
	0.01	1.00	1.00	0
0.01	0.02	2.00	2.02	1.0
	0.05	5.00	5.21	4.2
	0.10	10.00	11.00	10.0
	0.05	1.00	1.00	0
	0.10	2.00	2.11	5.6
0.05	0.15	3.00	3.35	11.8
	0.20	4.00	4.75	18.8
	0.50	10.00	19.00	90.0
	0.10	1.00	1.00	0
	0.15	1.50	1.59	5.9
0.10	0.20	2.00	2.25	12.5
	0.30	3.00	3.86	28.6
	0.40	4.00	6.00	50.0
	0.50	5.00	9.00	80.0
	0.20	1.00	1.00	0
	0.30	1.50	1.71	14.3
	0.40	2.00	2.67	33.3
0.20	0.50	2.50	4.00	60.0
	0.60	3.00	6.00	100.0
	0.80	4.00	16.00	300.0
	1.00	5.00	∞	∞

probabilities $P(D\vert E)$ and $P(D\vert \bar{E})$. Note that the table entries confirm that the Odds Ratio is always farther away from 1 than the Relative Risk, and that the two measures are relatively close until either the exposed or unexposed risk of D becomes large. Generally, the Odds Ratio is less than 10% larger than the Relative Risk (both are greater than 1 here) when the sum of the risks in the exposed and unexposed is less than 0.1.

4.4 Symmetry of roles of disease and exposure in the odds ratio

The Odds Ratio is notoriously confusing when first encountered, particularly in contrast to the simplicity of the interpretation for the Relative Risk. Why is the Odds Ratio then used so often? A fundamental reason is that the Odds Ratio is symmetric in the roles of D and E. Recall from Section 4.1 that the Relative Risk does not enjoy this symmetry. That reversing the roles of D and E makes no difference in computation of the Odds Ratio holds the key to estimating association between an exposure and disease in case-control studies, introduced in Chapter 5.3. To establish this property, note that

$$OR = \frac{P(D|E)}{P(\text{not } D|E)} \Bigg/ \frac{P(D|\text{not } E)}{P(\text{not } D|\text{not } E)}$$

$$= \frac{P(D\&E)/P(E)}{P(\text{not } D\&E)/P(E)} \Bigg/ \frac{P(D\&\text{not } E)/P(\text{not } E)}{P(\text{not } D\&\text{not } E)/P(\text{not } E)}$$

$$= \frac{P(D\&E)}{P(\text{not } D\&E)} \Bigg/ \frac{P(D\&\text{not } E)}{P(\text{not } D\&\text{not } E)}$$

$$= \frac{P(D\&E)}{P(D\&\text{not } E)} \Bigg/ \frac{P(\text{not } D\&E)}{P(\text{not } D\&\text{not } E)}$$

$$= \frac{P(D\&E)/P(D)}{P(D\&\text{not } E)/P(D)} \Bigg/ \frac{P(\text{not } D\&E)/P(\text{not } D)}{P(\text{not } D\&\text{not } E)/P(\text{not } D)}$$

$$= \frac{P(E|D)}{P(\text{not } E|D)} \Bigg/ \frac{P(E|\text{not } D)}{P(\text{not } E|\text{not } D)}. \tag{4.4}$$

The last expression is, of course, just the Odds Ratio for E associated with D. Thus the Odds Ratio for D associated with E is equivalent to the Odds Ratio for E associated with D.

4.5 Relative hazard

Referring back to the basic definitions of disease occurrence given in Chapter 2, we suppose that the interval of risk of interest is labeled by $[0, T]$ on the appropriate time scale relevant to an investigation. For any time t during this interval, we defined in Chapter 2, Section 2.2.1 the incidence proportion $I(t)$ over the time interval $[0, t]$, and the hazard function $h(t)$ at time t. Recall that $I(t)$ measures the cumulative incidence from time $t = 0$ to time t, whereas the hazard function measures the incidence rate at exactly time t. The two functions are linked through Equation 2.1.

With a simple binary exposure variable E, there are two incidence proportions (and two hazard functions) of interest. These are $I_E(t)$ and $I_{\bar{E}}(t)$, the incidence proportions over the interval $[0, t]$ for the exposed and unexposed, respectively. Similarly, we label the hazard functions for the two groups by $h_E(t)$ and $h_{\bar{E}}(t)$.

As a quantitative measure of the relative difference in incidence between the exposed and unexposed populations, we can use

$$RR(t) = \frac{I_E(t)}{I_{\bar{E}}(t)},$$

the Relative Risk of incidence over the interval $[0, t]$. (To this point we have focused on a fixed interval $[0, T]$.) An analogous definition can also be given for $OR(t)$, the Odds Ratio associated with cumulative incidence over the interval $[0, t]$ for the exposed and unexposed.

An alternative measure of the relationship between exposure and incidence is given by

$$RH(t) = \frac{h_E(t)}{h_{\bar{E}}(t)},$$

the *Relative Hazard* at time t. This provides an instantaneous measure of how exposure affects incidence of D. It is possible that the Relative Hazard could assume widely varying values at different ts within $[0, T]$, so that, at certain times, $RH(t_1) > 1$ (E increases the risk for D at t_1), and at other points in time, $RH(t_2) < 1$ (E decreases the risk for D at t_2). Of course, dramatic changes in the nature of $RH(t)$ over $[0, T]$ may be masked in consideration of $RR(T)$, the Relative Risk at the end of the interval. We return to this point in Chapter 17.

For now, suppose we are willing to assume that the Relative Hazard remains constant over the interval $[0, T]$; that is, the relative impact of exposure on the instantaneous incidence rate remains the same over time. In symbols, this is equivalent to

$$RH(t) = \frac{h_E(t)}{h_{\bar{E}}(t)} = RH, \tag{4.5}$$

where RH is a constant. This assumption is often referred to as *proportional hazards*, reflecting that the hazard functions for the exposed and the unexposed are proportional to each other, and thus have the same shape.

If $I_{\bar{E}}(T)$ is small, then it follows from Equation 2.1 that, with the proportional hazards assumption (Equation 4.5),

$$RR(T) \approx OR(T) \approx RH(T) \equiv RH. \tag{4.6}$$

Note that $I_{\bar{E}}(T)$ can be small either because the disease is rare or because the relevant interval of observation $[0, T]$ is very short. Also, the proportional hazards assumption means that $I_E(t)$ will also be small in these situations.

Figure 4.1 illustrates $RH(t)$, $RR(t)$, and $OR(t)$ in the very simple situation where the hazard functions for both the exposed and unexposed are constant. The baseline

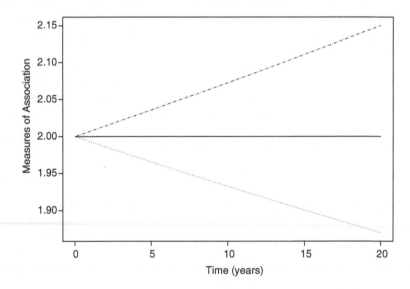

Figure 4.1 *Plot of three measures of association (Relative Hazard: solid line, Relative Risk: dotted line, Odds Ratio: dash-dotted line) as the risk period extends in time.*

hazard function is here chosen to be $h_{\bar{E}}(t) = 0.007$/year, an incidence or hazard rate that is roughly the rate for incidence of coronary heart disease in middle-age males. With a constant Relative Hazard of $K = 2$, the Relative Risk and Odds Ratio curves remain extremely close to 2 as the risk period extends, until about $t = 15$ years. With any risk interval shorter than 15 years of follow-up, there will be little difference anticipated in estimates of the three measures of association. In sum, with these low risks, if the proportional hazards assumption is valid, there is very little difference between choosing RH, $RR(15)$, or $OR(15)$ as a measure of the relative difference in incidence between the exposed and unexposed. Figure 4.1 is typical in showing that the Relative Hazard lies between the Relative Risk and the Odds Ratio (Greenland and Thomas, 1982).

4.6 Excess risk

Both the Relative Risk and Odds Ratio are *relative*, not absolute, measures of risk differences between the exposed and unexposed. To convey an absolute measure of the impact of exposure on risk, we use the *Excess Risk*, denoted by ER, and defined by:

$$ER = P(D|E) - P(D|\bar{E}). \tag{4.7}$$

The Excess Risk uses the same basic risk components as the Relative Risk (and the Odds Ratio, for that matter), but looks at the absolute, rather than relative, difference in risk levels. For example, the Relative Risk for lung cancer associated with cigarette smoking is about five times as great as the Relative Risk for CHD due to smoking. On the other hand, the Excess Risk for CHD is larger since it is the more common disease. Therefore, from a health policy or public health point of view, cigarette intervention programs may be more important in terms of their impact on CHD.

Note that ER must lie between -1 and $+1$; the value $ER = 0$ is the null value since this is equivalent to $P(D|E) = P(D|\bar{E})$, that is, independence of D and E. If $ER > 0$, then there is a greater risk for D when exposed (E) than when unexposed ($\bar{E}$); the opposite is true when $ER < 0$. The Excess Risk measure is the basis of an additive model for risk because the risk of disease among exposed individuals is obtained by taking the risk in the unexposed and then *adding* ER to this baseline risk.

One helpful interpretation of the Excess Risk relates to the difference in the number of cases in populations where either everyone is exposed or everyone is unexposed. For example, if the population size is N and there is no exposure in the population so that $P(D) = P(D|\bar{E})$, then the number of cases is simply $N \times P(D|\bar{E})$. Similarly, if in the same population everyone was exposed, so that $P(D) = P(D|E)$, the number of cases is $N \times P(D|E)$. The difference in these caseloads is then $N \times P(D|\bar{E}) - N \times P(D|E)$; expressing this as a fraction of the population size yields $P(D|\bar{E}) - P(D|E) = ER$. Thus, the Excess Risk can be seen as the excess number of cases, as a fraction of the population size, when population members are all exposed as compared to them all being unexposed.

The data in Table 3.1 allow computation of the Excess Risk for infant mortality in the U.S. in 1991 associated with the mother's marital status: $ER = (16,712/1,213,854) - (18,784/2,897,205) = 0.0138 - 0.0065 = 0.0073$. On the other hand, the Excess

Risk for infant mortality associated with low birthweight is $(21{,}054/292{,}323)$ − $(14{,}442/3{,}818{,}736) = 0.0720 − 0.0038 = 0.0682$. In this case, low birthweight is more influential than marital status on both the absolute and relative comparative scales. At face value, one interpretation of the Excess Risk is that we would expect the infant mortality percentage to increase by 7% if all births exhibited low birthweight as compared to all births being of normal birthweight. In the next section, we discuss and question the apparent assumption of a causal role for birthweight in infant death that underlies this statement.

4.7 Attributable risk

Discussion so far indicates that an individual may become diseased without exposure to the risk factor of interest, that is, $P(D|\bar{E})$ can be greater than 0. Since in that scenario not all disease can be due to exposure, it is appealing to ask how much of the disease D in the population can be explained by the presence of the risk factor E. The *Attributable Risk* is a measure of association designed to provide an answer to this question and is defined as the fraction of all cases of D in the population that can be attributed to E. In a population of size N, there are $NP(D)$ individuals with characteristic D. Now suppose that exposure to E is eradicated. Assuming the risk of D in the population is then given by $P(D|\bar{E})$, there would then be $NP(D|\bar{E})$ cases of D. The fraction of cases that would be removed, or thereby explained as due to E, is $[NP(D) − NP(D|\bar{E})]/NP(D)$. The common factor N cancels in the numerator and denominator, leaving the definition

$$AR = \frac{P(D) - P(D|\bar{E})}{P(D)}.$$

From Section 3.4, $P(D) = P(D|E)P(E) + P(D|\bar{E})P(\bar{E})$, so that

$$AR = \frac{P(D|E)P(E) + P(D|\bar{E})P(\bar{E}) - P(D|\bar{E})}{P(D)}$$

$$= \frac{P(D|E)P(E) + P(D|\bar{E})(P(\bar{E}) - 1)}{P(D)}$$

$$= \frac{P(D|E)P(E) - P(D|\bar{E})P(E)}{P(D)}$$

$$= \frac{P(E)[P(D|E) - P(D|\bar{E})]}{P(D|E)P(E) + P(D|\bar{E})P(\bar{E})}$$

$$= \frac{P(E)[RR - 1]}{P(E)RR + P(\bar{E})}$$

$$= \frac{P(E)[RR - 1]}{1 + P(E)(RR - 1)}. \tag{4.8}$$

This expression shows that the Attributable Risk depends on both the strength of the association between D and E and the prevalence of the risk factor E. Therefore, the Attributable Risk incorporates the advantages of both a relative and an absolute measure of association. The null value is $AR = 0$, which occurs if and only if $P(D) = P(D|\bar{E})$, that is, D and E are independent. When exposure to E raises the risk of D, $0 < AR \leq 1$; when exposure to E is protective, $AR < 0$. In the latter situation, however, AR can become an arbitrarily large negative number as the disease frequency becomes increasingly smaller.

The attractiveness of the Attributable Risk is the insight it promises into the potential impact of an intervention program designed to reduce exposure to a risk factor E. However, the assumption that the risk in the unexposed can be applied to individuals who are "changed" from Es to $\bar{E}$s through an intervention program assumes essentially that the $E - D$ relationship is causal. An additional tacit assumption is that modification of an individual's E status does not alter other risk factors; in the extreme it is possible that reducing exposure to E may actually increase exposure to other risk factors and thereby make the disease burden greater. For example, automobile drivers might respond to seat-belt laws by increasing their average speed, under a perception of increased safety, thereby offsetting mortality reductions introduced by higher seat-belt usage. Both of these concerns—causality and the effect of other factors—also apply to the Relative Risk and Odds Ratio, but are less apparent there, perhaps a disadvantage of these apparently simple measures. For the moment, we lay aside these misgivings, with the promise to address them head-on in Chapter 8.

We illustrate the computation of the Attributable Risk using the data from Table 3.1 on infant mortality. Here, when the risk factor is the mother's marital status (E is unmarried), $P(D) = 0.0086$, and $P(D|\bar{E}) = 18,784/2,897,205 = 0.0065$, so that $AR = (0.0086 - 0.0065)/0.0086 = 0.25$. We already observed, in Section 4.1, that $RR = 2.12$; with $P(E) = 1,213,854/4,111,059 = 0.2952$, the Attributable Risk associated with marital status can also be calculated through (4.8), again yielding $AR = 0.2952(2.12 - 1)/[1 + 0.2952(2.12 - 1)] = 0.25$.

Similarly, when E refers to a low-birthweight infant, $AR = (0.0086 - 0.0038)/0.0086 = 0.56$. The naive interpretation of this quantity is that infant mortality could be reduced by 25% if all mothers were married, or by 56% if we could eliminate low-birthweight infants. While it is plausible that a substantial fraction of infant mortality could be prevented by intervention programs designed to eliminate the risk of a low-birthweight child, it is not believable that 25% of infant deaths could be eradicated merely through a program to have single pregnant women marry before they give birth. In light of our comments above, this suggests that marital status does not, in fact, cause infant mortality; the apparent association, as captured by either the Relative Risk, Odds Ratio, or Attributable Risk, is likely due to the effect of other factors that are related to both marital status and infant mortality. We deal with this topic at length in Chapter 8.

One drawback in interpreting the Attributable Risk is that it does not behave as a conventional fraction when more than one risk factor is examined. That is, the Attributable Risks for two distinct exposures cannot be added to give the Attributable Risks for both factors considered simultaneously, even when the exposures are independently distributed. Table 4.2 provides hypothetical data on two binary exposures, E and F, that might have generated the infant mortality data of Table 3.1. The entries of the table give the frequency of infant deaths for the four possible exposure categories,

Table 4.2 *Hypothetical data on two independent risk factors for infant mortality*

Infant Mortality	$E \& F$	$E \& \bar{F}$	$\bar{E} \& F$	$\bar{E} \& \bar{F}$	Total
Death	25,497	5,561	4,084	354	35,496
Live at 1 year	1,002,268	1,022,204	1,023,681	1,027,410	4,075,563
Total	1,027,765	1,027,765	1,027,765	1,027,764	4,111,059

defined by the presence and absence of E and F. Note that the data have been set up so that E and F are independent. The Relative Risk for infant death associated with E is $0.0151/0.0022 = 7.0$, and associated with F is $0.0144/0.0029 = 5.0$. Further, $P(E) = P(F) = 0.5$, so that, using Equation 4.8, the Attributable Risk associated with E is 0.75 and with F is 0.67. With homage to Yogi Berra, it appears as if infant death is 75% due to E; the other 67% is due to F! These two factors are independent and certainly the attributable risk for both combined cannot be the sum of the individual ARs since this would greatly exceed 1. From another point of view, establishing the AR associated with E to be 0.75 cannot be interpreted as claiming that only 25% of infant mortality remains to be explained in the sense that Attributable Risks for other factors will be 0.25 or smaller. (Note that, using the data in Table 4.2, one can see directly that the fraction of cases "attributable" to both factors taken together is $[(35,496/4,111,059) - (354/1,027,764)]/(35,496/4,111,059) = 0.96$. Begg (2001) constructs a simpler example illustrating this issue and discusses its implication for cancer epidemiology.

The Attributable Risk is often used as a measure of how many diseased cases are "on the table" when evaluating the importance of a prevention program designed to reduce exposure to E. Note that, in this context, the Attributable Risk conceptually assumes a perfect intervention that will eradicate exposure to E. Because such an intervention is unlikely in practice, when comparing Attributable Risks for different risk factors we must be conscious that an exposure with a smaller Attributable Risk may yet be the more effective target for an intervention program if it is easier to modify in individuals.

4.8 Comments and further reading

Only a few of the possible measures of association between E and D have been defined, focusing on those most commonly used in the literature. With such a plethora of association measures, their names and usage can be easily misinterpreted. Most confusing is that the term Attributable Risk has sometimes been used to describe what we call the Excess Risk, which in turn is sometimes called the Risk Difference. The Attributable Risk is also called the Population Attributable Risk to differentiate it from other meaningful fractions that apply to subgroups of the population. One of these, termed the Excess Fraction (!), yields the fraction of cases *among the exposed* that are due to exposure. Rothman and Greenland (1998, pp. 53–56) gives a lengthy discussion of such attributable fractions.

With rare diseases, the Relative Risk, Odds Ratio, and Relative Hazard are approximately the same (see Sections 4.3 and (4.6)) and the names are thus often used interchangeably in this setting. There are sampling conditions, however, where an estimated Odds Ratio approximates the Relative Hazard or the Relative Risk, even with common outcomes, and this has led to confusion regarding the assumption of rare diseases in equating these measures of association. We discuss this further in the next chapter.

The media are often unable to discern the key difference between the Odds Ratio and the Relative Risk, and this is of particular import with common outcomes. One recent egregious error of this kind was the reporting of a study that showed videos of actors, posing as patients, to physicians to determine referral patterns for cardiac catheterization (Schulman et al., 1999). Sample referral proportions were 84.7% for blacks and 90.6% for whites, leading to an Odds Ratio of 0.57, or approximately 0.6. Such Odds Ratios were unnecessarily reported in the journal's summary of the article, and by the lead author on the television program *Nightline*—unnecessary because the simpler Relative Risk was available. Unfortunately, the Odds Ratio was misinterpreted by the media as a Relative Risk, leading to startling claims that blacks were only 60% as likely as whites to be referred for a crucial medical procedure, reported on the front pages of *The Washington Post* and *USA Today*. In fact, the Relative Risk is $0.847/0.906 = 0.93$, a much less striking number. (Full analysis of the data showed that only black women had a lower rate, and that these results largely depended on responses to two specific actresses.)

A final caution regarding the interpretation of the Attributable Risk is illustrated by our computations that link marital status to infant mortality. Even if the causal assumption was appropriate, the value $AR = 0.25$ for marital status, when applied to the total number of deaths, assumes that if all mothers were married the exact same pregnancies would occur as observed. It is entirely plausible that marital status increases the number of live pregnancies, thereby leading to a different population at risk and a greater number of infant deaths than anticipated.

4.9 Problems

Question 4.1

Illustrate two properties of the Odds Ratio using the 2×2 population table of Table 4.3; (1) Compute the Odds Ratio; (2) show that multiplying each row by a different constant does not change the Odds Ratio; (3) show that multiplying each column by a different constant does not change the Odds Ratio; (4) interchange the rows and then

Table 4.3 *Population 2 × 2 table for two characteristics, A and B*

	B	$\bar{B}$	
A	1005	1212	2217
$\bar{A}$	15	24	39
	1020	1236	2256

Table 4.4 *Deaths of Titanic passengers by sex*

		Outcome after Accident		
		Death	Survival	
Sex	Male	682	161	843
	Female	127	339	466
		809	500	1309

compute the Odds Ratio—what is the relationship between this value and the ones previously calculated? What is the relationship between the logarithms of these two Odds Ratios?

Question 4.2

Data on deaths of *Titanic* passengers after the disaster are given in Table 4.4, classified by sex of the passenger. Calculate the odds of dying for (1) men and (2) women. What is the Odds Ratio for death, associated with sex (i.e., being a man as opposed to a woman)? What is the Odds Ratio for survival, associated with sex? What is the Relative Risk for (1) death and (2) for survival, associated with sex? Which of these measures of association do you feel is the best way to summarize the differences between men and women, and why?

Question 4.3

Using the data provided in Table 3.5, calculate the Relative Risk for both childhood mortality and childhood suicide in Sweden associated with living with a single parent. What is the Attributable Risk of both these outcomes associated with the child's living arrangement?

Question 4.4

Suppose a study reports that an association between coffee drinking and oral cancer yields an Attributable Risk of 0.50. A lobbyist for tea importers claims that banning coffee would eliminate 50% of oral cancer cases. What is your reaction and why?

Question 4.5

Consider a 10-year follow-up study of the association between a measure of stress (E, dichotomized into two levels: high and low) and high blood pressure (D, dichotomized into two levels: high and normal). In the study, participants were treated at the appearance of high blood pressure to attempt to return them to normal levels. It was noted that the Relative Risk for having high blood pressure, associated with a high stress level, was 2 if incidence of D, during follow-up, was used as the outcome, but was 4 if prevalence of D at the end of the study was used as an alternative outcome. Qualitatively explain this discrepancy.

CHAPTER 5

Study Designs

Everything in the last chapter applied to properties of a population. But we almost always have to deal with samples with limited and varying information. With a random sample of births, how do we examine the relationship between birthweight and infant mortality? What kind of accuracy can we expect and how does it depend on the size of the sample? Does it matter how we select the births to be sampled? We must confront the following issues:

- How do we estimate a measure of association from a *random sample* from the population of interest?
- How do we assess the uncertainty inherent in a random sample estimate?
- How do we determine whether an observed association in a sample reflects a true association in the population rather than a chance variation (*statistical significance*)?

The methods for addressing these questions depend on how we draw the random sample from the population. In this chapter, we consider simple forms of random sampling and their broad impact on the answers to these questions. In the following chapters, we discuss both the statistical significance of an observed sample association and estimation of various measures of association.

Before discussing study designs, we describe nested components of the population of interest. The *Target Population* refers to the population to which we would like to apply our estimates and inferences regarding the relationship between disease and exposure. Sometimes, it can be extremely difficult to sample directly from the Target Population; in such cases, there is often a convenient subgroup of the population for which appropriate sampling frames are available. We call this subgroup the *Study Population*, the population from which we are able to sample. Finally, the *Sample* comprises the actual sampled individuals from the Study Population for whom we collect data on disease, exposure, and other factors. Figure 5.1 is a schematic of these three groups. Note that the figure is not intended to be representative of scale. Typically the Study Population is a very large fraction of the Target Population, whereas the Sample is extremely small relative to the Study and Target Populations. For example, in many studies, a telephone interview may be used to collect information on study subjects. In these surveys, the Study Population comprises individuals in families that possess a residential telephone. As another example (Section 3.5), the Target Population might be the general community from which one might be tempted—with great risk as we have seen—to use individuals with hospital or clinic records as a

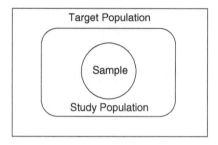

Figure 5.1 *Schematic of target population, study population, and the sample.*

convenient Study Population. The exercises at the end of this chapter contain several examples of epidemiological studies of various designs, illustrating possible choices of Study Populations within a given Target Population.

Intelligent choice of Study Populations will help us investigate our primary interest, the relationship between E and D. While selecting an appropriate Study Population is often predicated on the availability of sampling frames and other sampling mechanics, there are situations where the choice is based on the need to obtain valid comparisons for estimating an effect measure. This is particularly true in the cohort and case-control designs of Sections 5.2 and 5.3. On the other hand, differences between the Target Population and Study Population introduce *selection bias* in our results if the Study Population is not representative of the Target Population *with regard to the disease–exposure relationship* of concern. This does not necessarily require that the Study Population is representative of all aspects of the Target Population. However, when random sampling is used, differences between the Sample and the Study Population are entirely due to random, or sampling, variation associated with the sampling technique employed. We can then use statistical methods to assess and describe these differences based on a detailed understanding of sampling procedures and variation. If the study sample is not selected randomly, we can treat the data in the same manner but without the same confidence in the calculations. Substantial bias can be introduced at this point if factors, often unmeasured or unknown, influencing the sample selection are associated with exposure and disease.

How do we usually obtain a random study sample from the Study Population? Three basic forms of sampling schemes are most commonly used in epidemiological studies. In each, we restrict attention to the association between the presence and absence of two binary factors, the outcome D and the exposure E, since the basic concept and the primary statistical impact of the designs are all captured even in this simplest scenario. Note that the sample data from any of the designs can be summarized in the form of a 2×2 contingency table as illustrated in Table 5.1. The rest of this chapter describes the three typical designs in terms of their statistical characteristics, determined by how study participants are sampled.

Table 5.1 *Generic form of a* 2×2 *contingency table for data relating a disease (D) and (binary) exposure (E)*

		Disease	
		D	not D
Exposure	E	.	.
	not E	.	.

5.1 Population-based studies

The main steps of a *population-based* design are simply:

1. Take a simple random sample of size n from the Study Population.
2. Subsequently, measure the presence and absence of both D and E for all sampled individuals.

Note that the word "subsequently" here refers to the order of sampling individuals and measuring the factors, D and E, for the sample; there are no requirements on the chronological timing of events that determine D and E relative to the time of sampling. A further subclassification of the design is often used to differentiate the timing of measurements on D and E. Specifically, Rothman and Greenland (1998) refer to a *prospective* study as one in which measurement of exposure is made on an individual prior to the occurrence and thus measurement of disease. Conversely, in a *retrospective* study, measurement of exposure occurs after an individual's disease status has been determined. A population-based study is often loosely called a cross-sectional study, but I prefer the former name as the latter suggests that measurement of D and E always coincides with sampling.

Whether a study is prospective or retrospective is not relevant to the study design and therefore not of immediate concern to the development of statistical properties. However, this classification may have considerable influence on the quality and validity of exposure measurement. For example, exposure assessment in a retrospective design must (1) evaluate the relevant risk levels in place *before* disease, and not after, and (2) ensure that measurements are not influenced by an individual's disease status. Note that prospective measurement of D may require a 10- or 20-year follow-up period after sampling.

The various types of population probabilities that may be of interest to the investigator can be classified as follows:

- *Joint* probabilities: $P(D \& E)$, $P(D \& \bar{E})$, $P(\bar{D} \& E)$, $P(\bar{D} \& \bar{E})$
- *Marginal* probabilities: $P(D)$, $P(E)$, $P(\bar{D})$, $P(\bar{E})$
- *Conditional* probabilities: $P(D|E)$, $P(D|\bar{E})$, $P(E|D)$, $P(E|\bar{D})$.

Each of these kinds of probabilities can be estimated using data generated from a population-based sample: estimates are given by the observed proportion of the simple random sample that corresponds to the population probability of interest.

Table 5.2 *Possible data from a population-based study (n = 200) of a mother's marital status and low birthweight*

		Birthweight		
		Low	Normal	
Marital status at birth	Unmarried	7	52	59
	Married	7	134	141
		14	186	200

For example, the population probability $P(D \ \& \ E)$ is estimated by the observed proportion of the sample (of size n) that have both characteristics D and E.

5.1.1 Example—mother's marital status and infant birthweight

In Chapter 3, we introduced data on the role of a mother's marital status or her baby's birthweight on subsequent infant mortality. A natural follow-up question is the extent to which the impact of marital status on infant mortality might be explained by birthweight. That is, it is plausible that unmarried women may receive poorer nutrition and prenatal care than married mothers-to-be, and thus deliver lower birthweight babies on average, which, in turn, would raise the risk of infant mortality substantially. To examine the relationship between marital status and birthweight, an investigator needs to collect data on these two factors in the population of interest.

Suppose that a sample size of 200 has been chosen for a population-based study. That is, a simple random sample of 200 births is selected from the Study Population. Table 5.2 shows a possible outcome of such a study. From this population-based data, we can then estimate:

- Joint probabilities, such as $\hat{P}$(unmarried mother and low birthweight infant) = $7/200 = 0.035$
- Marginal probabilities, such as $\hat{P}$(low birthweight infant) = $14/200 = 0.07$
- Conditional probabilities, such as $\hat{P}$(low birthweight infant|unmarried mother) = $7/59 = 0.119$, or $\hat{P}$(low birthweight infant|married mother) = $7/141 = 0.050$.

Sensible estimates can be obtained of the Relative Risk, Odds Ratio, Excess Risk, and Attributable Risk for a low-birthweight infant associated with the mother's marital status using the relevant estimates of the conditional probabilities $P(D|E)$, $P(D|\bar{E})$, etc. in the definitions of a particular effect measure. We will discuss these estimates in more detail in the next chapter. For now, we see that

- $\widehat{RR} = (7/59)/(7/141) = 2.39$
- $\widehat{OR} = [(7/59)/(52/59)]/[(7/141)/(134/141)] = 2.58$
- $\widehat{ER} = (7/59) - (7/141) = 0.069$
- $\widehat{AR} = [(14/200) - (7/141)]/(14/200) = 0.29$.

Note the (by-now familiar) slightly higher value for the Odds Ratio as compared with the Relative Risk. The estimate of the Attributable Risk suggests that close to 30% of low birthweights in the population are attributable to the mother's marital status. Maternal marital status is presumably not casually associated with low birthweight but a proxy for poorer prenatal care and nutrition, as suggested earlier.

5.2 Exposure-based sampling—cohort studies

The primary feature of a *cohort* study is that sampling is carried out separately for subpopulations at different exposure levels, leading to distinct cohorts. The main steps of a cohort design are:

1. Identify two subgroups of the population on the basis of the presence or absence of E.
2. Take a simple random sample from each of these two subgroups (that is, the Es and not Es) *separately*, of sizes n_E and $n_{\bar{E}}$, respectively.
3. Measure subsequently the presence and absence of D for individuals in both random samples.

As for population-based studies, the timing and manner of measurement of the two factors D and E are not pertinent to the sampling characteristics of a cohort design. The key statistical property of the design is the separate identification and sampling of the exposure groups. When and how D and E are measured are important considerations in assessing the potential accuracy and bias in disease and exposure measurement, but are not germane to the direct statistical impact of the design itself.

Note that the investigator has to prespecify the sample sizes for the two separate samples taken from the exposure groups. This division of the overall sample size is important in determining the amount of information that a cohort study yields on the disease–exposure relationship, as we shall discuss further. For an extreme example, if one exposure group is allocated a very small sample size, then there will be little information available on the disease–exposure relationship.

Table 5.3 shows a possible outcome of a cohort study using the same population as for the population-based design in Section 5.1.1. Here, we have selected two random samples, each of size 100, the first from the population of unmarried mothers and the second from married mothers. This design assumes that, prior to sampling, one is able to divide the population by marital status into two distinct sampling frames.

Table 5.3 *Possible data from a cohort study ($n_E = n_{\bar{E}} = 100$) of a mother's marital status and low birthweight*

		Birthweight		
		Low	Normal	
Marital status at birth	Unmarried	12	88	100
	Married	5	95	100
		17	183	200

Data arising from such a cohort design have the following implications for estimation of population probabilities:

- Joint probabilities cannot be estimated—clearly, frequencies of joint characteristics such as unmarried mothers with low birthweight babies are artificially influenced by the exact allocation of the number of unmarried mothers sampled from the total sample of 200.

- Marginal probabilities are not estimable for the same reason.

- Only conditional probabilities that condition on exposure status can be estimated, such as $\hat{P}(D|E) = \hat{P}$(low birthweight infant|unmarried mother) $= 12/100 = 0.120$, or $\hat{P}(D|\bar{E}) = \hat{P}$(low birthweight infant|married mother) $= 5/100 = 0.050$.

The estimable conditional probability estimates provide essentially the same picture as those yielded by the population-based study of the same population (although the precision of these estimates may not be the same, but this is getting ahead of ourselves).

Although only some basic conditional probabilities are estimable from a cohort design, these are fortunately the basic building blocks of the Relative Risk, Odds Ratio, and the Excess Risk. The Attributable Risk is not directly estimable from a cohort study because we cannot estimate $P(E)$. From Table 5.3 we can estimate

- $\widehat{RR} = (12/100)/(5/100) = 2.40$
- $\widehat{OR} = [(12/100)/(88/100)]/[(5/100)/(95/100)] = 2.59$
- $\widehat{ER} = (12/100) - (5/100) = 0.070$.

Again, these estimates are compatible with those provided by the population-based data from the same population.

5.3 Disease-based sampling—case-control studies

A case-control study has the same specifications as a cohort study, except that the roles of E and D are reversed. Separate samples are thus selected from cases (D) and nondiseased individuals or controls ($\bar{D}$). The main steps of the design are:

1. Identify two subgroups of the population on the basis of the presence or absence of D.

2. Take a simple random sample from each of these two subgroups (that is, the Ds and not Ds) *separately*, of sizes n_D and $n_{\bar{D}}$, respectively.

3. Measure subsequently the presence and absence of E for individuals in both random samples.

As for cohort designs, the investigator must prespecify the number of cases and controls selected in the two separate random samples. Table 5.4 describes a possible outcome of a case-control study of mother's marital status and infant birthweight using samples of 100 cases (D) and 100 controls (not D). Here, implementing the design involves sampling first 100 low birthweight infants and then taking a further random sample of 100 normal birthweight infants. This again assumes that two sampling

Table 5.4 *Possible data from a case-control study ($n_D = n_{\bar{D}} = 100$) of a mother's marital status and low birthweight*

		Birthweight		
		Low	Normal	
Marital status at birth	Unmarried	50	28	78
	Married	50	72	122
		100	100	200

frames, one of low birthweight infants in the population and the other of normal birthweight infants, are accessible to the investigator.

For similar reasons as in cohort designs, only a limited set of probabilities can be estimated using case-control data:

- Joint probabilities cannot be estimated—frequencies of joint characteristics are again artificially influenced by the exact allocation of the number of low birthweight babies sampled from the total sample of 200.

- Marginal probabilities are not available for the same reason.

- Only conditional probabilities that condition on outcome status, here infant birthweight, can be estimated such as $\hat{P}(E|D) = \hat{P}$(unmarried mother|low birthweight infant) $= 50/100 = 0.500$, or $\hat{P}(E|\bar{D}) = \hat{P}$ (unmarried mother|normal birthweight infant) $= 28/100 = 0.280$.

At first glance, it seems unlikely that we can estimate any measure of association from a case-control design. This is indeed partly true in that it is impossible to estimate the Relative Risk or the Excess Risk with case-control data. However, we can directly estimate the Odds Ratio for E associated with D, given by $[P(E|D)]/[P(\text{not } E|D)]/[P(E|\text{not } D)]/[P(\text{not } E|\text{not } D)]$, and then take advantage of the fact that this is identical to the Odds Ratio for D associated with E (using the symmetry of the roles of disease and exposure in the definition of the Odds Ratio that we highlighted in Section 4.4). Thus, from Table 5.4,

$$\widehat{OR} = [(50/100)/(50/100)]/[(28/100)/(72/100)] = 2.57,$$

compatible with the estimates provided by the population-based and cohort data.

In a situation where the outcome D is rare in both exposed and unexposed populations, the Odds Ratio will closely approximate the Relative Risk so that the case-control estimate of the Odds Ratio can be used as an approximate estimate of the Relative Risk. It was, in part, this observation—that case-control studies can still be used to estimate Relative Risks in rare disease settings (Cornfield, 1951)—that led to their increased popularity as a study design over the past 50 years. The first modern use of the design was a study of the effect of reproductive history on the incidence of breast cancer (Lane-Claypon, 1926). The next section shows that the rare disease assumption is unnecessary for estimating the Relative Risk or Relative Hazard from case-control data if clever adjustments are made in the sampling of controls.

The Attributable Risk also appears to be unestimable from a case-control design. However, in the rare disease setting, we can again obtain an approximation; to see this, we first need some algebraic work to derive an alternative formulation for AR. Recall from Section 4.7 that $AR = [P(D) - P(D|\bar{E})]/P(D) = 1 - [P(D|\bar{E})/P(D)]$. Now,

$$P(D|\bar{E}) = P(D|\bar{E})(P(\bar{E}) + P(E))$$
$$= P(\bar{E})P(D|\bar{E}) + \frac{P(D|E)P(E)}{RR},$$

the last step following from the definition of RR. Hence,

$$AR = 1 - \frac{P(\bar{E})P(D|\bar{E})}{P(D)} - \frac{P(D|E)P(E)}{RR \times P(D)}$$
$$= 1 - P(\bar{E}|D) - \frac{P(E|D)}{RR},$$

using Bayes' formula twice (see Section 3.4). It follows that

$$AR = P(E|D)\left(1 - \frac{1}{RR}\right). \tag{5.1}$$

From case-control data we can estimate $P(E|D)$ directly, and then with the rare disease assumption estimate RR approximately by the estimate of the Odds Ratio. With the data of Table 5.4, this approach yields

$$\widehat{AR} = \frac{50}{100}\left(1 - \frac{1}{2.57}\right) = 0.31,$$

which is very similar to the estimate obtained from the population-based data of Table 5.2. Note that use of the rare disease assumption is questionable here since data from the population-based study reveal that $\hat{P}$(low birthweight infant|unmarried mother) = 0.119, and $\hat{P}$(low birthweight infant|married mother) = 0.050, suggesting that OR may be substantially larger than RR; in fact the estimates from either Table 5.2 or Table 5.3 show that OR is approximately 8% greater than RR. Again, use of the rare disease assumption can be avoided in using Equation 5.1 under a variant of case-control sampling described in Section 5.4.2.

5.4 Key variants of the case-control design

As was hinted in Section 5.3, it is possible to estimate the Relative Risk or Relative Hazard from case-control samples without the rare disease assumption by modifying the sampling scheme for the controls. On the surface, the rare disease assumption appears to preclude situations where either the disease frequency is high or, essentially equivalently, the interval of risk underlying the definition of disease incidence is sufficiently long so that the cumulative incidence over the entire interval is high. One way to evade the issue of high cumulative incidence is to divide the risk interval into smaller subintervals, chosen so that risk levels in each subinterval meet the rare disease assumption, and then to carry out separate case-control studies for each subinterval of risk. Odds Ratios can be calculated for each subinterval, and the possibility that these vary over time can be incorporated into the subsequent statistical analysis. In practice, it is natural to implement case-control designs in this fashion when cases can only be sampled as they accumulate in a population. With this in mind, we describe the two most useful and widely used variants of the case-control scheme, the first of which uses exactly the general strategy we just outlined. These modified designs are called *nested case-control studies* because they can be viewed as taking a subsample from a conceptual larger cohort or population.

5.4.1 Risk-set sampling of controls

In a case-control design with risk-set sampling of controls, it is common to select all cases that occur in a population in the defined risk period $[0, T]$, although it is perfectly acceptable for only a random sample to be chosen. For each incident case that is identified and sampled at time t, one or more controls are randomly drawn from the population of individuals still at risk of disease at t. Exposure measurements are taken for each case and for its corresponding set of sampled controls. In essence, this is a stratified, or matched, case-control design where the strata are defined by the times at risk over the interval $[0, T]$. There is no point in sampling controls at times where no disease occurs since they would have no comparative case group. This form of control sampling is widely referred to as *risk set sampling* or *density sampling*. Note that, unlike the traditional or classic case-control sampling of Section 5.3, it is possible for a control sampled at time t to later become a case and enter the sample a second time. Although this is unlikely in large populations unless the disease is common, such a participant must be included in the data set twice. Similarly, it is also theoretically possible that the same individual be selected as a control more than once at differing times, with the same admonition.

Further, note that risk-set sampling of controls accommodates the possibility that the study population is *dynamic* in that individuals may enter and leave the population during the risk interval. The key to the definition of controls in this situation is that they must be *at risk* of being a case (and thus being sampled through that path) at the time of sampling. In addition, the possibility that an individual's exposure level changes over time is also allowed, with the provision that exposure assessment applies *at the time of sampling* for both cases and controls.

To illustrate this form of control sampling, consider a study of the role of the herpes simplex virus type 2 (HSV-2) on the risk for cervical cancer (Lehtinen et al., 2002). In this investigation, the study population consisted of 550,000 women who had donated blood samples to population-based serum banks in Finland, Norway, and Sweden. These samples were collected for a variety of reasons, including first-trimester screening samples during pregnancy and samples from routine health examinations and health promotion projects. Cases of cervical cancer from this study population were identified, over an appropriate calendar risk period, from cancer registries with subsequent linkage to the serum bank using unique identifiers. For each case found, three controls were also chosen from the serum bank who were cancer-free *at the time of diagnosis of the case*. (Controls were also matched to cases by age, geographic

Table 5.5 *Expected cell entries in a 2 × 2 contingency table for data generated by risk-set sampling*

		Case	Risk-Set Control
	E	$N_E(t)h_E(t)$	$m \times \frac{N_E(t)}{N_E(t)+N_{\bar{E}}(t)}$
Exposure			
	not E	$N_{\bar{E}}(t)h_{\bar{E}}(t)$	$m \times \frac{N_{\bar{E}}(t)}{N_E(t)+N_{\bar{E}}(t)}$

subgroups of the bank, and length of storage time for the blood sample, but we defer discussion of this form of matching until Chapter 16.) The donated blood allowed assessment of prior infection with HSV-2 via identification of antibodies. In this case, one possible weakness of the study is that exposure assessment refers to infection status at the time of the donation rather than at the time of sampling. Improving exposure information to avoid this complication would have involved tracing all cases and controls for further blood testing.

With this variant of control sampling, we can calculate expected counts of exposed and unexposed participants in both case and control samples. At any time t, let $N_E(t)$ and $N_{\bar{E}}(t)$ be the number of individuals still at risk in the exposed and unexposed population, respectively; the dependence of these numbers on time allows for dynamic changes in the population. The number of cases expected in the exposed group at time t is then $N_E(t) \times h_E(t)$, by the definition of the hazard rate, $h_E(t)$, under exposure. Similarly, the number of cases expected in the unexposed group at the same time is $N_{\bar{E}}(t) \times h_{\bar{E}}(t)$, with the same notation. On the other hand, if m controls are sampled at t in the manner described, then the expected number of exposed and unexposed controls are simply $m \times N_E(t)/[N_E(t) + N_{\bar{E}}(t)]$, and $m \times N_{\bar{E}}(t)/[N_E(t) + N_{\bar{E}}(t)]$, respectively, since the proportion of exposed individuals at risk at time t is simply $N_E(t)/[N_E(t) + N_{\bar{E}}(t)]$. Table 5.5 shows these expected counts for each cell in the resulting 2 × 2 table at time t.

The Odds Ratio for this expected data table is quickly seen to be $h_E(t)/h_{\bar{E}}(t) = RH(t)$. If we assume proportional hazards, then $RH(t)$ does not depend on t, and so the Odds Ratios for each of these tables at differing times is a constant, equal to RH. In this way, a constant Relative Hazard can be derived from a case-control design with risk-set sampling, and can be estimated using methods for combining Odds Ratios across many 2 × 2 tables discussed later in the book, in particular in Chapters 9, 16, and 17.

Why does the (sample or data) Odds Ratio from Table 5.5 not estimate the population Odds Ratio? The answer is that, with risk-set sampling, the exposure distribution of the sampled controls does not reflect the exposure distribution of $\bar{D}$s as it does for the classic case-control sampling of Section 5.3. Happily, the distortion introduced by this form of sampling leads the sample Odds Ratio to estimate the Relative Hazard, arguably a more interpretable measure of association.

An important variation of density sampling involves selecting all cases as for risk-set sampling, but sampling controls throughout the risk interval $[0, T]$ without regard to the timing of the incident cases. The expected cell entries from the table that pools

Table 5.6 *Expected cell entries in a 2 × 2 contingency table for data generated by persistent sampling of controls*

		Case	Control
Exposure	E	$\int N_E(t)h_E(t)\,dt$	$\int m(t) \times \frac{N_E(t)}{N_E(t)+N_{\bar{E}}(t)}\,dt$
	not E	$\int N_{\bar{E}}(t)h_{\bar{E}}(t)\,dt$	$\int m(t) \times \frac{N_{\bar{E}}(t)}{N_E(t)+N_{\bar{E}}(t)}\,dt$

the cases and controls collected in this way are given in Table 5.6, where we have taken the liberty of using integral signs to reflect that we are pooling the case and control observations over time. If preferred, these integrals can be loosely interpreted as "sums" over distinct short time periods that span the entire risk interval. Note that we allow for the possibility that the number of sampled controls, $m(t)$, varies over the risk interval. The Odds Ratio from this table is complex, but can be simplified enormously if we assume that the Relative Hazard, $RH(t)$, is constant over time (see Equation 4.5) and that the proportion of exposed individuals, $N_E(t)/[N_E(t) + N_{\bar{E}}(t)] = p_E$, also does not vary with time. In this scenario, the Odds Ratio from Table 5.6 is then $OR = [RH \times \int p_E N(t)h_{\bar{E}}(t)\,dt \times \int(1 - p_E)m(t)\,dt]/[\int(1 - p_E)N(t)h_{\bar{E}}(t)\,dt \times \int p_E m(t)\,dt] = RH$, where $N(t) = N_E(t) + N_{\bar{E}}(t)$ is the total number at risk at time t. Thus again, the sample Odds Ratio, this time from a table pooled over time, estimates the Relative Hazard, albeit with the crucial assumption that the population prevalence of exposure remains constant over time even when the population size varies. Avoiding this assumption by stratifying the pooled table over the time at risk (or, equivalently, time of sampling) takes us back to a form of risk-set sampling, albeit without a fixed number of controls per case in each stratum.

Notice that we did not require any assumption about the frequency with which D occurs over the entire risk period (e.g., a rare disease assumption), under either form of density sampling, in showing that a sample Odds Ratio can be seen as an estimate of a constant Relative Hazard.

5.4.2 Case-cohort studies

Suppose n_D cases are selected as with risk-set sampling, or the traditional design for that matter. Now, m controls are chosen at random from the entire population at risk at $t = 0$ (of size N, say), the beginning of the risk period. Exposures are calculated for all sampled participants as usual. Here, the controls may, in fact, include a case and vice versa, so that the word control here means something slightly different from its usage in the traditional design; the sampled controls are often referred to as a subcohort of the original Study Population. The sampling scheme is known as the *case-cohort* design.

The Women's Health Trial used a case-cohort approach as part of a general investigation of the effects of a low fat diet on women's health, with particular interest in the risk of breast cancer. In this study, women were randomly assigned to a low fat intervention or control (no major intervention) group. At 2-year intervals, participants

Table 5.7 *Probabilities of cell entries in a* 2×2 *contingency table for data generated by case-cohort sampling*

		Case	Cohort
Exposure	E	$n_D P(E\|D)$	$m P(E)$
	not E	$n_D P(\bar{E}\|D)$	$m P(\bar{E})$

filled out 4-day food frequency questionnaires and blood samples were drawn and stored. Evaluation of disease incidence involved 10 years of follow-up. Assessment of the intervention depended on the full set of enrolled women, but investigation of the role of actual dietary information and blood lipid analyses used the case-cohort approach on a subgroup of 32,000 women of ages between 45 and 69, whose fat intake was high at entry and who possessed at least one known risk factor for breast cancer. In particular, all breast cancer cases were sampled, together with 10% of the original 32,000 as a subcohort. The case-cohort design minimized the expense of abstraction of the food diaries and laboratory tests. Self et al. (1988) provide a complete description of the study design.

Under case-cohort sampling, the expected total number of exposed (unexposed) controls in the subcohort is simply $m P(E)$ ($m P(\bar{E})$, respectively). On the other hand, the expected number of exposed (unexposed) cases is $n_D P(E|D)$ ($n_D P(\bar{E}|D)$). Table 5.7 gives the expected cell entries for the entire sample.

The data Odds Ratio for this table is $P(E|D)P(\bar{E})/P(E)P(\bar{E}|D) = P(D|E)/P(D|\bar{E}) = RR$, so that with this sampling scheme and control definition, the data Odds Ratio actually estimates the population Relative Risk. As for risk-set sampling, we often summarize by saying that in a case-cohort study the data Odds Ratio estimates the Relative Risk, again with no assumption of disease rarity. Similarly to risk-set sampling, the (data) Odds Ratio from Table 5.7 does not estimate the population Odds Ratio because, again, the exposure distribution of the sampled controls (i.e., the cohort) fails to reflect the exposure distribution of $\bar{D}$s. In fact, it yields the total population exposure distribution as can be seen in the right-hand column of Table 5.7. Nevertheless, the distortion introduced by case-cohort sampling leads the sample Odds Ratio to estimate the population Relative Risk. If we prefer to estimate the population Odds Ratio, we can always "remove" any cases from the cohort sample, so that then the right-hand column of Table 5.7 reverts to being a sample of disease-free ($\bar{D}$) controls, in which case the data now have the same structure as a traditional case-control design providing an Odds Ratio estimate as in Section 5.3.

In sum, cases are sampled in identical fashions in all three case-control design strategies, but the subtle differences in the way "controls" are sampled lead the sample Odds Ratio to estimate (1) the population Odds Ratio for classic case-control designs, (2) the Relative Hazard for risk-set sampling, and (3) the Relative Risk for case-cohort studies. This is but one sign that data analysis techniques and their interpretation depend in important ways on how the sample is selected from the Study Population.

That is, the design matters! In Chapter 7 and beyond, we will see repeatedly how the various case-control designs impact how we use the sample to both estimate a measure of association and the uncertainty surrounding such estimates.

5.5 Comments and further reading

The case-control design has traditionally been thought to suffer from increased exposure measurement error and selection bias through an inappropriate choice of a control population. However, modern case-control studies are usually designed with careful consideration of these potential problems. Further, the cohort study is also subject to potentially greater error in disease measurement since it often requires long periods of follow-up. Selection bias is also an issue if the exposure groups are not carefully defined. Forms of selection bias in either design are discussed at length in Kleinbaum et al. (1982, Chapter 11). We look at statistical reasons to prefer one of the three basic design strategies in the next chapter.

Case-cohort and nested case-control designs are particularly appealing when general exposure information is collected in a preliminary fashion for all sampled individuals in a large cohort—for example, serum samples or extensive diet histories—but exact exposure measurement from such sources is expensive. Other forms of density sampling are discussed in Langholz and Goldstein (1996). The case-cohort design is well suited to studies of multiple outcomes since the same control sample can be used for each comparison. Wacholder (1991) discusses practical issues concerning the choice of a nested case-control or case-cohort design. Rodrigues and Kirkwood (1990) give a very readable description of the various case-control designs, with practical suggestions for making a specific choice depending on the frequency and acuteness of the disease.

There is substantial literature on the appropriate choice of controls and methods for sampling in case-control designs. See Wacholder et al. (1992a,b,c) for an overview of control selection. Random digit dialing (Waksberg, 1978) is often used for control sampling when no convenient sampling frame is available, although this method is becoming increasingly problematic as nonresponse rates for telephone surveys have risen substantially in recent years. Choosing controls, whether in a cohort or case-control study, raises again the issue of how "representative" the Study Population is of the Target Population with regard to the validity of extrapolation of particular sample information to the Target Population. While "representativeness" is necessary in describing many aspects of the Target Population, it is often not required and may not even be desirable if our sole intent is estimation of a measure of association. For example, in case-control studies, we may have access to an accurate registry of cases for a well-defined subset—restricted, for example, by geography or the nature of the cases—that is not representative of all cases in the population. In this case, we are still able to implement a successful case-control design for estimating the Odds Ratio, say, by ensuring that disease-free individuals, or controls, are selected at random from a Study Population that adequately serves as the source population only for the restricted group of cases.

5.6 Problems

Question 5.1

Forastiere et al. (2002) investigated the possibility of increased risk of silicosis among female ceramic workers in Italy. Ceramic workers from about 100 plants in central Italy had been surveyed annually for occupational diseases since 1974. Of these, 814 were women, of whom 2 had baseline disease and were excluded, and 642 of the remaining 812 had at least one radiograph during an average follow-up period of 6.7 years. This excluded 172 women who had no follow-up, a group that was younger and worked in the ceramic industry for a shorter period than the study group. Follow-up examinations included an average of 5.9 radiographs used to determine incidence of silicosis. Incidence levels were compared according to the work histories of the women (whether their primary work area was in sanitary ware, crockery, or other).

What kind of study best describes this investigation? What are possible definitions of the Target and Study Populations? For a particular choice of each of these populations, indicate one possible source of selection bias. With regard to the timing of disease occurrence and exposure measurement, is the study prospective or retrospective? What is the most likely form of possible measurement error? Consult Forastiere et al. (2002) if you wish to read further.

Question 5.2

Feychting et al. (1997) investigated a possible association of residential and occupational magnetic field exposure with leukemia and central nervous system tumors in Sweden. The study group comprised approximately 400,000 individuals over 16 years of age, who lived for at least 1 year within 300 m of any 220- or 400-kV power lines in Sweden during the period 1960–1985. All individuals developing leukemia or a central nervous system tumor were sampled for detailed assessment of residential and occupational magnetic field exposure. For each case, two controls were selected at random from individuals who belonged in the study group during the year of diagnosis of the case and exposure measurements were taken for each of these individuals. (Controls were also matched to cases by sex, age, parish of residence, and location of power line, but we defer discussion of this form of matching until Chapter 16.)

What kind of study best describes this investigation? What are possible definitions of the Target and Study Populations? For a particular choice of each of these populations, indicate one possible source of selection bias. With regard to the timing of disease occurrence and exposure measurement, is the study prospective or retrospective? What is the most likely form of possible measurement error? Consult Feychting et al. (1997) if you wish to read further.

Question 5.3

The Pregnancy, Infection, and Nutrition Study (Dole et al., 2003) investigated risk factors for preterm birth (defined as less than 37 weeks of completed gestation). Women between 24 and 29 weeks gestation were recruited for study from two prenatal clinics in central North Carolina, beginning in August 1995; eligibility requirements included ability to speak English, no multiple gestation, over 16 years of age, planned to deliver at study site, and telephone access. Of the 3965 eligible women, 2444 were recruited and 2029 completed a self-administered mail-back psychosocial questionnaire, most between gestational weeks 24 and 30. A further telephone interview was administered around 29 weeks gestation. The questionnaires included standardized instruments to measure various forms of stress. Each enrolled woman's pregnancy was monitored, including medical chart review, to determine a preterm delivery.

What kind of study best describes this investigation? What are possible definitions of the Target and Study Populations? For a particular choice of each of these populations, indicate one possible source of selection bias. With regard to the timing of disease occurrence and exposure measurement, is the study prospective or retrospective? What is the most likely form of possible measurement error? Consult Dole et al. (2003) if you wish to read further.

Question 5.4

All children (under 19 years of age) diagnosed with neuroblastoma over the period May 1, 1992 to April 30, 1994 were contacted for parent interviews in a study conducted by Olshan et al. (2002). Interviews focused on parental occupational history, medication use, and pregnancy histories, with a particular interest in maternal vitamin use. Similar interviews were also administered to parents of healthy children who were ascertained by random digit-dialing. (Matching was also sought on a child's date of birth and the first eight digits of the telephone numbers. We defer further discussion of matching until Chapter 16.)

What kind of study best describes this investigation? What are possible definitions of the Target and Study Populations? For a particular choice of each of these populations, indicate one possible source of selection bias. With regard to the timing of disease occurrence and exposure measurement, is the study prospective or retrospective? What is the most likely form of possible measurement error? Consult Olshan et al. (2002) if you wish to read further.

Question 5.5

Helms et al. (2003) investigated the role of serious gastrointestinal infections on 1-year mortality by using Danish registry systems. The investigators sampled all cases of culture-confirmed infections with nontyphoidal *Salmonella, Campylobacter, Yersinia enterocolitica,* or *Shigella,* listed with the Danish national registry of enteric pathogens. For each case, another 10 randomly selected individuals were chosen from the Danish civil registration system that assigns a personal identification number to all citizens of Denmark. These control individuals had to be alive on the date the infection sample was received for the case. (Matching was also used on the case's age, sex, and county of residence. We defer further discussion of matching until Chapter 16.) The registration system was then used to obtain vital status and date of any death within 1 year from the infection date in both cases and controls.

What kind of study best describes this investigation? What are possible definitions of the Target and Study Populations? For a particular choice of each of these populations, indicate one possible source of selection bias. With regard to the timing of disease occurrence and exposure measurement, is the study prospective or retrospective? What is the most likely form of possible measurement error? Consult Helms et al. (2003) if you wish to read further.

CHAPTER 6

Assessing Significance in a 2×2 Table

Now that we have some ideas for collecting information on disease and exposure, we had better do some homework on what to do with the data, which probably cost a lot of money to collect! Specifically, we turn to the assessment of whether an observed association of D and E in a sample of data reflects a population in which D and E are truly associated or may have arisen from the vagaries of random variation. Before we spend too much effort trying to interpret a relationship between marital status and infant birthweight, we want to convince ourselves that we are not simply tilting at windmills, that is, making a fuss about these variables' apparent association if it could be just due to the chance variation of sampling. In the language of hypothesis testing, a suitable null hypothesis to address this question is that D and E are independent. This, of course, can also be stated in terms of any of the measures of association introduced in Chapter 4:

$$H_0 : D \text{ and } E \text{ are independent} \Leftrightarrow RR = 1 \Leftrightarrow OR = 1 \Leftrightarrow ER = 0$$

It will be convenient to summarize the sampled data by a 2×2 table, as in Table 6.1, and refer to cell entries using the given symbols. Thus, a refers to the number of exposed individuals who developed disease. For this discussion, we consider only the traditional case-control design, although we say more about the analysis of nested case-control and case-cohort designs in the next chapter.

6.1 Population-based designs

Independence of D and E is equivalent to stating that $P(D \ \& \ E) = P(D) \times P(E)$, as we saw in Section 3.4.1. With a population-based design, each of these three probabilities can be estimated directly from sample proportions of the various single or joint characteristics, which are immediately available from the 2×2 table that classifies sampled individuals. From Table 6.1, we have:

- $P(D \ \& \ E)$ can be estimated by a/n
- $P(D)$ can be estimated by $(a + c)/n$
- $P(E)$ can be estimated by $(a + b)/n$.

This suggests looking at the quantity $a/n - [(a + c)/n] \times [(a + b)/n]$ to examine the question of independence. If this number is large, it raises doubt about the validity of independence in the Study Population. Note that $a/n - [(a + c)/n] \times [(a + b)/n] = (ad - bc)/n^2$, since $n = a + b + c + d$. As n is fixed by the design, it makes sense to use the term $(ad - bc)$ to assess independence of D and E.

Table 6.1 *Symbols for entries in generic 2 × 2 table*

		Disease		
		D	not D	
Exposure	E	a	b	$a+b$
	not E	c	d	$c+d$
		$a+c$	$b+d$	$n=a+b+c+d$

Table 6.2 *Possible data from a population-based study (n = 200) of a mother's marital status and low birthweight*

		Birthweight		
		Low	Normal	
Marital status at birth	Unmarried	7	52	59
	Married	7	134	141
		14	186	200

There is nothing special about the a entry in Table 6.1. We could just as easily equate independence with the statement $P(D \text{ \& not } E) = P(D) \times P(\text{not } E)$. This in turn leads to examination of the quantity $c/n - [(a+c)/n] \times [(c+d)/n]$, which similarly simplifies to $(bc - ad)/n^2$, the negative of what we obtained by focusing on the a cell. This also occurs when we compare $P(\bar{D} \text{ \& } E)$ to $P(\bar{D}) \times P(E)$, or $P(\bar{D} \text{ \& } \bar{E})$ to $P(\bar{D}) \times P(\bar{E})$.

To avoid paying attention to the sign, we simply square our measure of noninde-pendence and compute $(ad - bc)^2$. Large values of this statistic will cast doubt on the hypothesis of independence of D and E. But what do we mean by "large"? For exam-ple, consider the population-based data from Table 5.2, repeated here in Table 6.2 for convenience. In this table, we have $(ad - bc)^2 = 329,476$; this seems large by any standard, but we really need a benchmark to assess "largeness." This is achieved by considering the sampling variation in the term $ad - bc$; in a population-based study, $ad - bc$ is a random variable with a sampling distribution that can be approximated by a Normal distribution when the sample size n is large. If the null hypothesis, H_0, that D and E are independent, is true, then the expectation of $ad - bc$ is zero, confirming our intuition that the size of $ad - bc$ provides a measure of evidence against independence. Furthermore, again supposing H_0 to be correct, the variance, V, of the approximating Normal distribution can be estimated by $\hat{V} = (a+b)(a+c)(b+d)(c+d)/n$. Note that the numerator of $\hat{V}$ is just the product of the four margin totals of the 2 × 2 table (see Table 6.1). It follows from this observation that, with a sufficiently large n, $(ad - bc)/\sqrt{\hat{V}}$ has an approximately *standard* Normal distribution, that is, $N(0, 1)$. Equivalently, $(ad - bc)^2/\hat{V} = n(ad - bc)^2/(a+b)(a+c)(b+d)(c+d)$ is closely approximated by a χ^2 distribution with one degree of freedom, $\chi^2_{(1)}$. Tables of the $\chi^2_{(1)}$

distribution can then be used to determine the chances of observing a value as large or larger than $n(ad - bc)^2/(a + b)(a + c)(b + d)(c + d)$, *assuming the null hypothesis,* H_0, *that* D *and* E *are independent, to be true.* This probability value is known as the *p-value,* associated with the null hypothesis H_0, generated by the observed data. As indicated, the p-value is the right-hand tail area, of the $\chi^2_{(1)}$ distribution, greater than the observed value of $n(ad - bc)^2/(a + b)(a + c)(b + d)(c + d)$. If the p-value is small, because $n(ad - bc)^2/(a + b)(a + c)(b + d)(c + d)$ is large, we are suspicious of the assumption that D and E are independent; conversely, if the p-value is not small, then the data do not provide convincing evidence that the assumption of independence is unreasonable.

To see this logic in action, look again at the data of Table 6.2. We already noted that $(ad - bc)^2 = 329,476$; $\hat{V} = (59 \times 141 \times 14 \times 186)/200 = 108,313$, so that $n(ad - bc)^2/(a + b)(a + c)(b + d)(c + d) = 3.04$. Comparison with a table of the $\chi^2_{(1)}$ distribution yields a p-value of 0.08. Thus, it turns out that the value $(ad - bc)^2 = 329,476$ is not very large at all, and, in fact, while suggestive of an association, is also somewhat compatible with the possibility that marital status and birthweight are independent in the underlying population.

6.1.1 Role of hypothesis tests and interpretation of p-values

In the introduction, we assumed familiarity with the basic ideas and interpretation of hypothesis tests, including the p-value, and confidence intervals. These concepts, while appealing, are surprisingly subtle and can be disturbingly misleading. Even the language we have just used to describe the interpretation of a p-value is somewhat sloppy and imprecise. While we cannot do justice to the literature surrounding these topics, there are a few comments worth noting, having encountered the first hypothesis test in the book.

The use of classical hypothesis testing, and associated p-values, has been roundly and deservingly criticized (Goodman and Royall, 1988). The p-value for a χ^2 test of independence does not represent the probability that the population Relative Risk is as far as or further from independence ($RR = 1$) as the observed sample Relative Risk. The p-value is certainly not the probability of H_0, given the data—this is almost the error of equating $P(A|B)$ with $P(B|A)$ discussed in Chapter 3.4—as the p-value depends rather on computing probabilities of possible observations, given H_0. Further, the p-value takes no account of the *power of the study* with regard to the hypothesis test, that is, the probability of accepting the null when it is actually false. Thus a small deviation from independence in a large study can have an identical p-value to a small study containing large deviations. In cynical moments, I find myself discarding a p-value as little more than an alternate measure of sample size since all null hypotheses will produce small p-values so long as enough data are collected.

How should we then interpret the p-values we report here? We use them as informal measures of the compatability of the data with the null hypothesis in question. This does not evade the criticisms outlined, or others for that matter (Goodman and

Royall, 1988), but it does reinforce that they cannot be treated in a formal manner and certainly should not be subject to an arbitrary cutoff value such as 0.05. In addition, p-values arise from calculations based on a null hypothesis that is unlikely to be exactly true. As such, p-values can only be considered as approximations. This is further supported by the fact that they usually do not account for sources of error beyond sampling variation, nor for the impact of multiple comparisons (performing many tests on the same set of data, an action rarely acknowledged in single p-value calculations).

One way to minimize the use of p-values is to focus on estimation of effects, rather than testing null values. We begin to look at this more closely in the next chapter. Uncertainty is often introduced into estimation through the use of confidence intervals. Although confidence intervals are subject to similar criticisms as p-values, they are better rough descriptors of the uncertainty involved in estimation because they avoid the more egregious misinterpretations associated with hypothesis testing, particular if more than one confidence level is used, as suggested in Chapter 3.3.

Alternative inference procedures are available that should be given serious consideration. These include the use of likelihood intervals (see Chapter 13.1.1 for an introduction to the likelihood function) and Bayesian methods. A brief introduction to both of these techniques can be found in Clayton and Hills (1993). In light of the above comments on p-values, it is interesting to note that p-values tend to overstate the evidence against the null hypothesis, as compared to likelihood or Bayesian intervals, particularly when the p-value is greater than 0.01 (Berger and Sellke, 1987).

6.2 Cohort designs

The logic used with population-based designs to investigate independence of D and E is not appropriate for data from a cohort design since it is not possible to estimate joint or marginal probabilities with this design. For example, consider the data in Table 5.3. Here the sample sizes in the random samples of unmarried and married mothers are preselected by the investigator; thus, the observed marginal frequency of unmarried mothers tells you nothing about the population frequency of this characteristic. Indirectly, the choice of the two sample sizes also determines the marginal frequency of low-birthweight infants so that the data again do not provide information regarding the occurrence of low birthweights in the population. By the same token, joint probabilities such as the probability of being an unmarried mother with a low-birthweight infant cannot be estimated from cohort data.

Nevertheless, it is still possible to investigate independence of D and E with cohort data through the equivalent formulation of independence as $P(D|E) = P(D|\text{not } E)$. Both of these conditional probabilities are immediately estimable from the two distinct exposure category samples, and the issue of independence then simplifies to the comparison of two separate population proportions or probabilities.

Specifically, we write the null hypothesis

$$H_0 : D \text{ and } E \text{ are independent} \Leftrightarrow P(D|E) = P(D|\text{not } E).$$

For simplicity write $p_1 = P(D|E)$ and $p_2 = P(D|\text{not } E)$. Using the notation of Table 6.1, we estimate p_1 and p_2 by

$$\hat{p}_1 = \frac{a}{a+b} = \frac{a}{n_1}$$

$$\hat{p}_2 = \frac{c}{c+d} = \frac{c}{n_2}$$

where n_1 and n_2 are the sample sizes of the E and $\bar{E}$ samples, respectively. The two estimates $\hat{p}_1$ and $\hat{p}_2$ are random variables whose sampling distributions can be approximated by Normal distributions when both n_1 and n_2 are large. The expectation of the approximating Normal sampling distribution for $\hat{p}_1$ is p_1, with variance given by $p_1(1 - p_1)/n_1$, and an analogous result holds for the approximate Normal sampling distribution of $\hat{p}_2$. Thus, the difference between the two estimates, $\hat{p}_1 - \hat{p}_2$, has an approximate Normal sampling distribution with expectation $p_1 - p_2$ and variance $[p_1(1 - p_1)/n_1] + [p_2(1 - p_2)/n_2]$.

Now, if we assume the null hypothesis, that D and E are independent, is true, then $p_1 = p_2$. We can then use the difference of our estimates, $\hat{p}_1 - \hat{p}_2$, as a measure of the dependence of D and E. If D and E are independent—that is, H_0 is true—then the parameters of the approximate Normal sampling distribution of $\hat{p}_1 - \hat{p}_2$ simplify; its expectation is then 0 and its variance is given by $p(1 - p)[(1/n_1) + (1/n_2)]$, where $p = p_1 = p_2$. The latter variance can be estimated by $\hat{V} = \hat{p}(1 - \hat{p})[(1/n_1) + (1/n_2)]$, with $\hat{p} = (a + c)/n$, the observed proportion of Ds in the whole sample.

A reasonable test statistic is thus given by $(\hat{p}_1 - \hat{p}_2)/\sqrt{\hat{V}}$, which is expected to follow a standard Normal sampling distribution if D and E are independent. If this statistic is large, there is evidence that D and E are associated. As before, "large" is interpreted in terms of the sampling distribution assuming independence. Alternatively, we can compute the square of this statistic, given by $(\hat{p}_1 - \hat{p}_2)^2/\hat{p}(1 - \hat{p})[(1/n_1) + (1/n_2)]$, which is approximately $\chi^2_{(1)}$ under H_0.

Some simple algebra shows that this test statistic is, in fact, equivalent to the χ^2 test statistic described in Section 6.1 for population-based data. To see this, observe that

$$(\hat{p}_1 - \hat{p}_2)^2 = \left(\frac{a}{n_1} - \frac{c}{n_2}\right)^2 = \frac{(n_2 a - n_1 c)^2}{n_1^2 n_2^2}$$

$$= \frac{(ac + ad - ac - bc)^2}{n_1^2 n_2^2}$$

$$= \frac{(ad - bc)^2}{n_1^2 n_2^2},$$

and

$$\hat{p}(1 - \hat{p})\left(\frac{1}{n_1} + \frac{1}{n_2}\right) = \frac{(a + c)}{n}\frac{(b + d)}{n}\frac{(n_1 + n_2)}{n_1 n_2}$$

$$= \frac{(a + c)(b + d)}{n n_1 n_2}.$$

Table 6.3 *Possible data from a cohort study ($n_E = n_{\bar{E}} = 100$) of a mother's marital status and low birthweight*

		Birthweight		
		Low	Normal	
Marital status at birth	Unmarried	12	88	100
	Married	5	95	100
		17	183	200

Thus,

$$\frac{(\hat{p}_1 - \hat{p}_2)^2}{\hat{p}(1 - \hat{p})(\frac{1}{n_1} + \frac{1}{n_2})} = \frac{(ad - bc)^2}{n_1^2 n_2^2} \times \frac{n n_1 n_2}{(a + c)(b + d)}$$

$$= \frac{n(ad - bc)^2}{n_1 n_2 (a + c)(b + d)}$$

$$= \frac{n(ad - bc)^2}{(a + b)(c + d)(a + c)(b + d)},$$

as claimed.

To illustrate the computation in this setting, we use the data of Table 5.3, repeated in Table 6.3 for convenience, which yields the observed test statistic of $200(12 \times 95 - 88 \times 5)^2 / 100 \times 100 \times 17 \times 183 = 98{,}000{,}000/31{,}110{,}000 = 3.15$, with an associated p-value of 0.08.

6.3 Case-control designs

As for cohort designs and for the same reasons, it is not possible to estimate either joint or marginal probabilities from a case-control design. Further, with case-control data, we cannot obtain information about the conditional disease proportions, $P(D|E)$ and $P(D|\text{not } E)$, either, since the disease frequencies in the data are determined by the sample sizes of cases and controls as prespecified by the investigator. In fact, the only probabilities that are estimable are exposure probabilities, conditional on disease status; that is, $P(E|D)$, $P(E|\bar{D})$. Here H_0, that D and E are independent, can then be given as $P(E|D) = P(E|\bar{D})$, an alternate specification of independence. Thus, in an analogous fashion to that used for cohort designs, we can assess the hypothesis of independence by comparing the observed sample frequency of exposed individuals among cases against that among controls. Using identical algebra to that used in Section 6.2, this comparison then yields the exact same χ^2 statistic used to test independence in both population-based and cohort designs. In sum, although based on differing justifications, we see that the identical χ^2 test of independence applies to each of the three designs we have considered.

Table 6.4 *Possible data from a case-control study* $(n_D = n_{\bar{D}} = 100)$ *of a mother's marital status and low birthweight*

		Birthweight		
		Low	Normal	
Marital status at birth	Unmarried	50	28	78
	Married	50	72	122
		100	100	200

Table 6.5 *Comparison of* χ^2 *test statistic from data generated from various study designs*

	Population-Based	Cohort	Case-Control
χ^2 statistic	3.04	3.15	10.17
p-value	0.08	0.08	0.002

Using the data given in Table 5.4, repeated in Table 6.4 for convenience, we illustrate the by-now familiar calculation of the χ^2 statistic for case-control data. Here, the observed test statistic is given by $200(50 \times 72 - 50 \times 28)^2/100 \times 100 \times 78 \times 122 = 968,000,000/95,160,000 = 10.17$. This is a very large value in terms of the $\chi^2_{(1)}$ distribution and yields a p-value of 0.002. Thus, the case-control data provides quite striking evidence that a mother's marital status is related to the possibility of having a low-birthweight infant. In the next section, we explain the marked difference between the results of the χ^2 test for data generated by each of the three design strategies applied to the same population and with the same sample size.

6.3.1 Comparison of the study designs

Table 6.5 summarizes the results of the χ^2 test of independence on the data from Tables 6.2 to 6.4. Note that the results of the three tests are not entirely incompatible with each other. However, while both the population-based and cohort data are merely suggestive of an association between a mother's marital status and infant birthweight, the case-control data appear to provide sufficient evidence to reject the notion that these two factors are unrelated.

The explanation of the differences between the designs can be found in terms of the *power* of the χ^2 test, that is, the probability that the test will reject independence given a population association between the two factors of interest. Although we cast doubt on the value of hypothesis testing in Section 6.1.1, the power of the χ^2 test remains a useful proxy for the amount of information in a data set regarding the question of independence of D and E. As with most hypothesis tests, the power of the χ^2 test depends on the extent of the true unknown population association and the sample size. This does not explain the different results generated by the three study designs since these factors are the same in each case.

Additional factors influence the power of the χ^2 test, namely, the *balance* of the two marginal totals for D and E, respectively. First, let us compare the population-based and cohort designs. Recall that, for either design, the χ^2 test is based on the (square of the) statistic $(\hat{p}_1 - \hat{p}_2)/\sqrt{\hat{V}}$ where $p_1 = P(D|E)$, $p_2 = P(D|\bar{E})$, and $\hat{V} = \hat{p}(1 - \hat{p})[(1/n_1) + (1/n_2)]$ where n_1 and n_2 are the sample sizes for the Es and $\bar{E}$s, respectively. If the null hypothesis is false, then D and E are related, and $p_1 - p_2 \neq 0$. The power of the χ^2 test increases with the size of $p_1 - p_2$, but, in a given population, this difference is fixed and therefore not influenced by choosing either a population-based or cohort design. Similarly, near the null hypothesis, $p = p_1 = p_2$ is also fixed. The variance term is, however, affected by the design through the term $[(1/n_1) + (1/n_2)] = n/n_1 n_2$. As this term decreases, the precision of our estimate $\hat{p}_1 - \hat{p}_2$ increases, and the χ^2 test statistic also increases. With the total sample size n fixed, $n/n_1 n_2$ is minimized when $n_1 n_2$ is maximized, which occurs when $n_1 = n_2 = n/2$. From this we can infer that, for a cohort design with fixed sample size n, the best sample size allocation, in terms of statistical power of the χ^2 test, is to take $n_1 = n_2 = n/2$. Further, since the sample sizes of Es and $\bar{E}$s are random in a population-based design, they will be essentially determined by the population $P(E)$, and will almost always be unequal, even if $P(E) = 0.5$. Hence, for large samples, a population-based design always yields a less powerful χ^2 test than a cohort design with equal sample sizes of Es and $\bar{E}$s.

By the same token, comparison of the case-control design to the population-based design can be considered in terms of $p_1 - p_2$, where now $p_1 = P(E|D)$ and $p_2 = P(E|\bar{D})$. According to the logic of the last paragraph, the most powerful choice of sample sizes for the case-control design is $n_1 = n_2 = n/2$, where n_1 and n_2 are now the sample sizes for the Ds and $\bar{D}$s, respectively. And, if equal (large) sample sizes of cases and controls are used, the case-control design always leads to a more powerful χ^2 test than a population-based design of the same population.

Finally, the cohort and case-control designs are compared, assuming that both use the optimal equal allocation of the overall sample size to their respective two random samples. This removes the influence of sample size so that differences in power now depend solely on the expected value of the part of the χ^2 statistic given by $(\hat{p}_1 - \hat{p}_2)/\sqrt{\hat{p}(1 - \hat{p})}$, where $\hat{p} = (\hat{p}_1 + \hat{p}_2)/2$ since $n_1 = n_2$. In large samples, this expectation is approximately $d = (p_1 - p_2)/\sqrt{p(1 - p)}$, where for cohort designs $p_1 = P(D|E)$, etc., and for case-control designs $p_1 = P(E|D)$, etc., and in either design $p = (p_1 + p_2)/2$. The power of the χ^2 test will be greater when d is larger, and this scaled difference grows as the average of p_1 and p_2, that is, p, gets closer to 0.5. Figure 6.1 illustrates this graphically for three different population Odds Ratios. Thus, in comparing a cohort to a case-control design, the greater power will belong to the design for which the average, p, of the relevant conditional probabilities lies closer to 0.5. That is, if $[P(E|D) + P(E|\bar{D})]/2$ is nearer to 0.5 than $[P(D|E) + P(D|\bar{E})]/2$, then the case-control design will have higher power than the cohort design for any population Odds Ratio that differs from 1, and vice versa. With $n_1 = n_2$, $P(E)$ closer to 0.5 than $P(D)$ implies that $[P(E|D) + P(E|\bar{D})]/2$ is nearer to 0.5 than $[P(D|E) + P(D|\bar{E})]/2$, and that therefore the case-control design is more powerful with large samples; when $P(E)$ is closer to 0.5 than $P(D)$, the converse of this statement is true by the same reasoning.

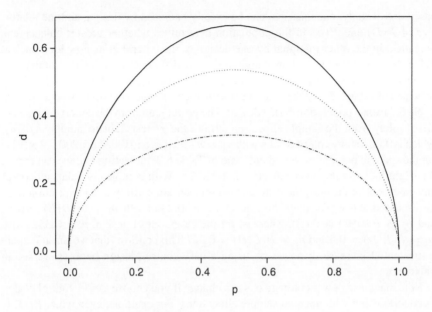

Figure 6.1 *Variation of the scaled difference in proportions, d, against the average of the proportions, p, at various fixed odds ratios (solid: OR = 4, dotted: OR = 3, dash-dot: OR = 2).*

In summary, we have learned that for large samples,

- In a cohort design with a fixed sample size, the χ^2 test of independence is most powerful when the exposed and unexposed samples are of equal size.

- A cohort design with equal samples of exposed and unexposed yields a more powerful χ^2 test of independence than a population-based study with the same overall sample size.

- In a case-control design with a fixed sample size, the χ^2 test of independence is most powerful when the case and control samples are of equal size.

- A case-control design with equal samples of cases and controls yields a more powerful χ^2 test of independence than a population-based study with the same overall sample size.

- When $P(E)$ is closer to 0.5 than $P(D)$, the case-control design with equal samples of cases and controls will give a more powerful χ^2 test of independence than the cohort design with equal numbers of exposed and unexposed.

- When $P(D)$ is closer to 0.5 than $P(E)$, then the cohort design with equal numbers of exposed and unexposed will give a more powerful χ^2 test of independence than the case-control design with equal samples of cases and controls.

These conditions all point to greater power being achieved when *both* disease and exposure marginal frequencies are closer to being balanced. In either a cohort or case-control study, one marginal can be exactly balanced by design, and the relative size of $P(D)$ and $P(E)$ in the population determines whether greater balance can be gained in the other marginal by one design or the other. Let us now look back at Tables 6.2 to 6.4 to observe how marginal balance differences explain the comparison of the χ^2 test statistics of Table 6.5. The exposure (marital status) marginal is exactly balanced in Table 6.3, and the outcome (birthweight) marginal is slightly better than in Table 6.2 from a population-based design. The power gain from the cohort design here arises solely from the sample allocation term of the χ^2 test statistic, namely $n/n_1 n_2$, which is 0.02 for any cohort design with $n_1 = n_2 = 100$, and $0.024 (= 200/59 \times 141)$ for the specific population-based outcome of Table 6.2, indicating that we can expect the slight increase in power reflected in Table 6.5. With completely balanced cohort and case-control designs, the differences in power are entirely due to variation in d, as discussed above. For the cohort design, $d = 0.240$ (with $p_1 = P(D|E) = 0.12$ and $p_2 = P(D|\bar{E}) = 0.05$), whereas, for the case-control design, $d = 0.352$ (with $p_1 = P(E|D) = 0.5$ and $p_2 = P(E|\bar{D}) = 0.28$). This confirms that we can anticipate a substantial increase in power by using a case-control design here, as we see in Table 6.5.

Note that these power comparisons can change if you choose a case-control design or cohort design with unequal sample allocations. For example, even when $P(D)$ is much smaller than $P(E)$, it is possible that the case-control design will yield less power than the cohort design if you allocate the total sample poorly. Further, remember that increasing the total sample size will increase power for all designs (again assuming a sensible allocation of this sample size in both the case-control designs and cohort designs). Thus, even if the available sample size of cases is limited in a case-control design (say, to 100, for example), it still adds power if we sample more than 100 controls as compared to balancing the sample sizes at 100. The gain in power comes from the decline in the sample size factor, $ssf = n/n_1 n_2$, as n increases, even though n_1, the number of cases, stays fixed. If $n_2 = kn_1$, say, then $ssf = (k + 1)/kn_1$. The relative size of ssf for $k = 1$ compared to $k > 1$ is $R = 2k/(k + 1)$, with the value of R then reflecting the ratio of the sample size factor with k controls per case to that with one control per case. Figure 6.2 plots R against k, the ratio of the number of controls to number of cases. With a fixed number of cases, the figure shows the growth in the sample size factor—and thus the power of the χ^2 test—as you increase the number of controls selected per case; however, as a rule of thumb, it is clear that you gain relatively little by adding extra controls, after you have four times as many controls as cases. The primary gain in power comes from increasing the number of controls per case from 1 to 4.

6.4 Comments and further reading

The power comparisons between the various designs, with resulting sample size implications given in Section 6.3.1, are appropriate at the null, that is, assuming independence between D and E. Different recommendations for sample size allocation are necessary when estimating a relationship away from the null. We return to this briefly in Chapter 7.1.1. Also, note that the χ^2 test is not immediately applicable

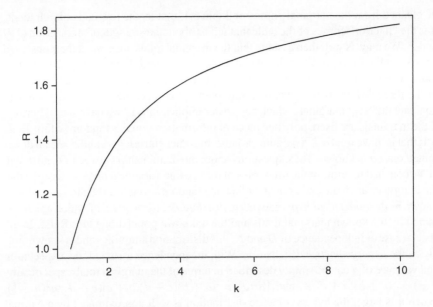

Figure 6.2 *Relative size of sample size factor, R, compared to the ratio of number of controls to cases, k, for a case-control design.*

to case-control data with risk-set sampling except under restrictive conditions. For a case-cohort design, the χ^2 test of independence can be directly applied, not to the data as represented in Table 5.7, but to the version where the cohort sample is modified by removal of any cases.

6.4.1 Alternative formulations of the χ^2 test statistic

For population-based designs, the a entry in Table 6.1 is a random variable with expectation $E(a) = nP(D\&E)$. Be careful not to confuse "Expectation" and "Exposure." If independence of D and E is assumed, then $E(a) = nP(D)P(E)$. Similar formulae can be developed for the b, c, and d entries. It is then easy to show that the χ^2 statistic can also be written as

$$\chi^2 \text{ statistic } = \sum_{i=1}^{2}\sum_{j=1}^{2}\frac{(O_{ij} - E_{ij})^2}{E_{ij}}, \tag{6.1}$$

where i and j index the four cells of the 2×2 tables so that $O_{11} = a$ etc., and E_{ij} denotes the estimated expectation of the relevant cell *under the assumption of independence*. That is, E_{11} is the estimate of $E(a) = nP(D)P(E)$ given by $E_{11} = n[(a + b/n)(a + c/n)]$. Equation 6.1 also holds under both cohort and case-control sampling schemes.

Yet another derivation of the χ^2 test for independence can be based on the following argument. Very little, if any information, about the relationship between D and E can be gleaned from the marginal entries of Table 6.1, that is, the row and column totals. It is the "interior" entries of the table that tell us about the strength of association of D and E. We may as well then assume that the marginal totals are *fixed* at their observed values, and then try to determine whether the a, b, c, and d entries suggest possible independence or otherwise. With fixed marginal totals, analysis of the data from any of the three designs is then identical (although, of course, the different designs will generate different marginals which has power implications as we have seen). Further, if the marginals are fixed, only one piece of information remains random within Table 6.1; that is, if we treat a as a random variable, the other entries, b, c, and d, are all determined once a is known. Thus, questions about the relationship between D and E can all be couched in terms of the properties of the random variable a once we assume that the marginals are fixed and known. In fact, the random variable a then follows what is known as the *noncentral hypergeometric distribution*, parameters of which are determined by the known marginal totals and the unknown population Odds Ratio. In the special case of independence of D and E, this distribution simplifies and is known simply as the *hypergeometric distribution*. With independence assumed, the expectation and variance of a can be simply described in terms of the marginal totals; specifically, $E(a) = (a+b)(a+c)/n$, and $Var(a) = (a+b)(c+d)(a+c)(b+d)/n^2(n-1)$. When n is large, the hypergeometric distribution is well approximated by a Normal distribution with the same expectation and variance. Thus under the null hypothesis, H_0, of independence, the random variable $[a - E(a)]/\sqrt{Var(a)}$ should approximately follow a standard Normal distribution, or equivalently, $(a - E(a))^2/Var(a)$ is approximately $\chi^2_{(1)}$. This then provides the basis for a test of independence of D and E. In fact, the test statistic, $(a - E(a))^2/Var(a)$, differs from the χ^2 statistic, $n(ad - bc)^2/(a+b)(c+d)(a+c)(b+d)$, only in that the term n in the numerator is replaced by $(n-1)$. This is irrelevant when n is large, and the two approaches will then give almost identical results. However, this difference between n and $(n-1)$ in these two versions of the χ^2 statistic will have important implications when we study the combination of many 2 × 2 tables with small sample sizes in Chapters 9 and 16.

6.4.2 When is the sample size too small to do a χ^2 test?

In discussing the χ^2 test of independence of D and E, we frequently referred to "large" samples or "large" n in order to invoke the approximation of the sampling distribution of the test statistic by the $\chi^2_{(1)}$ distribution. Just how large does n have to be? In fact, the quality of the approximation does not depend solely on n; extensive examination has determined that it is accurate so long as the expectation (assuming independence) of each entry inside Table 6.1 is greater than 1 (Larntz, 1978). We can check this by using estimates of these expectations for each entry in the 2 × 2 table; that is, by examining whether $(a+b)(a+c)/n$ is greater than 1 for the a entry, and so on. For example, Tables 6.2 to 6.4 meet these criteria easily.

The exact sampling distribution of cell entries can be used to construct a test of independence when the sample size is so small that use of the approximating $\chi^2_{(1)}$ distribution is questionable. With the assumption of fixed marginals, the relevant exact distribution is the hypergeometric as noted in Section 6.4.1, whose use as the null

sampling distribution of *a* leads to the *Fisher exact test*. Further discussion of this test
can be found in either Fleiss (1981) or Breslow and Day (1980). For either cohort or
case-control designs, an alternative exact test is based on the binomial distributions for
each of the two samples generated by the design. This exact test has somewhat greater
power than Fisher's exact test (D'Agostino et al., 1988). The widespread availability
of such exact tests precludes the need to use a continuity correction to improve the
adequacy of the χ^2 approximation; if we face a 2×2 table where use of the continuity
correction makes a noticeable difference, then proceed with an appropriate exact test
and avoid use of the χ^2 test altogether.

6.5 Problems

Question 6.1

When a risk factor is rarer in the population than a disease, which kind of study design
is usually more powerful for studying the possible association between the factor and
the disease?

Question 6.2

Table 6.6 provides data from a case-control study of oral cancer in females and
employment in the textile industry. Using the χ^2 test, evaluate whether employment
in the textile industry is associated with oral cancer.

Question 6.3

Using the data provided in Question 3.1, evaluate the association between fish consumption and 25-year mortality from CHD using the χ^2 test.

Question 6.4

Perez-Padilla et al. (2001) conducted a case-control study on biomass cooking fuel
exposure and tuberculosis in Mexico. The authors hypothesized that exposure to
cooking fuel smoke would increase the risk of developing tuberculosis. Cases were
288 patients with active smear or culture positive tuberculosis, and controls were 545
patients with ear, nose, and throat ailments from the same hospital, seen at the same
time. Current and past exposure to biomass smoke was obtained by interview.

Table 6.6 *Case-control data on textile industry employment and oral cancer*

| | | Oral Cancer | | |
		Cases	Controls	
Employment history	10 years or more in textile industry	22	9	31
	Other work history	35	48	83
		57	57	114

Table 6.7 *Case-control data on biomass fuel exposure and tuberculosis*

| | | Tuberculosis | | |
		Cases	Controls	
Biomass fuel exposure	Yes	50	21	71
	No	238	524	762
		288	545	833

Table 6.8 *Cohort data on hair loss experience and CHD*

| | | CHD | | |
		Heart Disease	No Heart Disease	
Hair loss experience	Balding	127	1,224	1,351
	No hair loss	548	7,611	8,159
		675	8,835	9,510

Table 6.7 gives the data for the association between current exposure to biomass smoke and TB. Calculate the χ^2 test statistic and associated p-value to examine the issue of independence of these two variables.

Question 6.5

The Physicians' Health Study (Lotufo et al., 2000) is a (retrospective) cohort study of 22,071 U.S. male physicians aged 40 to 84 years. Of these, 9,510 were free of coronary heart disease and had no hair loss at baseline; these individuals subsequently completed a questionnaire after 11 years of follow-up to determine their experience of hair loss when they were 45 years old. The cross-classification of individuals by hair loss at 45 years and subsequent incidence of CHD is given in Table 6.8. Calculate the χ^2 statistic to examine the association between hair loss experience at 45 years of age and subsequent incidence of CHD.

Question 6.6

Suppose two investigators are planning case-control studies, and both determine to randomly select 100 cases and 100 controls from their populations of interest. The first investigator believes that exposure probabilities in the cases and controls ($P(E|D)$ and $P(E|\text{not } D)$) are roughly 0.4 and 0.1, respectively (so an Odds Ratio of about 6 is expected). The second investigator believes that, in her situation, the exposure probabilities in the cases and controls are roughly 0.2 and 0.04, respectively (so that again an Odds Ratio of about 6 is anticipated). Which study has the greater power to detect a significant association between the relevant exposure and disease?

CHAPTER 7

Estimation and Inference for Measures of Association

As argued in Section 6.1.1, the goal of an epidemiological study is estimation of effects rather than mere assessment of the independence or nonindependence of an exposure and disease outcome. How large is the effect of prenatal care on the incidence of low birthweight babies? How effective is a vaccine in preventing a communicable disease? How strong is the association between elevated dietary fat and heart disease? We now focus on estimation of the measures of association introduced in Chapter 4 using data arising from any of the designs discussed in Chapter 5. A key component of our analysis is determination of the level of uncertainty associated with proposed estimators, expressed via calculation of confidence intervals. We again use the notation for entries in a 2×2 table given in Table 6.1.

7.1 The odds ratio

For both population-based and cohort designs, a straightforward estimate of the Odds Ratio is available through its definition, Equation 4.2. This formula shows that estimation of the Odds Ratio only requires estimates of the conditional probabilities $P(D|E)$ and $P(D|\text{not } E)$, both of which can be estimated directly for both population-based and cohort studies. For example, the estimate for $P(D|E)$ in both designs is simply the observed proportion of exposed individuals who are Ds, that is $a/(a+b)$. Substituting this estimate and the analogs for the other conditional probabilities yields the following estimate for the Odds Ratio:

$$\widehat{OR} = \left[\frac{a/(a+b)}{b/(a+b)}\right] \bigg/ \left[\frac{c/(c+d)}{d/(c+d)}\right]$$
$$= \frac{ad}{bc}.$$

For case-control data, we rely on the expression of the Odds Ratio in terms of the conditional probabilities that condition on disease status, as described in Section 4.4. These conditional probabilities, such as $P(E|D)$ and $P(E|\text{not } D)$, are directly available from case-control data, again estimated by the respective sample proportions; for example $P(E|D)$ is estimated by the observed proportion of cases who are Es, that is, $a/(a+c)$. Substituting these estimates into (4.4) then gives

$$\widehat{OR} = \left[\frac{a/(a+c)}{c/(a+c)}\right] \bigg/ \left[\frac{b/(b+d)}{d/(b+d)}\right]$$
$$= \frac{ad}{bc}.$$

Table 7.1 *Possible data from a cohort study ($n_E = n_{\bar{E}} = 50$) with OR = 1*

		Disease Status		
		D	$\bar{D}$	
Exposure status	E	8	42	50
	$\bar{E}$	11	39	50
		19	81	100

Thus, the estimate of the Odds Ratio does not depend on the study design employed; we can infer this directly from our earlier observation (Section 4.4) that the Odds Ratio is symmetric in the roles of D and E in its definition.

7.1.1 Sampling distribution of the odds ratio

The estimate, ad/bc, of the Odds Ratio is a random variable and, as such, has an associated sampling distribution describing the probabilities that the estimate will fall in specified ranges of values for a given sample size and study design. Equivalently, the sampling distribution of $\widehat{OR}$ describes the frequency with which ad/bc takes on certain values after repeated samples under identical sampling conditions. To illustrate the sampling distribution of ad/bc, consider a cohort study of a population for which, unknown to the investigator, $P(D|E) = P(D|\text{not } E) = 0.2$, so that the true Odds Ratio is 1.0. For example, imagine that D again refers to a low birthweight infant, and E denotes use of a vitamin supplement, both factors measured in a population of women with no health insurance. Table 7.1 gives a typical result of the outcome, if the investigator randomly samples 50 exposed and 50 unexposed individuals.

The estimate of the Odds Ratio from Table 7.1 is $\widehat{OR} = (8 \times 39)/(11 \times 42) = 0.68$; the χ^2 test for independence of D and E yields a test statistic of 0.58 with a p-value of 0.44. This result seems compatible with what might be expected given the population information.

Now imagine repeating this study over and over again. Each time the results will be slightly different reflecting sampling variation—the differing values of $\widehat{OR}$ will exhibit the properties underlying the sampling distribution of $\widehat{OR}$. Figure 7.1 displays a frequency histogram of 1000 repeated versions of this cohort study. If we repeated this study an infinite number of times, then this histogram would be the sampling distribution (assuming a small enough bin size for the histogram).

It is obvious from Figure 7.1 that the sampling distribution of $\widehat{OR}$ is skewed to the right. This is typical of sampling distributions of Odds Ratio estimates, particularly with moderate sample sizes that often occur in epidemiological studies. In part, the skewness arises from the restriction on the range of an Odds Ratio—Odds Ratios must always be nonnegative—that we noted in Section 4.2. From another point of view, the Odds Ratio estimate is a quotient of random quantities which tend to have skewed sampling distributions (as compared to quantities resulting from adding or subtracting random quantities). The skewness has important implications for using $\widehat{OR}$ as the basis of statements about the true unknown OR in a population.

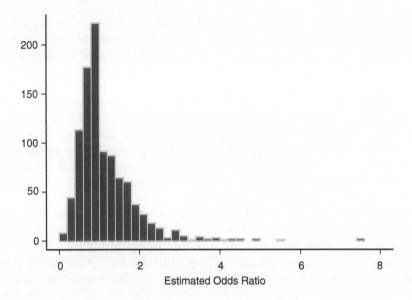

Figure 7.1 *Frequency histogram of 1,000 estimated odds ratios for data generated from a cohort design with OR = 1 and 50 exposed and 50 unexposed.*

First, note that the smallest value of $\widehat{OR}$ in the 1000 studies was 0.15, and the largest was 7.58. (Can you imagine the confusion when one study reports an over sevenfold increase in the risk of low birthweight and another about a sevenfold decrease in risk, both associated with vitamin use! We must always be conscious of the impact of sampling variation.) The average and median of the 1000 $\widehat{OR}$s was 1.16 and 1, respectively. A reflection of the skewness of its sampling distribution, $\widehat{OR}$ tends to be a little too large "on the average" (16% in this example). On the other hand the median of the sampling distribution is exactly the true value of OR, showing that half the time a single study will yield an estimated OR that is bigger than the population OR, and half the time it will be smaller. This is an attractive property of the sampling distribution, but the "average" result indicates that when $\widehat{OR}$ is bigger than OR it tends to be farther away from OR than when it is smaller than OR. This is an example of *statistical bias* in the estimator $\widehat{OR}$ of OR—this bias decreases as the sample size increases. We return to this issue briefly in Section 7.1.4 when discussing small sample estimators.

Of greater importance is that it does not seem reasonable to approximate the sampling distribution of $\widehat{OR}$ by a Normal distribution; that is, the histogram in Figure 7.1, approximately the sampling distribution, cannot be reproduced effectively by any Normal density curve, the familiar bell-shape. This is disturbing, because approximating sampling distributions by Normals is the basis of the construction of confidence intervals for many estimation problems, at least in large samples where exact sampling distributions may be difficult to compute.

Fortunately, there is a simple way around the complications caused by a skewed sampling distribution through use of a *transformation*. We seek to transform the estimate $\widehat{OR}$ so that the sampling distribution of the transformed result has a more symmetric sampling distribution. Then we can calculate confidence intervals on the transformed scale, and transform back at the end to give results on the original and familiar Odds Ratio scale. For the Odds Ratio, a successful transformation to achieve reasonable symmetry is the logarithmic or "log" transformation. (Recall that taking logarithms of products and quotients is just the summation or subtraction of the logs of the individual components.) It does not matter which base is used for the logarithm, that is $\log_{10}$ (logs to base 10) will be just as useful in this regard as $\log_2$ or any other base. Throughout, we will use the so-called *natural* logarithm, $\log_e$, but denote this simply by log. Many books and calculators use the notation *ln* to refer to a natural logarithm. We reiterate that the choice of base is irrelevant so long as we consistently use the same base throughout our calculations.

Now look at the impact of the (natural) log transformation on the results of our 1000 cohort studies. Figure 7.2 illustrates the frequency histogram of the 1000 estimates, $\log(\widehat{OR})$, of the log Odds Ratio, $\log(OR)$. Now, the smallest value of $\log(\widehat{OR})$ is -1.90 [i.e., $\log(0.15)$], and the largest is 2.03 [i.e., $\log(7.58)$]. The average and median of the 1000 replicated $\log(\widehat{OR})$s are -0.011 and 0, respectively. The frequency histogram is now considerably more symmetric, and the average value of $\log(\widehat{OR})$ over the 1000 studies is very close to the true $\log(OR) = 0$. Thus, the bias in the estimator $\log(\widehat{OR})$ of $\log(OR)$ is much smaller than we found with $\widehat{OR}$, and it now looks reasonable to approximate the sampling distribution of $\log(\widehat{OR})$ by a Normal distribution. In the next section, we therefore construct confidence intervals for $\log(OR)$ on the logarithm scale, and then transform back, by taking an exponential, to find the analogous confidence

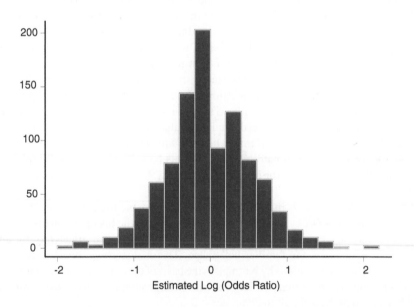

Figure 7.2 *Frequency histogram of 1,000 estimated log odds ratios for data generated from a cohort design with OR = 1 and 50 exposed and 50 unexposed.*

intervals for the Odds Ratio. (Recall that the inverse of the natural logarithm of a number is the exponential of that number; that is, $e^{\log(OR)} = OR$.)

Before turning to inference techniques, note that the general shape of the sampling distribution of $\widehat{OR}$ will be the same if the data are generated from either a population-based or case-control study. If the sample size n is increased, this shape persists (although eventually skewness starts to diminish), while the variability or spread of the sampling distribution declines. However, as our discussion of the power of the χ^2 test in Chapter 6.3.1 revealed, for a fixed total sample size n, the variability of the sampling distribution of $\widehat{OR}$ is considerably influenced by which design is used. But the comparison between the designs and recommendations for sample size allocation is not as simple if the population Odds Ratio is not at the "null," that is $OR \neq 1$. For both cohort and case-control designs, an optimal allocation of the total sample size can be determined (Robinson, 1991): specifically, when $OR > 1$, it is better to sample fewer exposeds than unexposeds in the cohort design, and fewer cases than controls in the case-control design. "Better" here means better in terms of reducing the variance of the estimate of the Odds Ratio. Unfortunately, the optimal allocation depends on the measure of association, so that different recommendations apply for estimation of the Relative Risk and Excess Risk in cohort studies. Even more disconcertingly, the optimal allocation for the Excess Risk is in the opposite direction from that for the Odds Ratio; that is, for a smaller variance of the estimate of the Excess Risk, when $ER > 0$, it is better to select more exposeds than unexposeds! It is therefore possible that a sample allocation favorable for estimation of the Odds Ratio is unfavorable for estimation of the Excess Risk. Other results are more akin to those of Chapter 6.3.1; for example, the optimal case-control allocation provides greater precision in estimating the Odds Ratio than the optimal cohort sampling scheme under exactly the same conditions in which the power of the χ^2 test of independence is higher for a case-control study, and vice versa. Further, the optimal allocation for either the cohort or case-control design always leads to at least as much precision as a population-based study. These comparisons are discussed in full detail in Robinson (1991).

7.1.2 Confidence interval for the odds ratio

In the previous section, we determined that the sampling distribution of $\log(\widehat{OR}) = \log(ad/bc)$ is more symmetric than that of $\widehat{OR}$, and is thus better approximated by a Normal distribution in large samples. Since the mean of $\log(\widehat{OR})$ is close to the true $\log(OR)$ when the sample size, n, is large, it follows that $\log(\widehat{OR}) - \log(OR)$ has an approximately Normal sampling distribution with zero expectation and variance, V, say.

To understand the variance V in a cohort study, we use the notation of Chapter 6.2, writing $\log(\widehat{OR}) = [\log \hat{p}_1/(1 - \hat{p}_1)] - [\log \hat{p}_2/(1 - \hat{p}_2)]$, where $\hat{p}_1$, the observed proportion of Ds among the exposed, estimates $p_1 = P(D|E)$, and so on. We know that the variance of $\hat{p}_1$ is just $p_1(1 - p_1)/n_1$ where n_1 is the number of exposed in the sample (Chapter 3.3). The key to estimating V is then to get a simple approximation of $\log \hat{p}_1/(1 - \hat{p}_1)$ in terms of $\hat{p}_1$. Properties of the logarithm function reveals that

$$\log \frac{\hat{p}_1}{1 - \hat{p}_1} \approx \log \frac{p_1}{1 - p_1} + (\hat{p}_1 - p_1) \times \frac{1}{p_1(1 - p_1)}.$$

Since the first term on the right-hand side of this expression is constant, this immediately shows that

$$Var\left(\log \frac{\hat{p}_1}{1 - \hat{p}_1} \right) \approx Var(\hat{p}_1) \times \frac{1}{[p_1(1 - p_1)]^2} = \frac{1}{n_1 p_1(1 - p_1)}.$$

We estimate this variance by plugging in $\hat{p}_1$ for p_1 as usual, giving

$$\widehat{Var}\left(\log \frac{\hat{p}_1}{1 - \hat{p}_1} \right) \approx \frac{1}{n_1 \hat{p}_1(1 - \hat{p}_1)} = \frac{1}{a} + \frac{1}{b}.$$

Exactly the same calculation leads to $\widehat{Var}(\log \hat{p}_2/(1 - \hat{p}_2)) \approx 1/c + 1/d$. Since the exposed and unexposed are independent samples, we then get an estimate of V by adding these two formulae so that an effective estimator of the sampling variance of $\log(\widehat{OR})$ is:

$$\widehat{Var}(\log(\widehat{OR})) = \frac{1}{a} + \frac{1}{b} + \frac{1}{c} + \frac{1}{d},$$

applicable to all three designs. In sum, the approximate sampling distribution of $[\log(\widehat{OR}) - \log(OR)]/[\sqrt{\widehat{Var}(\log(\widehat{OR}))}]$ is standard Normal, so that two-sided $100(1 - \alpha)\%$ confidence limits for $\log(OR)$ are given by

$$\log(\widehat{OR}) \pm z_\alpha \sqrt{\widehat{Var}(\log(\widehat{OR}))}$$

where z_α is the $(1 - \alpha/2)$th percentile of the standard Normal distribution. For example, for a 95% confidence interval, we use $z_\alpha = 1.96$. For a 90% confidence interval, $z_\alpha = 1.644$, etc.

This provides confidence limits for $\log(OR)$, but we wish to make statements in terms of the more readily understood OR. To obtain the relevant confidence limits for OR we simply antilog—that is, exponentiate—the limits for $\log(OR)$.

7.1.3 Example—coffee drinking and pancreatic cancer

MacMahon et al. (1981) report on a traditional case-control study of pancreatic cancer and its relationship to various lifestyle habits including consumption of tobacco, alcohol, tea, and coffee. Table 7.2 gives the resulting data on coffee drinking and incidence of pancreatic cancer, for men and women separately. Cases were recruited from 11 hospitals in Boston and Rhode Island over a 5-year period; controls were then sampled from the patient populations of physicians who treated the selected pancreatic cancer cases, excluding patients who had any pancreatic disease, or who suffered from other smoking or alcohol-related conditions. Further description of the study can be found in MacMahon et al. (1981).

For the moment we ignore the role of sex and the dose-related information on coffee drinking (given in terms of average daily coffee consumption in cups per day). Table 7.3 displays the simplified data on cases and controls in terms of whether they are regular coffee drinkers, providing a simple binary exposure factor.

Table 7.2 *Data from a case-control study of pancreatic cancer*

Sex	Disease Status	Coffee Drinking (Cups per Day)				Total
		0	1–2	3–4	≥5	
Men	Case	9	94	53	60	216
	Controls	32	119	74	82	307
Women	Case	11	59	53	28	151
	Controls	56	152	80	48	336
	Total	108	424	260	218	1010

Table 7.3 *Grouped case-control data on coffee drinking and pancreatic cancer*

		Pancreatic Cancer		
		Cases	Controls	
Coffee drinking (cups per day)	≥1	347	555	902
	0	20	88	108
		367	643	1010

The Odds Ratio is estimated by $\widehat{OR} = (347 \times 88)/(555 \times 20) = 2.75$. The corresponding estimate of $\log(OR)$ is then $\log[(347 \times 88)/(555 \times 20)] = 1.01$. The variance of the sampling distribution of $\log(OR)$ is estimated by $1/347 + 1/555 + 1/20 + 1/88 = 0.066$. Thus, the 95% confidence interval for $\log(OR)$ is $1.01 \pm 1.96\sqrt{0.066} = (0.508, 1.516)$. The corresponding 95% confidence interval for OR is then $(e^{0.508}, e^{1.516})$, that is, $(1.66, 4.55)$. Note that the χ^2 test statistic arising from Table 7.3 is 16.60, with an associated p-value of 0.5×10^{-4}. There thus appears to be a substantial, and statistically significant, increase of risk at somewhere between 1.5 to 4.5 times the risk of pancreatic cancer for coffee drinkers compared with abstainers (since pancreatic cancer is sufficiently rare, we can interpret an Odds Ratio as a Relative Risk). This data is further examined in later chapters to assess whether this conclusion holds up under a more detailed analysis.

7.1.4 Small sample adjustments for estimators of the odds ratio

Already noted is that the estimate $\widehat{OR} = ad/bc$ is somewhat biased in small samples in that the expectation of the sampling distribution of $\widehat{OR}$ is somewhat different than OR. This effect disappears when the sample size (or sizes in a cohort or case-control study) is large. Nevertheless, for small samples, it is intriguing to see whether there is an improved estimator that reduces this bias. Various simple modifications to the estimator for OR have been examined to see which is most effective in reducing small sample bias. The most effective of these yields the small sample estimator of OR

given by Jewell (1986) as

$$\widehat{OR}_{SS} = \frac{ad}{(b+1)(c+1)}.$$

(Of particular importance when $\widehat{OR} < 1$, this should not be used to estimate $1/OR$; instead use $bc/(a+1)(d+1)$—see Jewell, 1986.)

We can make similar small sample adjustments to the method of constructing a confidence interval for OR. Recall that we work on the log scale by first constructing a confidence interval for $\log(OR)$, centered at a point estimate of $\log(OR)$. Since bias is *not invariant* under the log transformation, we cannot simply take the logarithm of OR_{SS} and expect that this will necessarily reduce bias in the estimate of $\log(OR)$. Although, as we have noted, bias is less of an issue on the log scale, seeking to reduce whatever bias remains leads to the estimator given by

$$(\log \widehat{OR})_{SS} = \log\left(\frac{\left(a+\frac{1}{2}\right)\left(d+\frac{1}{2}\right)}{\left(b+\frac{1}{2}\right)\left(c+\frac{1}{2}\right)}\right),$$

obtained by adding $1/2$ to each cell entry in the original 2×2 table. The mean of the sampling distribution of the small sample estimator, $(\log \widehat{OR})_{SS}$, is closer to the true population $\log(OR)$ than the mean of the sampling distribution of $\log(ad/bc)$. The same trick also reduces the bias in the estimator, $\hat{V}$, of the sampling variance, yielding

$$\widehat{Var}((\log \widehat{OR})_{SS}) = \hat{V}_{SS} = \frac{1}{\left(a+\frac{1}{2}\right)} + \frac{1}{\left(b+\frac{1}{2}\right)} + \frac{1}{\left(c+\frac{1}{2}\right)} + \frac{1}{\left(d+\frac{1}{2}\right)}.$$

This estimator is less biased as an estimate of the variance of the sampling distribution of $(\log \widehat{OR})_{SS}$ than $1/a + 1/b + 1/c + 1/d$. The estimates $(\log \widehat{OR})_{SS}$ and $\hat{V}_{SS}$ are then used to construct an adjusted confidence interval for $\log(OR)$, and then for OR, as before. The small sample estimators have the added advantage that they can be computed when a cell of the 2×2 table has a zero entry.

From Table 7.3, the small sample estimate of OR is $(347 \times 88)/(556 \times 21) = 2.62$, and for $\log(OR)$ is $\log[(347.5 \times 88.5)/(555.5 \times 20.5)] = 0.993$. The small sample estimate of the variance of $(\log \widehat{OR})_{SS}$ is $1/347.5 + 1/555.5 + 1/20.5 + 1/88.5 = 0.065$. Thus, the small sample 95% confidence limits for $\log(OR)$ are $0.993 \pm 1.96\sqrt{0.065} = (0.495, 1.492)$, yielding $(1.64, 4.45)$ as the associated 95% confidence interval for OR.

Small sample adjustments should be treated with caution, as they only have a noticeable impact in situations where, by definition, the sample is small so uncertainty is great. The suggested adjustments for confidence interval calculations are generally accepted, although there is controversy over appropriate modifications to the point estimate, $\widehat{OR}$. The estimator $\widehat{OR}_{SS}$ is conservative in the sense that it is smaller than the estimate provided by adding $1/2$ to each cell before computing the usual Odds Ratio estimate. The latter approach provides an estimator that is almost *median unbiased*—that is, half the time it is bigger than the unknown OR and half the time it is smaller; however, as for the estimator $\widehat{OR} = ad/bc$, it tends to be further away from OR when it is bigger than OR than when it is smaller than OR. On the other hand,

$\widehat{OR}_{SS}$ is usually closer to the true OR on the average, but tends to give a smaller (than OR) estimate more often than a larger estimate. In any case, there is only substantial difference between the two approaches when the sample size is very small, and then random variation is of much greater concern than this difference.

The principal value of a small sample adjustment is in its alerting us to situations where the sample size is small enough to have a noticeable impact on an estimator, thereby suggesting that large sample approximations may be suspicious. In these situations, exact sampling distribution calculations should be employed both in testing independence and in the construction of a confidence interval, whatever choice of point estimator is preferred. As in Section 6.4.2, exact confidence interval results for the Odds Ratio are based on numerical calculation of the exact sampling distribution of $\widehat{OR}$ using either the noncentral hypergeometric or binomial distributions. With the data of Table 7.3, the former technique gives an exact confidence interval for OR of (1.64, 4.80).

7.2 The relative risk

The ingredients of the Relative Risk are the two conditional probabilities $P(D|E)$ and $P(D|\text{not } E)$, both of which can be directly estimated from either a population-based or a cohort study. We reiterate that the Relative Risk is not directly estimable with the traditional case-control design, although it can be indirectly approximated through estimation of the Odds Ratio if the outcome is rare (see Chapters 4.3 and 5.3). Alternatively, the Relative Risk can be estimated directly from a case-cohort design (Chapter 5.4.2). To estimate RR from population-based or cohort data, we simply substitute the sample estimates of $P(D|E)$ and $P(D|\text{not } E)$ into the formula (4.1) for RR. This yields

$$\widehat{RR} = \frac{a/(a+b)}{c/(c+d)}.$$

For the same reasons underlying the estimator of the Odds Ratio, the sampling distribution of $\widehat{RR}$ is skewed, particularly when samples are small. We again can use the log transformation to reduce this skewness, thereby ameliorating the inherent distortion from using $\widehat{RR}$ as the center of a confidence interval. As before, the log transformation also allows for improved approximation of the sampling distribution by a Normal distribution. To center a confidence interval, we estimate $\log(RR)$ by $\log \widehat{RR} = \log[a/(a+b)]/[c/(c+d)]$. Using the same notation as in Section 7.1.2, we derive an estimate of the variance of the sampling distribution of $\log \widehat{RR}$ by again approximating $\log \hat{p}_1$ in terms of $\hat{p}_1$ (where $p_1 = P(D|E)$, etc.). Via the properties of the logarithm function, we have

$$\log \hat{p}_1 \approx \log p_1 + \frac{(\hat{p}_1 - p_1)}{p_1}.$$

With the first term on the right-hand side being constant, this leads to

$$Var(\log \hat{p}_1) \approx \frac{Var(\hat{p}_1)}{p_1^2} = \frac{1 - p_1}{n_1 p_1}.$$

Substituting $\hat{p}_1$ for p_1 gives

$$\widehat{Var}(\log \hat{p}_1) \approx \frac{1 - \hat{p}_1}{n_1 \hat{p}_1} = \frac{b}{a(a+b)}.$$

Exactly the same calculation leads to $\widehat{Var}(\log \hat{p}_2) \approx d/c(c+d)$. Since the exposed and unexposed are independent samples, and $\log \widehat{RR} = \log \hat{p}_1 - \log \hat{p}_2$, adding these two variance estimates yields

$$\widehat{Var}(\log(\widehat{RR})) = \frac{b}{a(a+b)} + \frac{d}{c(c+d)}.$$

Then, using the fact that $[\log(\widehat{RR}) - \log(RR)]/\sqrt{\widehat{Var}(\log(\widehat{RR}))}$ is approximately a standard Normal, we have that two-sided $100(1 - \alpha)\%$ confidence limits for $\log(RR)$ are given by

$$\log(\widehat{RR}) \pm z_\alpha \sqrt{\widehat{Var}(\log(\widehat{RR}))}$$

where z_α is the $(1 - \alpha/2)$th percentile of the standard Normal distribution. As for the Odds Ratio, we exponentiate to get the corresponding confidence interval for RR. This approach is equally applicable to data arising from a population-based or a cohort design.

As with the Odds Ratio, there is a small sample adjustment to our estimate of the Relative Risk given by

$$\widehat{RR}_{SS} = \frac{a/(a+b)}{(c+1)/(c+d+1)}.$$

The comments in Section 7.1.4 regarding the appropriate use of small sample estimators apply here for the Relative Risk.

7.2.1 Example—coronary heart disease in the Western Collaborative Group Study

Rosenman et al. (1975) report on the Western Collaborative Group Study (WCGS), a form of population-based study that collected follow-up data on a group of employed men from 10 Californian companies, aged 39 to 59 years old, regarding the onset of coronary heart disease (CHD). Interest focused on several possible risk factors including lifestyle variables, such as smoking; physiological measurements, such as blood pressure and cholesterol level; and certain behavioral characteristics. In the third category, particular attention was paid to behavior type, a binary variable whose two levels are referred to as Type A and Type B. Type A behavior is characterized by aggressiveness and competitiveness, whereas Type B behavior is considered more relaxed and noncompetitive. After recruitment, from 1960 to 1961, participants were monitored for around 9 years, although a few were lost to follow-up. Occurrence of coronary heart disease was determined by expert diagnosis and usually was due to some form of heart attack. Table 7.4 provides data on 3154 men whose follow-up was deemed complete, in terms of their behavior type and whether they suffered a CHD event during follow-up.

Table 7.4 *Coronary heart disease and behavior type*

		Yes	No	
		Occurrence of CHD Event		
Behavior type	Type A	178	1411	1589
	Type B	79	1486	1565
		257	2897	3154

The χ^2 test statistic from Table 7.4 is 39.9 with p-value smaller than 10^{-8}, suggesting a clear association between behavior type and occurrence of CHD. The estimate of RR is $\widehat{RR} = (178/1589)/(79/1565) = 2.22$; the associated estimate of log(RR) is $\log(178/1589)/(79/1565) = 0.797$. The estimated sampling variance of log($\widehat{RR}$) is $1411/(178 \times 1589) + 1486/(79 \times 1565) = 0.017$, so that 95% confidence limits for log(RR) are $0.797 \pm 1.96\sqrt{0.017} = (0.542, 1.053)$. The corresponding 95% confidence interval for RR is then $(1.72, 2.87)$, suggesting anywhere from twice to close to three times the risk for CHD in Type A individuals. The small sample estimate of RR is $\widehat{RR}_{SS} = (178/1589)/(80/1566) = 2.19$, essentially unchanged from the standard estimate.

7.3 The excess risk

Estimation of the Excess Risk from population-based or cohort data parallels that of the Relative Risk, since ER also depends solely on $P(D|E)$ and $P(D|\text{not } E)$. Substituting the sample estimates for $P(D|E)$ and $P(D|\text{not } E)$ into the definition of ER of Equation 4.7 gives

$$\widehat{ER} = \frac{a}{a+b} - \frac{c}{c+d}.$$

Note that this estimate simply involves *subtraction* of two proportion estimates, suggesting that the sampling distribution of $\widehat{ER}$ may not be plagued by the skewness that occurs with $\widehat{OR}$ and $\widehat{RR}$. This can be seen directly from the observation that the two proportion estimates, $P(D|E) = a/(a+b)$ and $P(D|\text{not } E) = c/(c+d)$, have symmetric sampling distributions, both closely approximated by Normal distributions. Since the E and $\bar{E}$ samples are independent in both population-based design and cohort designs, it follows that $\widehat{ER}$ has an approximately Normal sampling distribution with expectation given by $P(D|E) - P(D|\bar{E}) = ER$. Since a proportion estimate $\hat{p}$ has a sampling variance estimated by $\hat{p}(1 - \hat{p})$ divided by the relevant sample size, it follows that the sampling variance of $\widehat{ER}$ is estimated by $[\hat{P}(D|E)(1 - \hat{P}(D|E))/n_E] + [\hat{P}(D|\bar{E})(1 - \hat{P}(D|\bar{E}))/n_{\bar{E}}]$; that is,

$$\widehat{Var}(\widehat{ER}) = \frac{ab}{(a+b)^3} + \frac{cd}{(c+d)^3}.$$

The resulting two-sided $100(1 - \alpha)$% confidence limits for ER are given by

$$\widehat{ER} \pm z_\alpha \sqrt{\widehat{Var}(\widehat{ER})},$$

where z_α is the $(1 - \alpha/2)$th percentile of the standard Normal distribution. No small sample adjustments to these estimates are required, because the symmetry of the sampling distribution of $\widehat{ER}$ means that the expectation of $\widehat{ER}$ is exactly ER.

Using the data of Table 7.4, the estimate of ER for CHD, associated with behavior type, is $(178/1589) - (79/1565) = 0.062$. The variance of $\widehat{ER}$ is estimated by $[(178 \times 1411)/1589^3] + [(79 \times 1486)/1565^3] = 0.000093$. Thus, a 95% confidence interval for ER is simply $0.062 \pm 1.96\sqrt{0.000093} = (0.043, 0.080)$.

7.4 The attributable risk

For a population-based study, an estimate of the Attributable Risk is easily derived by substituting sample estimates for $P(D)$ and $P(D|E)$ into the definition of AR, or, equivalently, sample estimates of $P(E)$ and RR into the (equivalent) formulation for AR given in Equation 4.8. So, with $\hat{P}(D) = (a + c)/n$, and $\hat{P}(D|\bar{E}) = c/(c + d)$,

$$\widehat{AR} = \frac{\frac{a+c}{n} - \frac{c}{c+d}}{\frac{a+c}{n}}$$
$$= \frac{(a + c)(c + d) - nc}{(a + c)(c + d)}$$
$$= \frac{ac + ad + c^2 + cd - ac - bc - c^2 - cd}{(a + c)(c + d)}$$
$$\Rightarrow \widehat{AR} = \frac{ad - bc}{(a + c)(c + d)}.$$

The sampling distribution of $\widehat{AR}$ is skewed, but in the opposite direction of and not as severely as the sampling distributions of $\widehat{OR}$ and $\widehat{RR}$. Most investigators suggest using $\log(1 - \widehat{AR})$ as a transformation scale on which to base confidence interval calculations. Without giving full details this time, the variance of $\log(1 - \widehat{AR})$ is estimated by

$$\widehat{Var}(\log(1 - \widehat{AR})) = \frac{b + \widehat{AR}(a + d)}{nc}.$$

Confidence intervals for $\log(1 - AR)$ are then constructed in the standard manner. The corresponding confidence limits for AR are then obtained by exponentiating the limits for $\log(1 - AR)$, subtracting 1, and then multiplying by -1, thereby inverting the transformation $\log(1 - AR)$.

Using the data from Table 7.4, $\widehat{AR} = [(178 \times 1,486) - (1,411 \times 79)]/(257 \times 1,565) = 153,039/402,205 = 0.38$. In addition, $\widehat{Var}(\log(1 - \widehat{AR})) = [1,411 + (0.38 \times (178+1,486))]/(3,154 \times 79) = 2,044.2/249,166 = 0.0082$, and a 95% confidence interval for $\log(1-AR)$ is $\log(1-0.38)\pm1.96\sqrt{0.0082} = (-0.656, -0.301)$. The corresponding interval for $1 - AR$ is then $(e^{-0.656}, e^{-0.301}) = (0.52, 0.74)$; for $-AR$, it is $(-0.48, -0.26)$; and, finally, a 95% confidence interval for AR is $(0.26, 0.48)$. We reiterate that the interpretation of these results, that 38% of CHD is due to behavior type, should be treated with caution as we have not yet thought through the issue of the causal nature of the relationship between behavior type and CHD.

For a cohort study, it is not possible to estimate the Attributable Risk since we cannot estimate $P(E)$. For case-control studies, however, an equivalent formulation of the Attributable Risk is given in Equation 5.1 as

$$AR = P(E|D)\left(1 - \frac{1}{RR}\right).$$

With case-control data we can directly estimate $P(E|D)$ from the sample of cases and, with the rare disease assumption, an estimate of the Odds Ratio can be used to approximate RR. Specifically, using $\hat{P}(E|D) = a/(a+c)$, and $\widehat{OR} = ad/bc$, we have

$$\widehat{AR} = \frac{a}{a+c}\left(1 - \frac{bc}{ad}\right)$$
$$= \frac{(ad - bc)}{d(a+c)}.$$

Under case-control sampling, an estimate of the variance of $\log(1 - \widehat{AR})$ is given by

$$\widehat{Var}(\log(1 - \widehat{AR})) = \frac{a}{c(a+c)} + \frac{b}{d(b+d)}.$$

Using this estimate of the variance of the sampling distribution of $\log(1 - \widehat{AR})$, confidence intervals for $\log(1 - AR)$, and subsequently for AR, are then obtained as before.

This procedure is illustrated using the case-control data of Table 7.3 on coffee drinking and pancreatic cancer. With this data, we have $\widehat{AR} = (347 \times 88) - (555 \times 20)/(88 \times 367) = 19,436/32,296 = 0.60$. This gives $\log(1 - \widehat{AR}) = -0.9208$ with an estimate of the sampling variance of $\log(1 - \widehat{AR})$ of $347/(20 \times 367) + 555/(88 \times 643) = 0.0473 + 0.0098 = 0.0571$. A 95% confidence interval for $\log(1 - AR)$ is then $-0.9208 \pm 1.96\sqrt{0.0571} = (-1.3891, -0.4525)$. The corresponding 95% confidence interval for AR is $(0.36, 0.75)$. This suggests, though naïvely, that somewhere between 36 and 75% of pancreatic cancer cases may be attributed to coffee drinking. The implausibility of the large value of the estimated Attributable Risk strongly hints that the observed association between coffee and pancreatic cancer may not be causal; we return to this issue in later chapters.

7.5 Comments and further reading

Because of the different sampling schemes, the methods of Section 7.1 cannot be directly applied to the sample Odds Ratio for data arising from either nested case-control sampling or a case-cohort study. In the nested case-control design, the pooled sample Odds Ratio only estimates the Relative Hazard (Chapter 5.4.1) in restrictive scenarios that include unlikely conditions, such as the hazard rates for both the exposed and unexposed being constant over time. In general, it is necessary to account for the stratification (or matching) by time at risk that is inherent to the design; methods to accommodate this sampling feature will be discussed in Chapters 16 and 17.

For case-cohort data, the sample Odds Ratio can be used to estimate the Relative Risk although the variance estimate in Section 7.1.2 is generally incorrect because of possible overlap between cases and controls—that is, the possibility that the control group contains individuals who are subsequently sampled as cases. While correcting the variance estimate is straightforward, Sato (1992a) describes a modified estimator of the Odds Ratio that takes into account the information in the overlapping group to improve precision (a slightly different estimator is relevant if one knows the size of, and the number if cases in, the larger cohort from which the case-cohort data was sampled (Prentice, 1986; Sato, 1992a). If there is very little overlap, these modifications can be ignored and the methods of this chapter directly applied, although this essentially returns us to the rare disease setting. In addition, if the "overlapping" cases are removed from the cohort sample, the methods of Section 7.1 directly apply to estimation of the Odds Ratio as for traditional case-control studies.

In this chapter we have considered quantifying uncertainty in a study of a particular design and sample size(s). Turning these techniques on their heads, we can determine the size of the sample(s) required to achieve a given level of precision for a specific design. Such calculations are referred to as *sample size planning*. There is a substantial literature on this topic, and we refer to Schlesselman (1982) and Greenland (1988) as good places to start. There are also chapters on this topic in many other books including Woodward (1999) and Newman (2001). For a straightforward introduction and review, see Liu (2000). I find sample size computations somewhat artificial. Usually, available resources for a study are constrained, and sample size calculations are often used to justify the value of a study, given fixed resources, as compared with precision assessment driving appropriate fund allocations. Further, sample size planning rarely accounts for all sources of error, some of which may be a far greater threat than sampling variability. For example, it may be more effective to expend a greater fraction of resources ensuring the quality of measurement of exposure and disease than to merely increase the sample size for a study with inaccurate data. It is particularly dangerous to blindly resort to sample size tables without fully understanding the statistical nuances of a planned design and analysis strategy.

7.5.1 Measurement error or misclassification

As indicated at the beginning of Chapter 2, we have been assuming exact measurement of both disease and exposure so far, particularly in this chapter. However, bias introduced by both systematic and random errors in measurement of these quantities leads often to far greater distortion of a disease-exposure association than is introduced by sampling. Thus, any epidemiological study must assess the possible impact of measurement error before drawing definitive conclusions. Even relatively small amounts of measurement error can have major effects on estimation of a measure of association. The direction of the association can be reversed, as is easily seen if we imagine, for example, that coffee drinking is completely miscoded in Table 7.3; that is, if coffee drinkers were actually abstainers and vice versa, the estimated Odds Ratio for the true coffee exposure would be $\widehat{OR} = 1/2.75 = 0.36$.

For binary measures of both exposure and disease, measurement error entails classifying an individual as $\bar{E}$ instead of E (or vice versa) or $\bar{D}$ instead of D (or vice versa). In this simple situation, measurement error is often referred to as *misclassification*; a study may be subject to exposure or disease misclassification, or both. As a first step in considering misclassification, it is important to distinguish *nondifferential* errors, where, for example, the misclassification of exposure is not influenced by an individual's disease status, from *differential* errors, where exposure misclassification rates vary by disease category. A similar issue applies to disease measurement, where misclassification may or may not depend on exposure. Differential misclassification of exposure is more likely in retrospective studies (Chapter 5.1) since exposure level is measured after disease identification. By the same token, differential misclassification of disease is more common in prospective studies (see Chapter 17.5.2 for an example).

There is an enormous amount of literature on the effects of measurement error, and several books, including Carroll et al. (1995), provide elegant introductions to the topic. In many situations, nondifferential misclassification of either exposure or disease biases an effect measure towards its null value (possibly even beyond it, as shown above), meaning that a measure of association would be even greater were there no measurement error; measurement error cannot therefore "explain away" an observed effect. However, there are enough common scenarios where this is not true—including (1) exposures with multiple levels (Chapter 11), (2) studies with multiple risk factors all subject to error (Chapters 8 and beyond), and (3) correlated errors in measuring both exposure and disease—for it to be very dangerous to assume this as a mantra.

What can be done if you suspect random measurement? Gaining information about the sizes of these random errors is a key first step. For example, validation studies can provide information about exposure misclassification probabilities when comparing a study's measurement technique to a "gold standard" method (i.e., one that gives an exact measurement). This assumes that it is either too expensive, impractical, or not ethical to use the "gold standard" method in the study. Sometimes, a form of validation study is built into the main study by requiring that the "gold standard" method is applied to a subsample of study participants in addition to a cruder measure which is used throughout. In simple scenarios, knowledge of misclassification probabilities from validation studies can be used to adjust estimates of measures of association and estimates of their variability (Kleinbaum et al., 1982). Even if these probabilities are not known exactly, it is valuable to carry out *sensitivity analyses* that assess the impact of various plausible levels of misclassification on a study's conclusion (Greenland and Kleinbaum, 1983). Use extreme care when applying these methods to case-control data with disease misclassification; due to the oversampling of apparent cases, misclassification rates in the study differ substantially from those found in the general population (Greenland and Kleinbaum, 1983).

One powerful and simple way to adjust for known levels of measurement error is illustrated by a very simplistic extension of our analysis of Table 7.4. Suppose it

Table 7.5 *Coronary heart disease and behavior type subject to additional misclassification*

		Occurrence of CHD Event		
		Yes	No	
Misclassified behavior type (E^*)	Type A	169	1342	1511
	Type B	88	1555	1643
		257	2897	3154

is known from testing studies that the measurement of behavior type in the Western Collaborative Group Study suffers from misclassification in that $P(E|\text{true Type A}) = 0.9$ and $P(\bar{E}|\text{true Type B}) = 1$. In this notation, E refers to measured behavior type, whereas "true Type A" is the actual behavior type. Thus, we assume that Type B behavior type is measured exactly, but Type A individuals are misclassified as Type B 10% of the time. In other words, the *sensitivity* of our Type A measurement is 90%, and the *specificity* is 100%. How should this information change our estimate of the Relative Risk from 2.22 (Section 7.2.1)? The simulation extrapolation (SIMEX) method provides a simple way to answer this question and is a technique that is easily extended to more complex scenarios.

The basis of the SIMEX technique is to systematically *increase* the amount of misclassification by different amounts, study the dependence of our estimate on the amount of additional misclassification, and then extrapolate backward to the case with no misclassification. In the WCGS example, suppose we generate a "new" measure of exposure, E^*, which is a reclassification of the E according to the following random rules: $P(E^*|E) = p$, $P(\bar{E}^*|\bar{E}) = 1$, where p is selected to be a value close to but less than 1. Table 7.5 shows an example of a new version of the data generated in this way, with $p = 0.95$, that yields an estimated Relative Risk of 2.088, slightly smaller than our original estimator.

This simulation is repeated many times for a fixed choice of p, and the estimated Relative Risks from each version are averaged. These repetitions allow us to remove sampling variability from the extra random misclassification. The simulation is then repeated for a different choice of p, and so on. Figure 7.3 shows a plot of the average estimated Relative Risks (for each choice of p) against p, for $0.8 \le p \le 1$. The average estimated Relative Risk when $p = 1$ is, of course, just $\widehat{RR} = 2.22$. Note that, using the ideas of conditional probabilities of Chapter 3.4, for a given p

$$P(E^*|\text{true Type A}) = P(E^*|E, \text{true Type A})P(E|\text{true Type A})$$
$$+ P(E^*|\bar{E}, \text{true Type A})P(\bar{E}|\text{true Type A})$$
$$= P(E^*|E)P(E|\text{true Type A}) + P(E^*|\bar{E})P(\bar{E}|\text{true Type A})$$
$$= 0.9p + 0$$
$$= 0.9p.$$

The second line of this calculation follows since the simulated value of E^* depends only on E, and not additionally on behavior type. The next step uses our assumption on

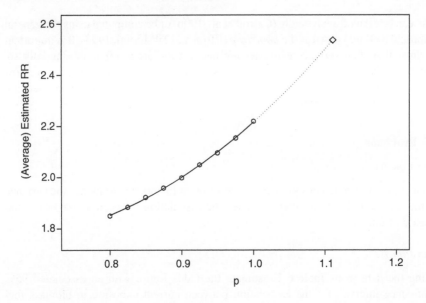

Figure 7.3 *Plot of the average estimated relative risks against p for data subject to additional misclassification (of amount p) of type A individuals in the Western Collaborative Group Study.*

the misclassification of behavior type as exposure E. Similarly, $P(E^*|\text{true Type B}) = 1$. Thus, the new simulated exposure variable, E^*, has sensitivity $90p\%$, and specificity 100% for measuring true Type A. We desire an estimate of the Relative Risk, based on the actual behavior type, that is, an exposure measurement with both sensitivity and specificity equal to 100%. In Figure 7.3, this corresponds to a $p = 1/0.9$, so that $90p\% = 100\%$. We therefore need to estimate the relationship between the average estimated Relative Risk and p, and then extrapolate to $p = 1/0.9$.

The pattern of estimated Relative Risks as p changes is clearly curved; so we fit this relationship (which we need for extrapolation) via a quadratic regression model of the form $E(y) = a + bp + bp^2$, using least squares (Moore and McCabe, 1998, Chapter 11). With the data of Figure 7.3, this fitted curve is shown as the solid line; extrapolating the curve to $p = 1/0.9$ yields an estimated Relative Risk of 2.54. This provides our assessment of what $\widehat{RR}$ would be if there were no misclassification of Type A individuals. This example shows that a small amount of nondifferential mis-classification of the exposure leads to an attenuation of the estimated effect of a little more than 10%. A similar result is easy to achieve using algebra with the straight-forward assumptions underlying this example, but the SIMEX method extends to far more complicated situations. In particular, we can perform a bivariate extrapolation with the SIMEX method if we assume that both the sensitivity and specificity of our measurement of behavior type are less than 100%. We can also incorporate misclas-sification of the disease outcome. In addition, the method extends to more detailed exposure measurements of the kind we consider in Chapters 11 and beyond.

The SIMEX method was first introduced by Cook and Stefanski (1995) and later analyzed by Carroll et al. (1996). Variance estimates of the final "adjusted" Relative

Risk can be derived analytically (Carroll et al., 1996) or be computed using the general empirical method known as the *bootstrap* (Efron and Tibshirani, 1993). It is important to stress that such variance estimates are necessarily larger, often substantially so, than those that ignore the possibility of misclassification, reflecting that we are now accounting for two sources of random error: first, random sampling error, and second, random measurement error.

7.6 Problems

Question 7.1

For a population-based design, name four different factors that influence the variance of the sample Odds Ratio that estimates the association between a risk factor and disease of interest.

Question 7.2

Using the data from Table 6.7, estimate the Odds Ratio, with an associated 95% confidence interval, for the association between current exposure to biomass fuel and tuberculosis. Repeat your analysis using the small sample adjustments for an estimate and confidence interval for an Odds Ratio. Compare the results from the two approaches and comment.

Question 7.3

Tuyns et al. (1977) carried out a case-control study of esophageal cancer in the region known as Ille-et-Vilaine in Brittany, France. The data set, *oesoph*, can be found at *http://www.crcpress.com/e_products/downloads/* and is also examined in detail in Breslow and Day (1980). One risk factor of interest was daily alcohol consumption, measured in grams per day, given in the data set in four levels: 0 to 39, 40 to 79, 80 to 120, and >120 g/day. Dichotomize this risk factor according to whether an individual's alcohol consumption is less than or greater than or equal to 80 g/day. With this binary measure of alcohol consumption, estimate the Odds Ratio with an associated 95% confidence interval. Also, examine the relationship between incidence of esophageal cancer and the dichotomized measure of alcohol consumption using the χ^2 test.

Question 7.4

Using the data from Question 3.1, compute the Relative Risk for 25 years mortality from CHD associated with eating no fish. Give a 95% confidence interval. Compute the small sample adjusted estimate of Relative Risk.

Question 7.5

Suppose a large cohort study follows 100,000 persons who smoke and 200,000 who do not smoke for incidence of bladder cancer, yielding the data in Table 7.6. Estimate the Excess Risk and Relative Risk, and associated 95% confidence intervals. Using your

Table 7.6 *Hypothetical cohort data on smoking and bladder cancer*

		Bladder Cancer		
		Cases	Controls	
Smoking status	Smokers	250	99,750	100,000
	Nonsmokers	125	199,875	200,000
		375	299,625	300,000

estimate of Relative Risk, plot a graph of Attributable Risk against P(smoking), the proportion of smokers in the general population. What Attributable Risk corresponds to P(smoking) = 0.2? Compute the maximum possible Attributable Risk.

Question 7.6

Using the data in Table 6.8 from the Physicians' Health Study, estimate the Relative Risk for CHD associated with experiencing hair loss at 45 years old. Provide a 95% confidence interval. Assuming that the sample proportion of physicians who suffered hair loss reflects the population frequency of this characteristic, estimate the Attributable Risk for CHD associated with experiencing hair loss by 45 years of age, and give a 95% confidence interval.

CHAPTER 8

Causal Inference and Extraneous Factors: Confounding and Interaction

This is the time to temper the exuberance of the last few chapters and catch our breath for a moment. We seem to have solved many problems: we have learned how to sample populations to collect useful information about the relationship between a risk factor and a disease outcome using a variety of measures of association; we have discussed how to assess whether an observed association may be simply due to chance and, of more importance, discussed methods to quantify both the association and the uncertainty surrounding its estimation. But what do these procedures really tell us about how exposure influences the risk of disease in practice? I am reminded here of the scene in *The Sound of Music* when the children, having learned to sing by merely using the names of the notes, complain that the song, however beautiful, doesn't mean anything! Notice that the statistical techniques we have introduced pay no attention to the nature of the exposure and disease variables. At the extreme, the methods do not even acknowledge whether E occurs before D in chronological time or not. If we define smoking to be our outcome D and having a lung tumor to be our exposure E, are we possibly establishing that lung cancer is a risk factor for smoking? In Section 7.1.3, why is the possibility that diagnosis with pancreatic cancer leads to increased coffee consumption not an equally plausible interpretation of our calculations? The point is that the statistical tools of Chapter 7 do not, in and of themselves, differentiate between the possibility that E causes D or D causes E.

Now that we have slowed down, there is yet a further complication that we have also been ignoring, namely the role of other factors in the association between exposure and disease outcome. For example, the analysis of data on a mother's marital status and her infant's 1-year mortality in Chapter 4.2 does not consider the possibility that other factors, such as health insurance coverage, may be associated with marital status and with infant mortality (for instance, from improved prenatal care in insured pregnant women). In particular, the Odds Ratio of 2.14, associating marital status with infant mortality, may be "due," in part, to the role of insurance coverage. This effect of extraneous factors is known as *confounding*, and such variables are referred to as *confounding factors*. A careful explication of confounding immediately allows us to understand why carrying a cigarette lighter does not cause lung cancer despite the fact that more lung cancer sufferers have just such a behavior history than the average person. In addition, this chapter unravels much more subtle ways in which confounding arises, or can even be introduced to a problem by an unsuspecting investigator.

When a confounding factor, which we denote by C, is ignored in our analysis, assessment of the direct relationship between E and D is distorted due to the association of C with both D and E. In addition to confounding, there is the further possibility that the effect of exposure, E, may depend on the level of C. For example, the association between marital status and infant mortality may be quite different for mothers with health insurance as compared with those without. This issue underlies what is known as *statistical interaction*, a separate concern from confounding.

At this point, all of these issues stop us in our tracks and must be considered before proceeding any farther on our journey. We first address the fundamental question of the causality of the relationship between D and E, as this discussion provides the conceptual framework to approach the problems of confounding and interaction later in the chapter. It is worth noting here that sampled data, in and of itself, cannot provide the key to causal issues. The use of *counterfactuals* in Section 8.1 and *causal graphs* in Section 8.2 requires that we bring a sophisticated understanding of the roles of various factors in the etiology of the disease in question. A major contribution of these methods is that they bring to the fore assumptions, largely untestable with observed data, that are nevertheless crucial for causal interpretations.

8.1 Causal inference

Forgetting for the moment that most epidemiological data arise from observations of humans, let us imagine the best possible world for experimentation if we wanted to know if, and by how much, changes in exposure, E, cause changes in the risk of the outcome, D. In a laboratory setting, we would run an experiment first where the experimental unit has exposure (E), and then, *under identical "conditions,"* when the unit is unexposed ($\bar{E}$). We would then attribute the observed difference in response under the two scenarios to the change in exposure. If we repeated this on a sample of different experimental units, the average response difference over the units would provide a summary measure of the causal effect of exposure on the outcome. This experimental strategy explicitly requires that the level of exposure is determined before (in chronological time) the occurrence of the outcome. We must also be able to hold fixed other relevant "conditions" when changing E, tacitly assuming, for example, that factors that determine such conditions are not the direct consequence of exposure.

8.1.1 Counterfactuals

Now try to conceive of the same experimental procedure applied to humans, using one of the examples of the last chapter for concreteness. If we want to understand the causal effect of coffee drinking on pancreatic cancer, we would ideally like to take each subject, sampled from a population, "expose" them to coffee drinking, and observe whether pancreatic cancer occurs over an appropriate follow-up period. Then, *on the same individual*, imagine turning back the clock to run the same experiment once more, but this time making the subject a coffee abstainer, measuring again if they develop pancreatic cancer or not. The possible hypothetical results of such an experiment on a population on N individuals are illustrated in Table 8.1. The fact that observations are repeated on the same individual corresponds to maintaining

Table 8.1 *Distribution of possible pancreatic cancer responses to the presence/absence of coffee in a population of size N*

Group	Coffee (E)	No Coffee ($\bar{E}$)	Number
1	D	D	Np_1
2	D	$\bar{D}$	Np_2
3	$\bar{D}$	D	Np_3
4	$\bar{D}$	$\bar{D}$	Np_4

"identical conditions" in our notional lab experiment. Two points are crucial to keep clear. First, as noted above, in even conceiving this experiment, what we define as coffee exposure must occur *prior* to incidence of pancreatic cancer. (We require a quite different experiment to establish whether incidence of pancreatic cancer causes changes in coffee consumption.) Second, factors determined before we set coffee exposure are held fixed; an individual's sex is certainly one of these fixed conditions. On the other hand, other factors fluctuate *after the experiment is set in motion*—in this case any variable, such as frequency of urination (caffeine is a diuretic), that is influenced by coffee drinking. These factors are not controlled identical conditions since they change in response to the experimental setting.

Which factors are controlled and which are not is a crucial feature of this hypothetical experiment and has an important impact on the interpretation of a causal impact. For example, imagine that some chemical in tea is, in fact, a causative agent in pancreatic cancer. If tea consumption is not considered one of the fixed conditions of the experiment, then when individuals are "exposed to coffee" they may subsequently drink less or no tea, thereby reducing their risk of pancreatic cancer in comparison to the experiment where they do not drink coffee. In this case, coffee drinking will correctly appear to cause a decrease in pancreatic cancer risk, albeit the pathway is through changes in tea consumption. On the other hand, if tea drinking is held fixed in both experimental settings for coffee, we might see no changes in the risk of pancreatic cancer when comparing the presence or absence of coffee drinking.

Returning to our experiment and Table 8.1, Group 1 individuals develop pancreatic cancer both when they drink coffee and when they do not. In a population of size N, there are exactly Np_1 individuals with these characteristics; equivalently, p_1 is the proportion of the population that develops pancreatic cancer under either exposure condition. It makes no difference whether they drink coffee or not. On the other hand, Group 2 individuals develop cancer when they drink coffee but not when they abstain. In this case, drinking coffee clearly made the difference between getting pancreatic cancer or not. Analogous explanations apply to Group 3 and Group 4 individuals, with p_2, p_3, and p_4 representing the fraction of the population in the respective groups. Clearly, $p_1 + p_2 + p_3 + p_4 = 1$, since every individual must conform to one, and only one, of the four different groups. Assuming that we know these population proportions, we can now easily calculate the causal effect of coffee drinking using any of the measures defined in Chapter 4. Before we continue with such calculations, we reiterate that the protocol for such experiments requires that exposure occurs prior to the outcome in time. It is conceptually impossible to envision this experimental strategy if exposure is determined by circumstances after the outcome has occurred.

We return to computation of causal effects. Specifically, Table 8.1 shows that in the population the probability of D, when all individuals drink coffee, is just $p_1 + p_2$; similarly, the probability of D if everyone abstained from coffee is $p_1 + p_3$. Differences between these two risks or probabilities allow us to define causal versions of our measures of association. First, the causal Relative Risk is just the ratio of these two risks:

$$RR_{causal} = \frac{p_1 + p_2}{p_1 + p_3}. \tag{8.1}$$

The difference between this quantity and RR, which we defined in Equation 4.1, is that the latter compares the risk of disease in two different subpopulations (those who drink coffee and those who do not), whereas RR_{causal} compares the same population under the two exposure possibilities. Similarly, the causal Excess Risk and Odds Ratios are defined by

$$ER_{causal} = (p_1 + p_2) - (p_1 + p_3);$$

$$OR_{causal} = \frac{\frac{p_1+p_2}{1-(p_1+p_2)}}{\frac{p_1+p_3}{1-(p_1+p_3)}}.$$

The null value of any of these three causal effect measures reflects a population characteristic, namely that over all individuals, the population risk of pancreatic cancer when everyone drinks coffee is the same as when everyone does not; in symbols, this occurs if and only if $p_2 = p_3$. It does not mean that coffee has no causal effect on any individual; there may be individuals of either Group 2 or 3 where coffee drinking makes the difference as to whether they contract pancreatic cancer or not. However, the number of Group 2 individuals exactly matches the number of Group 3 individuals so that the net result is that drinking coffee does not change the *population* risks of pancreatic cancer.

Now we return to reality by recognizing that it is impossible to observe the results of both experiments for even a single individual in the population; that is, it is logically impossible for us to watch a person's experience with the cancer twice, once when we expose them to coffee and once when they are unexposed (this is the essence of Milan Kundera's "unbearable lightness of being"). For a single person in any of the groups described in Table 8.1, we only observe the outcome under one exposure condition. Their response under the other exposure possibility is merely postulated—in princi-pal, we could have observed it if we changed the experimental conditions—but it is never observed. For this reason, the unobserved response is called a *counterfactual*. So, for an individual who drinks coffee, whether he would develop pancreatic cancer had he abstained from coffee is a counterfactual. Nonetheless, the causal effect mea-sures depend on these counterfactuals, specifically on the distribution of the various counterfactual patterns listed in Table 8.1. Note that there is more involved in Table 8.1 than merely assuming the existence of counterfactuals; for example, our discussion has tacitly assumed that the counterfactuals for one individual are unrelated to those of another, an assumption that may be violated when studying infectious diseases.

Given that we are able to observe individuals under only one exposure condition, is there any hope of being able to estimate causal effects between E and D? In particular, how does the Relative Risk, RR, defined in Equation 4.1 relate to the causal Relative Risk, RR_{causal}, defined in Equation 8.1? This is a crucial question because the estimation procedures of Chapter 7 are designed to measure RR and not RR_{causal}. In short, to claim that estimates of RR describe causal effects, we need to know if and when $RR = RR_{causal}$.

There is certainly no guarantee that these quantities will even be close to each other. For example, referring to Table 8.1, recall that in practice, for each individual we only get to observe one of the experiments; that is, we either see his cancer incidence if he drinks coffee or if he does not, but not both. Suppose for Group 1 and 3 individuals we observe their responses to coffee drinking, and for Group 2 and 4 individuals we observe their response to coffee abstention. In other words, in our realistic study it turns out that all coffee drinkers are Group 1 or 3 individuals, and all abstainers are Group 2 or 4 individuals. The resulting observable 2×2 table for the entire population is then given in Table 8.2. The Relative Risk, RR, from this table is infinite, as is the Odds Ratio, OR, because the observed risk of cancer among coffee abstainers is zero! Of particular concern, this is true whatever the actual causal Relative Risk or Odds Ratio may be! It is just as easy to rearrange the scenario leading to a modified version of Table 8.2 with $RR = OR = 0$. In sum, the value of the Relative Risk from an observable table like Table 8.2 may bear little relationship to the causal Relative Risk determined by the distribution of unobservable counterfactual patterns as given in Table 8.1. The observable Relative Risk is largely determined by the mechanism that "decides" which exposure condition is available for observation for each individual.

The situation seems hopeless until we notice that there is one situation that forces a connection between RR and RR_{causal}. As we have just seen, the key issue is which exposure condition is "observed" for individuals in each group (as defined in Table 8.1), a choice that is not under our control. However, suppose the chances of "observing" the coffee drinking response are identical across all four groups of individuals. As a special case, suppose for each group the toss of a fair coin determines whether, for a given individual, we observe coffee drinking or abstention (this would happen, for example, if individuals decide to drink coffee by tossing a fair coin). On average,

Table 8.2 *Population data on coffee drinking and pancreatic cancer under nonrandom counterfactual observation*

		Pancreatic Cancer	
		D	$\bar{D}$
Coffee drinking (cups per day)	$\geq 1\ (E)$	Np_1	Np_3 $N(p_1 + p_3)$
	$0\ (\bar{E})$	0	$N(p_2 + p_4)$ $N(p_2 + p_4)$
		Np_1	$N(p_2 + p_3 + p_4)$ N

Table 8.3 *Population data on coffee drinking and pancreatic cancer under random counterfactual observation*

		Pancreatic Cancer		
		D	$\bar{D}$	
Coffee drinking (cups per day)	≥ 1	$\frac{N(p_1+p_2)}{2}$	$\frac{N(p_3+p_4)}{2}$	$N/2$
	0	$\frac{N(p_1+p_3)}{2}$	$\frac{N(p_2+p_4)}{2}$	$N/2$
		$\frac{N(2p_1+p_2+p_3)}{2}$	$\frac{N(p_2+p_3+2p_4)}{2}$	N

the observable 2×2 table would look like Table 8.3, from which we immediately see that $RR = (p_1 + p_2)/(p_1 + p_3) = RR_{causal}$.

Although this equivalence of RR and RR_{causal} is only true on the average, any difference between the two quantities diminishes rapidly as the population size N grows larger. In most settings, our Target Population is essentially infinite, in which case the described mechanism for determining the observed exposure will lead to $RR = RR_{causal}$. In the above logic, it does not matter if the chances of seeing a particular exposure is exactly 0.5, nor in fact if the mechanism that determines the observed exposure is even random. The fundamental assumption that yields $RR = RR_{causal}$, called the *randomization assumption*, is that the process that determines which exposure condition is observed for an individual is *independent* of the outcomes for that individual under either exposure; in other words, the probability of observing a specific exposure condition does not depend on the group, as defined in Table 8.1, to which the individual belongs. In the example, the randomization assumption implies that the choice of an individual to drink coffee or not does not depend in any way on their future (pancreatic cancer) responses to coffee drinking or abstention.

Confounding can now be broadly defined. For any setting where $RR \neq RR_{causal}$, we say that confounding is present. This definition could just as easily and equivalently be based on our other measures of association, since they are all simple combinations of the risks of disease under different exposure conditions. When confounding is present, we cannot infer a causal effect from the crude measures of association of Chapter 4. In summary, confounding describes a situation where the causal population parameters RR_{causal}, OR_{causal}, and ER_{causal} differ from the respective population parameters RR, OR, and ER that are based on observable exposure conditions and not on counterfactuals. The randomization assumption implies no confounding, thereby allowing us to infer causal effects from the methods of Chapters 6 and 7.

Can we ever really invoke the randomization assumption? One major advantage of randomized studies is that if exposure is randomly assigned to individuals, the randomization assumption necessarily holds. That is, if your exposure is determined at random by the experimental design, it cannot depend on information connected to your outcome. Thus, randomized studies remove the possibility of confounding, and are therefore extremely appealing as a means to determine causal effects. Of course, we assume here that exposure randomization can be implemented without error. For example, in randomizing dietary interventions to individuals, we cannot be certain that subjects comply with their assigned diet; because of this, we can only guarantee a lack of confounding for the assigned intervention and not for the actual diet consumed; see Question 8.9(3). In the next chapter we also discuss reasons why you may wish to consider confounding even in a randomized study with perfect compliance. Nonetheless, randomization is a great idea in principle as far as avoiding the deleterious effects of confounding.

The primary vulnerability of human epidemiological studies of risk factors is that randomization of exposure is simply not possible most of the time; without it, the randomization assumption is usually not testable from study data. (How can we know why people choose to drink coffee or not, or exactly what influences this decision?) Furthermore, all of the above discussion begs the question of how large the discrepancies between causal and observed effects are when confounding is present, although the discussion surrounding Table 8.2 shows that the impact can be arbitrarily large and in either direction (that is, RR can either be smaller or greater than RR_{causal}). How can we gauge the effect of confounding in a study? To better understand the randomization assumption and factors influencing the amount of confounding, let us see how it easily fails due to the influence of an extraneous factor C.

8.1.2 Confounding variables

In the example on coffee and pancreatic cancer, let C denote the sex of an individual. First, note that the risk of pancreatic cancer is known to be higher for males than females. Now suppose, plausibly, that men are also more likely to be coffee drinkers than females (or vice versa, for that matter). In this situation, the randomization assumption does not hold; to see this, note that we are more likely to "observe" the coffee drinking exposure for males, which in turn means that the response is more likely to be cancer since it is more common among males. This conclusion is true regardless of any effect of coffee itself. This thus violates the necessary independence between the "observed" exposure condition and the outcomes for individuals. Here, confounding has occurred due to the role of the extraneous factor, sex.

A helpful schematic illustrates this phenomenon clearly. Figure 8.1 illustrates the associations between the three factors, represented as "pipelines." Imagine that water can arise from any variable and flow in either direction on any pipeline. The direction of the arrow on a pipeline represents a causal effect, and the strength of such a relationship can be thought of as the flow rate in the relevant pipeline (or equivalently, the diameter of the pipe); that is, a high flow rate in the pipeline linking C and D

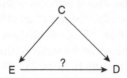

Figure 8.1 *Schematic describing confounding.*

symbolizes a large (causal) association between C and D. Our interest focuses on the existence and size of a pipeline between E and D: one can imagine starting a flow of water at "source" E to see if any water, and how much, appears subsequently at D. If this happens, this would, at first blush, indicate a pipeline between E and D with the strength of flow measuring the strength of the relationship. However, now we see the presence of C and the possibility that some of the water arriving at D may have made its way via the pipeline that links E to C and then to D, casting doubt on even the existence of a direct link from E to D. At the very least, we cannot be sure how much of the flow rate measured at D should be attributed to the pipeline from E to D, and how much to the other pipeline through C. It is this indirect association of E with D (through C) that violates the randomization assumption as noted, thereby leading to confounding. The amount of confounding (that is, the difference between RR and RR_{causal}, for example) depends on the size of the two associations between C and D and between C and E.

In this simple situation, the variable C must possess two properties to be a confounder:

- C must be causally associated with D.
- C must be causally associated with E.

Loosely speaking, these two conditions indicate that the two component pipelines in the path $E–C–D$ must exist for C to be a confounder. Formally, the conditions directly imply that the randomization assumption fails, so that confounding exists. It is crucial that both pipelines from C exist; otherwise any water showing up at D from the source E must have followed the direct pipe from E to D, the causal path. The insistence that C be causally associated with D, denoted by the direction of the pipeline from C to D, is important; without this restriction, the above conditions for confounding are not sufficient, meaning that a factor C can be associated with both D and E without being a confounder. Similarly, the requirement that C causes E rather than E causes C is critical; if E causes C, then both pipelines from E to D in Figure 8.1 reflect causal effects of E. We address these issues more carefully when we expand our discussion of Figure 8.1 into a more formal introduction to causal graphs and confounding in Section 8.2.

8.1.3 Control of confounding by stratification

Now that we have some understanding of how confounding is introduced via one or more confounding variables, we return to the question of how to derive causal information in the presence of one or more confounding factors. That is, in our example, we want to estimate the causal effect of coffee consumption on pancreatic cancer, allowing, for the moment, that the sex of an individual may be a confounder. This is usually only possible if after individuals have been sampled, by whatever design, data are collected on the set of potential confounding variables of concern, sex in this specific case; the exception is when so-called *instrumental variables* for the exposure are measured (see Section 8.5). We are unable to remove confounding effects due to unmeasured factors, so that considerable care must be taken in the design phase to ascertain factors that might have a substantial confounding effect on the relationship of interest.

The simplest strategy to eliminate confounding effects is the removal of variation in the confounding factor C. If there is no variation in C, then it cannot influence the association between E and D. Or, in the language of counterfactuals, if C is fixed, then the observed exposure counterfactual cannot be influenced by the level of C. Since the variation of C is not under our control in the design approaches of Chapter 5, one method to achieve no variation in C is to *stratify* the population and data into separate groups that share a common value for the confounding factor C. Here, we assume that C is discrete, allowing for the possibility of a distinct set of strata within each of which there is no variation in the level of C. We briefly discuss the issue of continuous confounding variables in Section 8.5.

At each level of C there is a causal measure of association between E and D; for example, the causal effect of coffee on pancreatic cancer for (1) males and (2) females. Imagine two versions of Table 8.1, one for males and one for females. For these strata causal effects to be estimable, we must invoke the randomization assumption within subgroups of the population in each of which C is constant. Formally, we are now claiming the randomization assumption, *conditional* on levels of C; in terms of counterfactuals, we assume that, at each distinct level of C, whichever exposure condition is "observed" is independent of the outcomes of the counterfactuals. In essence, this new conditional randomization assumption requires that there be no other confounding variables beyond those accounted for by C. The development of Section 8.1.1 now allows us to estimate the causal effect of E on D, holding C fixed (for example, for males and females separately), using the part of the sampled data that can be allocated to this particular level or stratum.

Dividing the population into strata based on C immediately raises a new issue, namely that our causal measure of E and D association may vary between levels of C; for example, the Relative Risk associating E and D at one level of C may be different from the Relative Risk at a different C level. The causal effects of coffee on pancreatic cancer for males may differ from those for females. If the causal measure of $E-D$ association is the same across all C levels, we say that there is no *statistical interaction* between C and E with regard to the outcome D *for this particular measure of association*. If the measures of $E-D$ association vary across levels of C, that is, interaction is present, we say that C *modifies the effect* of E on D as captured by this measure of association. Therefore, an extraneous factor C can have two impacts on the relationship between E and D: it can confound the relationship and it can also have an interactive effect. That is, C can be a confounder and/or an effect modifier. Whereas the definition of confounding does not depend on whether we use the Relative Risk, Odds Ratio, or Excess Risk, the notion of statistical interaction is extremely dependent on the selected measure of association. We discuss this observation and its interpretation at length in Chapter 10.

It should now be obvious that by conditioning on a confounding factor C, we have introduced a possibly different causal effect of E at each level of C (two causal effects for coffee, when C is just sex). With the randomization assumption now conditional on C, we can estimate each of these causal effects separately using any of our designs and accounting for sampling uncertainty with the methods of Chapters 6 and 7. When there is no statistical interaction for our chosen measure, the underlying stratum causal effects are assumed to be all the same, suggesting that we should be able to combine the separate strata estimates into one summary estimate of the "common" causal effect. Statistical techniques for achieving this goal are explored in the next chapter.

Note here that we have "solved" the effect of confounding by stratifying on C or, in other words, by controlling or conditioning on the value of C, and then invoking a weaker condition that the randomization assumption holds in strata of C even if it does not hold in the entire population. This, as we have discussed, yields causal effects within each stratum of C. This may meet our needs in describing the causal effect of E, but be aware that we can also get the overall causal effect of E on D by piecing together our estimates in each C stratum, as long as we have information on how C is distributed in the population. Overall effects are obtained by first calculating the risks for the exposed and unexposed, in each C stratum separately and then computing the "average" risk by weighting these according to the C distribution. Any overall causal effect measure can then be calculated from these "averaged" risks for the two exposure groups.

8.2 Causal graphs

Although the use of counterfactuals provides us with a firm basis for discussing causation and confounding, a large number of confounding variables leads to a complicated scenario. In such cases, we may wish to minimize the number of confounding variables to measure or consider in the analysis. Further, we would like to refine the thinking about conditions on the directions of association in Figure 8.1 that are necessary for confounding. Causal graphs shed considerable light on both of these issues.

We frame our discussion in the context of a new example on the possible effects of an early childhood vaccine on a subsequent child heath condition such as autism. We are cognizant that access to medical care may prevent such health conditions in a manner totally unrelated to the issue of vaccines. However, simultaneously, availability of medical care will increase the chances of a child receiving vaccination. Further, a family's socioeconomic status (SES) influences their access and ability to pay for medical care and thereby their likelihood of vaccinating their child. Finally, a family's health history, potentially including genetic information, is suspected of affecting the risk of the childhood condition, and is also associated with options for medical care. Here, the primary interest is on the causal implications of a population-wide childhood vaccination program. What would be the total number of children with the condition under review in the population if every child, as opposed to no child, were vaccinated? In estimating the causal effects of vaccination, which of these extraneous variables, access to medical care, SES, and family history, are confounders? Will it be sufficient to stratify solely on access to medical care? Do we need to adjust for all three of these factors? Causal graphs provide a framework to address such questions conceptually.

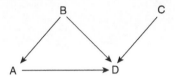

Figure 8.2 *A simple directed causal graph.*

Some simple terminology to describe graphs is needed. Unfortunately, many mixed metaphors have infiltrated common terms used in causal graphs, perhaps because they are widely used in fields varying from traffic engineering to pedigree analysis in human genetics; we will do our best to clarify any confusion. First, each variable for individuals in our study defines a *node* of the graph. The edges of the graph connecting any two nodes represent relationships between these variables. An edge with an arrow connects causal variables to their effects. This, of course, represents prior knowledge about how the variables operate in the population, particularly that the outcome of a causal variable must chronologically follow the effect. A *directed graph* is a causal graph where every edge has a single directed arrow, representing that no variable can be a cause and an effect of another variable at the same time. Figure 8.2 illustrates a simple directed graph. Note the assumption here that B causes D directly and also through A. On the other hand, C causes D but does not cause A or B either directly or indirectly.

Within a directed graph, a *directed path* between two nodes is a path connecting the nodes where each edge of the path is an arrow that always follows the direction of the path. In Figure 8.2, B–A–D is a directed path, whereas both B–D–A and C–B–D are not.

A directed graph is called *acyclic* if no directed path forms a closed loop, that is, starts at a node and returns to that node, implementing the restriction that no variable can "cause itself." This definition seems overly restrictive at first as we can imagine causal effects between an exposure and an outcome in both directions. For example, suppose that D represents a respiratory condition in a child, and E, the mother's smoking status. We can guess that the mother's smoking causes changes in the child's respiratory condition and that a mother might change her smoking habits in light of her child's health. This suggests the Figure 8.3(a) graph, which is not acyclic. Such feedback loops can often be avoided by considering chronological time; Figure 8.3(b) provides a directed acyclic graph where we carefully define two distinct variables for D and E, one for each of two chronological times, say, $t = 0$ and $t = 1$. Note that this causal graph allows the possibility that E at $t = 0$ causes D at $t = 1$ and that D at $t = 0$ causes E at $t = 1$, without forcing a feedback loop.

Not all intermediate variables on an edge need to be represented in full detail on the graph. In Figure 8.2, it is possible that C causes other variables on the path to D that do not connect to any other nodes. These intermediate variables do not need to be included, as their action does not alter our understanding of all the other causal pathways represented at the level of detail given in the figure.

(a)

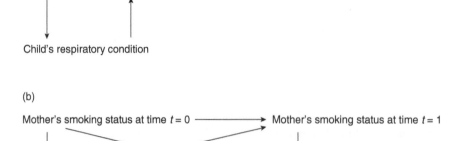

Figure 8.3 *Simple examples of a (a) cyclic, and (b) acyclic directed causal graph.*

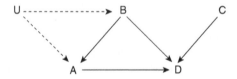

Figure 8.4 *A directed acyclic causal graph that includes unmeasured variables U.*

Usually, the nodes represent only measured variables on individuals under study. However, the impact of unmeasured variables is often of concern, and should be included in the graph when their presence is strongly suspected. When variables have not been measured, it is helpful to denote pathways in and out of their node by dashed edges. Figure 8.4 extends Figure 8.2 to allow for the presence of unmeasured variables that cause both A and B.

Some additional definitions that apply to directed acyclic graphs follow. First, a backdoor path, from node A to node B, say, is a path that begins by leaving A along an edge whose arrow points into A (i.e., against the flow), and then continues onto B along edges without regard to the direction of the arrows. For example, in Figure 8.2, $D–B–A$ is a backdoor path from D to A. On the other hand, there is no backdoor path from C to any of the other nodes.

A node A on a specific path is called a *collider* if the edges of the path entering and leaving A both have arrows pointing into A. A path is *blocked* if it contains at least one collider. Figure 8.5 illustrates a directed acyclic graph where the node D is a collider in the path $C–D–A–F–B$; the path is blocked due to the presence of the collider D.

Finally, a node A, at the end of a single directed edge originating at a node B, is called the *child* of B; B is then the *parent* of A. Similarly, any node A at the end of a

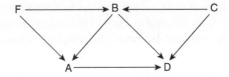

Figure 8.5 *A directed acyclic causal graph with a collider.*

directed path originating at *B* is referred to as a *descendant* of *B*; equivalently, *B* is an *ancestor* of *A*. As is logical, children of a node are a subset of descendants of that node. In Figure 8.5, the node *A* is the child of both *F* and *B*; it is also the descendant of node *C*. Similarly, node *F* has three descendants, *A*, *B*, and *D*; node *D* has four ancestors, *A*, *B*, *C*, and *F*. In any directed acyclic graph, the only pathways between two distinct variables are either (1) a directed path or (2) a backdoor path through a common ancestor.

8.2.1 Assumptions in causal graphs

Up to this point, we have constructed some simple causal graphs containing directed edges, without being very careful about what this structure actually assumes. How do we relate a causal graph to our previous definitions of causal effects and to observable associations between variables included in the graph?

As indicated, the directed edges of a causal graph already carry basic assumptions about cause and effect that are based on prior knowledge of the context, and not necessarily inferred from observed data in our study of interest. In particular, if *A* is the parent of *B*, then this assumes that *A* causes *B* as defined by counterfactuals in Section 8.1.1; that is, *A* has a direct effect on *B* not mediated by other variables represented in the graph. In general, different direct paths from *A* to *B* represent different causal pathways. Just as importantly, the absence of a directed path from *A* to *B* assumes the lack of any cause and effect. For example, in Figure 8.5, the variable *F* directly causes *A* and *B*, and causes *D* through both *A* and *B*. On the other hand, *F* does not cause *C*, directly or indirectly. This is a good place to emphasize that the use of a particular causal graph assumes that all relevant causal effects are represented, even those due to unmeasured variables, at least at the appropriate level of detail. Causal graph interpretations can be severely misleading if key variables are missing.

The presence and absence of paths between variables invoke certain assumptions about the observable population association, or independence, between the variables represented by the nodes. Specifically, a population association between variables *A* and *B*, say, implies the existence of at least one unblocked path between *A* and *B*; equivalently, no unblocked paths between *A* and *B* implies their independence. Thus, in Figure 8.5, the variables *C* and *F* are assumed independent. Conversely, the existence of an unblocked path between *A* and *B* almost always has the consequence that *A* and *B* are associated or dependent. That this is not always true follows from the unusual possibility that associations arising from different (unblocked) pathways between *A* and *B* might cancel out, leading to independence. For example, in Figure 8.5, there is the direct path from A to D and three unblocked paths (A–B–D, A–F–B–D, A–B–C–D); the associations inferred by each of these paths could cancel each other out, leaving A and D independent. However, this phenomenon is extremely unlikely to happen in practice.

In general, these assumptions can be summarized as: variable A is conditionally independent of any nondescendant, given its parents. While it is not important for our immediate purposes to dissect this statement further, it is important to note that these association assumptions are not sufficient in and of themselves, as they provide no information about the causal *direction* of the links between variables; that is, if coffee causes pancreatic cancer or vice versa. Direction of the edges is provided by causal assumptions, which cannot be directly verified from the data. Without these assumptions, though, any attempt at causal inference is futile. The assumptions about association and direction let us see whether causal associations can be inferred from observed associations, thereby also deducing the presence of confounding. This is the topic of the next section.

While these assumptions behind a causal graph provide important insight into the relationships between variables, we note that the graph provides no information about the strength of association, or even whether a factor increases or decreases the risk of disease. Nor does it give information about the form of the relationship in cases where at least one of the variables has a continuous scale (in contrast, *structural equation models* superimpose linear, or other highly specified, relationships between variables on a causal graph).

8.2.2 Causal graph associating childhood vaccination to subsequent health condition

Return to the motivating example introduced at the beginning of Section 8.2. Figure 8.6 provides a directed acyclic graph that captures our assumptions about the relationships between various factors. Note that in addition to including specific causal links, the graph also assumes absences of other links. For example, it is assumed that SES only affects the health condition through vaccination and access to medical care, and that family history does not directly influence SES. In order to assess confounding, it is important to include all relevant causal effects at the appropriate level of detail. In addition, the graph assumes that there are no unmeasured variables that may be causally related to any of the described factors.

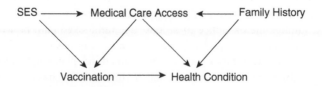

Figure 8.6 *A directed acyclic causal graph associating childhood vaccination with a subsequent health condition.*

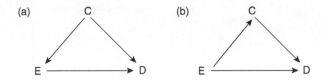

Figure 8.7 *Causal graphs indicating both the presence (a) and absence (b) of confounding.*

With the graph definitions in hand, we are now in a position to answer the questions posed earlier. Is the relationship between vaccination and the health condition confounded by these other factors? If so, which of these should we control for by stratification to ensure the removal of confounding? We address both of these issues in the following sections.

8.2.3 Using causal graphs to infer the presence of confounding

One of the most attractive features of a causal graph is that it allows us to directly infer whether the marginal association between an exposure, E, and outcome, D, is confounded; that is, whether $RR \neq RR_{causal}$ or not, etc. First, consider the simplest situation introduced in Sections 8.1.1 and 8.1.2, where there is a single potential confounding variable, C. Figure 8.7(a) shows the classic causal graph describing C as a confounder; note again that C is assumed to be a common cause of both E and D. On the other hand, Figure 8.7(b) describes a situation where C does not confound the E–D relationship, since it is directly caused by E; in this case, both pathways E–D and E–C–D describe two distinct causal effects of E on D. The key difference between these two situations is the presence of an unblocked backdoor path from E to D in Figure 8.7(a) in addition to the direct causal pathway (the path E–C–D is not a backdoor path in Figure 8.7(b)). The presence of this backdoor path causes the randomization assumption to fail, as we discussed in Section 8.1.2, leading to confounding when C is ignored. The role of backdoor paths in detecting the presence of confounding is easily generalized to more complex graphs.

To determine whether confounding exists, we follow two simple steps. Given any directed acyclic graph:

- Delete all arrows from E that point to any other node.

- In this reduced graph, determine whether there is any unblocked backdoor path from E to D. If such a path exists, the causal E–D relationship is confounded by the effects of the other variables; if there is no such path, there is no confounding.

The first step removes from the graph any causal pathways from E to D that represent the effects of E on D that we are trying to measure. As we have just seen, applying this rule to the two graphs of Figure 8.7 immediately distinguishes between (a) when there is confounding and (b) where there is no confounding. The latter case illustrates the classic epidemiological maxim that an extraneous variable on the pathway between exposure and disease should not be considered a confounder. In this scenario, *both* pathways from E to D represent causal effects of E. For example, one would not

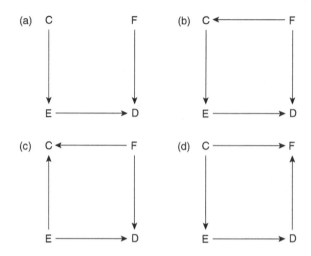

Figure 8.8 *Causal graphs indicating both the presence (b) and absence (a,c,d) of confounding.*

usually consider the occurrence of colon polyps as a confounder of the association between dietary fiber intake and incidence of colon cancer. The second step amounts to checking whether exposure, E, and disease, D, share a common ancestor.

Now consider the graphs of Figure 8.8, which represent a variety of other causal graphs involving E and D, now with two extraneous factors C and F. Applying the above steps shows immediately that there is no confounding of the causal relationship between E and D in Figures 8.8(a,c,d), but that confounding exists in Figure 8.8(b). We know this because in Figure 8.8(a) there is no causal relationship between C and F, in Figure 8.8(c) the edge from E to C is removed as it reflects a causal effect of E, and in Figure 8.8(d) there is no unblocked backdoor path since F is a collider. The case in Figure 8.8(d) indicates that confounding cannot arise from the presence of variables that are caused by the outcome D. The confounding in Figure 8.8(b) arises either when F causes C as shown, or C causes F (not shown). As mentioned in Section 8.1.2, the quantitative amount of confounding distortion depends on the strength of association represented in *each* edge of an unblocked backdoor path that is the source of confounding.

The distinctions between the four cases of Figure 8.8 demonstrate the need to consider causal pathways in appropriately assessing whether control of extraneous factors is needed to remove confounding. In particular, mindless stratification on all extraneous variables may be unnecessary and can introduce confounding where none previously existed, a phenomenon we unravel in the next section.

This section ends by reviewing the causal graph, Figure 8.6, that describes the assumed causal relationships between childhood vaccination and a subsequent health condition and related factors. Notice here that the presence of the three factors—SES, medical care access, and family history—leads to confounding of causal association from vaccination to health condition. In particular, there are several backdoor paths from vaccination to health condition including (1) vaccination to medical care access to health condition and (2) vaccination to medical care access to family history to health condition. Note that medical care access is a collider on one path from SES to family history (through medical care access), so that no backdoor path can include this as a segment. We now extend these ideas to figure out which of these variables need to be controlled for, in order to remove this confounding.

8.3 Controlling confounding in causal graphs

As noted in Section 8.1.3, one successful strategy for handling confounding involves stratification of the population (and thus the data) into groups where all confounders share the same level. Given the ease with which we can use casual graphs to identify confounders, it is natural to ask if we can employ a similar approach to determine whether stratification on a particular set of confounders is sufficient to eliminate *all* confounding associated with the graph. Let us see exactly how this is achieved.

Note first that stratification on a single variable is equivalent to removing that variable or node from the graph, since the absence of variation in a variable means that it can no longer influence other variables in the graph. Metaphorically, stratification on C places a "stopcock" or "valve" at node C that makes it impossible for water to flow through C on any path. From another point of view, when we stratify on C, we are considering the causal graph for other variables *at a fixed value of C*, our interest then focusing on whether there is still confounding of the causal effect of E on D within strata defined by common levels of C.

These ideas suggest examining the issue of continued confounding after stratification on C by simply removing the node corresponding to C from the graph (and thereby all edges into and out of C), and then examining whether there is still any unblocked backdoor path from E to D using the methods of Section 8.2.3. Unfortunately, this does not quite work if C is a collider, for reasons we turn to next.

8.3.1 Danger: controlling for colliders

An important subtle idea arises when colliders are included in a set of stratifying variables: by placing a stopcock at a collider, new pathways are "opened." Consider the part of the causal diagram in Figure 8.6 representing the role of a vaccine in causing a childhood condition, namely, the section involving SES, family history, and access to medical care. If we seek to remove confounding by stratifying the population solely on levels of health care access (thereby removing this node), a new pathway is inadvertently opened between SES and family history.

That stratification on a collider induces an unanticipated association is most easily illustrated by looking at some hypothetical data, as in Table 8.4. From this hypothetical scenario, observe that dietary sugar content is associated with tooth decay under either condition of fluoridation; similarly, fluoridation is associated with the risk of tooth decay at two fixed levels of sugar in the diet (high and low, say). (There is no statistical interaction with regard to the Odds Ratio or Excess Risk in either case.)

Table 8.4 *Hypothetical data on water fluoridation, high-sugar diet, and tooth decay*

Fluoridation (A)			Tooth Decay (D)			
			D	$\bar{D}$	OR	ER
A	High-sugar diet (B)	B	160	40	2.67	0.2
		$\bar{B}$	120	80		
$\bar{A}$	High-sugar diet (B)	B	80	120	2.67	0.2
		$\bar{B}$	40	160		

High-sugar diet (B)			Tooth Decay (D)			
			D	$\bar{D}$	OR	ER
B	Fluoridation (A)	A	160	40	6.00	0.4
		$\bar{A}$	80	120		
$\bar{B}$	Fluoridation (A)	A	120	80	6.00	0.4
		$\bar{A}$	40	160		

Pooled table			Fluoridation (A)			
			A	$\bar{A}$	OR	ER
	High-sugar diet (B)	B	200	200	1.00	0.00
		$\bar{B}$	200	200		

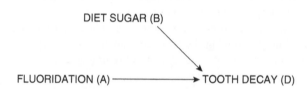

Figure 8.9 *A simple directed causal graph linking fluoridation and diet sugar to tooth decay.*

Further, the pooled table, obtained by ignoring the outcome D, demonstrates that fluoridation and a high-sugar diet are independent in this population, as shown in the causal graph of Figure 8.9. If we now stratify the population on levels of tooth decay, an association between fluoridation and diet sugar appears (Table 8.5). Qualitatively, we can understand this induced association as follows: among individuals with tooth decay, if we know that an individual was exposed to fluoridated water, we are more likely to believe that they have a high-sugar diet as it provides an alternative explanation of tooth decay.

The lesson from this section is that stratification on a collider variable inadvertently introduces a new pathway in our causal graph. This new pathway must be accounted for in determining whether stratification on a set of variables is sufficient to remove confounding.

Table 8.5 *Hypothetical data (from Table 8.4) relating water fluoridation to high-sugar diet, after stratification by tooth decay*

Tooth Decay (D)

| | | \multicolumn{2}{c}{Fluoridation} | | |
High-sugar diet		A	$\bar{A}$	OR	ER
	B	160	80	0.67	−0.083
	$\bar{B}$	120	40		

No Tooth Decay ($\bar{D}$)

| | | \multicolumn{2}{c}{Fluoridation} | | |
High-sugar diet		A	$\bar{A}$	OR	ER
	B	40	120	0.67	−0.083
	$\bar{B}$	80	160		

8.3.2 Simple rules for using a causal graph to choose the crucial confounders

Now turn to the use of causal graphs in determining whether controlling a particular set of confounders is sufficient to remove *all* confounding of the causal effects of exposure on the disease outcome. We refer to the proposed set of stratification factors as the set $S = \{C_1, \ldots, C_s\}$. Now that we understand the implication of stratification by a collider in S, we can describe a simple set of steps that allow us to determine whether any confounding remains after stratification on all factors in S. We refer back to the causal graph, Figure 8.6, to illustrate the method. The steps are as follows:

- Delete all arrows from E that point to any other node.
- Add in new undirected edges between nodes, for any pair of nodes that have a common descendant in the set of stratification factors S.
- In this new graph, determine whether there is any unblocked backdoor path from E to D that avoids passing through any node in the set of stratification factors. If no such path is found, confounding is controlled by the proposed stratification factors; if there is such a path, stratification by these factors is insufficient to remove all confounding.

Applying this procedure to Figure 8.7(a) trivially shows that stratification on C removes its confounding effect in this scenario. Similarly, in Figure 8.8(b), control of either C or F, or both, is sufficient to remove confounding. Turning to our example, Figure 8.6, suppose we consider stratifying solely on medical care access, in response to the confounding we noted in Section 8.2.3. With $S = \{\text{medical care access}\}$, performing the first two steps of the method yields the causal graph of Figure 8.10. For visual simplicity, we have removed medical care access from the graph. An undirected connection between SES and family history appears since medical care access is a collider and a stratification factor. From this graph we immediately see that an unblocked backdoor path from vaccination to health condition still exists; so the causal relationship between them remains confounded. However, from similar analyses we

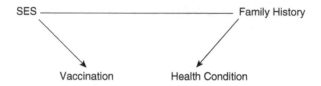

Figure 8.10 *A directed acyclic causal graph associating childhood vaccination with a subsequent health condition, after stratification on medical care access.*

see that, to remove all confounding, it would be sufficient to stratify on medical care access and SES, on medical care access and family history, or on all three. Since family history data may be difficult to collect, it is valuable to note here that confounding is removed when we control solely for medical care access and SES.

This section illustrates that indiscriminate stratification may introduce confounding where none was originally present. Recall that there is no confounding of the causal E–D relationship in Figure 8.8(c) because the variable C is a collider. Here, the observable unadjusted Relative Risk can be interpreted as the causal Relative Risk. On the other hand, if we inadvertently stratify on C, an undirected edge is created that links E and F, now creating an unblocked path from E to D through F that does not pass through C. Thus, controlling for C now introduces confounding and the Relative Risk, in strata of C, do *not* have a causal interpretation.

8.4 Collapsibility over strata

Having grown accustomed to stratification as a mechanism to control the confounding influence of a factor C, we recall that this introduces the possibility of statistical interaction. How do we relate the ideas of confounding and interaction to properties of our measures of association both within strata of C, and in the entire population when C is ignored? Is there a definition of confounding that can be based simply on these observable Relative Risks, the ones obtained within C strata and from ignoring C altogether, without recourse to counterfactuals and the complexity of causal graphs? The answer, even in the simplest situation of a single extraneous factor C, is almost, but not quite.

With the Relative Risk as the chosen measure of association, Table 8.6 illustrates four different scenarios distinguished by the presence and absence of confounding and/or interaction. Example 1 demonstrates the simplest case, where the Relative Risk for the E–D relationship has the same value, 2.00, at the two levels of a binary extraneous factor C. There is thus no statistical interaction between C and E, at least in terms of RR. In addition, the Relative Risk in the pooled table when C is ignored is also 2.00, the same as seen for each stratum. With no confounding of the E–D relationship by C, the pooled table does not distort the association between E and D in the subtables where there is no C variation.

In Example 2 of Table 8.6, there is again no interaction between C and E because the Relative Risk for D associated with E remains 2.00, both when C is present and when it is absent, for all individuals. On the other hand, in the pooled table we see

Table 8.6 *Examples illustrating the presence and absence of confounding and interaction*

Example 1: No Confounding and No Interaction

	C				not C				Pooled		
	D	$\bar{D}$			D	$\bar{D}$			D	$\bar{D}$	
E	120	280	400	E	14	86	100	E	134	366	500
$\bar{E}$	60	340	400	$\bar{E}$	7	93	100	$\bar{E}$	67	433	500
	$RR_C = 2.00$				$RR_{\bar{C}} = 2.00$				$RR = 2.00$		

Example 2: Confounding and No Interaction

	C				not C				Pooled		
	D	$\bar{D}$			D	$\bar{D}$			D	$\bar{D}$	
E	216	504	720	E	14	86	100	E	230	590	820
$\bar{E}$	12	68	80	$\bar{E}$	7	93	200	$\bar{E}$	19	161	180
	$\widehat{RR}_C = 2.00$				$\widehat{RR}_{\bar{C}} = 2.00$				$RR = 2.66$		

Example 3: No Confounding and Interaction

	C				not C				Pooled		
	D	$\bar{D}$			D	$\bar{D}$			D	$\bar{D}$	
E	60	340	400	E	14	86	100	E	74	426	500
$\bar{E}$	120	280	400	$\bar{E}$	7	93	100	$\bar{E}$	127	373	500
	$RR_C = 0.50$				$RR_{\bar{C}} = 2.00$				$RR = 0.58$		

Example 4: Confounding and Interaction

	C				not C				Pooled		
	D	$\bar{D}$			D	$\bar{D}$			D	$\bar{D}$	
E	108	612	720	E	14	86	100	E	122	698	820
$\bar{E}$	24	56	80	$\bar{E}$	7	93	100	$\bar{E}$	31	149	180
	$RR_C = 0.50$				$RR_{\bar{C}} = 2.00$				$RR = 0.86$		

a Relative Risk of 2.66, notably higher than observed in the C strata, indicating the considerable confounding of the E–D relationship by C. Here the pooled table that ignores C overstates the relationship observed between E and D when there is no variation in C.

Examples 3 and 4 display a striking difference in the Relative Risk for D associated with E when C is present ($RR = 0.50$) as compared with when C is absent ($RR = 2.00$). In fact, for individuals with C, exposure to E is protective against D, whereas for individuals without C, exposure to E raises the risk of D. In each of these examples, there is substantial statistical interaction between C and E in terms of the Relative Risk. Some might argue that it makes little sense to distinguish these two examples, which both feature unusual statistical interaction. However, in Example 3, which lacks confounding, the pooled Relative Risk of 0.58 is equal to the causal Relative Risk. This pooled value is an "average" of the stratum-specific Relative Risks and is much closer to the value in the C stratum (0.50), which contains substantially more of the population and is therefore weighted more in the "averaging." On the other hand, in Example 4 the averaging process is confounded so that the pooled Relative Risk of 0.86 has no causal interpretation. Although the causal understanding of the pooled Relative Risk in Example 3 may not be of value here because of the properties of the stratum Relative Risks, in other situations it is helpful to know if and when the pooled value can be given a causal interpretation.

Returning to the issue raised at the beginning of this section, can we delineate when confounding is present or absent by merely examining the stratum-specific and pooled Relative Risks? The answer appears to be straightforward, at least when there is no interaction (Examples 1 and 2): with a common stratum-specific Relative Risk (no interaction), confounding is present only when the stratum-specific Relative Risk differs from the pooled Relative Risk. In cases such as Example 1, we say that the strata, or subtables, are *collapsible* since the Relative Risk observed from the pooled table agrees with that of each stratum.

Now consider the relationships between a potential confounding variable C and the exposure and outcome variable under studies, E and D, that must exist in order for the strata to not be collapsible with regard to the Relative Risk. Assuming that there is no interaction with C in the E–D relationship in terms of the Relative Risk, the conditions that lead to the Relative Risk in the pooled population differing from the Relative Risk from any fixed C stratum are:

- C and D are associated in both the Es and the $\bar{E}$s.

- C and E are associated.

Both of these conditions have to hold for the tables to not be collapsible. These are similar conditions to those for confounding in terms of counterfactuals (introduced in Section 8.1.2), but here there is no requirement that the C–E and C–D relationships be causal. In particular, the question of collapsibility does not distinguish the two situations of Figure 8.7 or, for that matter, similar causal graphs where D causes C rather then the other way around. However, if we are willing to assume the basic causal graph structure of Figure 8.7(a), then collapsibility of the Relative Risks is equivalent to no confounding.

The issues of confounding and interaction in Table 8.6 in terms of the Relative Risk have been discussed. Similar examples can be produced using other measures of association. While noting that the absence of statistical interaction with regard to the Excess Risk means something quite different (see Chapter 10) we come to exactly the same conclusions regarding the conditions for collapsibility if we use the Excess Risk. On the other hand, with the assumption that the Odds Ratios for D associated with E are constant across the C strata, then the pooled table Odds Ratio equals the common stratum-specific Odds Ratio if and only if

Table 8.7 *Example showing that randomization does not imply collapsibility for the odds ratio*

	C			not C			Pooled		
	D	$\bar{D}$		D	$\bar{D}$		D	$\bar{D}$	
E	50	50	100	80	20	100	130	70	200
$\bar{E}$	20	80	100	50	50	100	70	130	200
	$OR_C = 4.00$			$OR_{\bar{C}} = 4.00$			$OR = 3.45$		

- C and D are associated in both the Es and the $\bar{E}$s.
- C and E are associated (i.e., not independent) in both the Ds and the $\bar{D}$s.

Now, the association between C and E, necessary for noncollapsibility, is conditional on D, so that even with the causal structure of Figure 8.7(a), collapsibility is not equivalent to the absence of confounding. This leads to the curious consequence that randomization of an exposure variable, guaranteeing no confounding, is not sufficient to ensure collapsibility with regard to the Odds Ratio (although there are limits to the size of the difference between the pooled and stratum-specific Odds Ratios). For example, imagine a population of size 400 for which the exposure E is randomized with equal probability to individuals. In each C stratum we would then expect roughly the same number of exposed as unexposed individuals. Table 8.7 illustrates a hypothetical situation with exact balance of E and $\bar{E}$, where it is easily seen that E and C are independent, i.e., there is no confounding. On the other hand, the pooled Odds Ratio of 3.45 is somewhat smaller than the common stratum-specific Odds Ratio of 4.00.

If the outcome is rare, we need not be too troubled by this oddity. In this case, Odds Ratios are close to the analogous Relative Risks so that, with no confounding, any discrepancy between the pooled Odds Ratio and the stratum-specific Odds Ratio will be very small. As a result, we can interpret collapsibility of tables with regard to the Odds Ratio in terms of confounding in essentially the same way as we did above for the Relative Risk.

In summary, for either the Relative or Excess Risk, noncollapsible tables, while suggestive of confounding, do not guarantee its existence without further assumptions on the causal graph linking C, E, and D, in particular the assumption that C is causally associated with D. This is approximately true for the Odds Ratio when D is rare. Another drawback of this approach to confounding is that, unlike with counterfactuals or causal graphs, it is limited to situations with no interaction, and this restriction varies depending on the particular measure of association (as we examine in further detail in the next chapter). We reiterate the final remark of Section 8.3.2, that collapsibility of tables can be misleading when the stratification variable is a collider. In this case, apparent noncollapsibility may suggest the presence of confounding when there is none. This situation illustrates the value of using causal graphs, as a complement to examining collapsibility, for a proper assessment of confounding, as it can prevent us from making this kind of mistake.

8.5 Comments and further reading

Great lengths have been taken to develop a conceptual understanding of confounding using both counterfactuals and causal graphs but have barely scratched the surface of the extensive, and often subtle, literature on causation. The idea of counterfactuals, or potential outcomes, dates to early work of the great philosopher David Hume, but found application in statistics and epidemiology only in the last century. Significant research has occurred in the past decade, in part motivated by application of the ideas to longitudinal studies, where additional difficulties and opportunities arise for exposures that change over time. These advances have been paralleled by similar developments in causal graphs. Pearl (2000) gives an excellent overview of graphical causal models; a more concise introduction is given in Pearl (1995). Greenland and Brumback (2002) contrast the counterfactual and causal graph approaches to other causation models. Greenland and Morgenstern (2001) review various definitions of confounding in health research. Halloran and Struchiner (1995) extend the ideas of causal inference to infectious disease outcomes where there is dependence among individuals' responses to exposure conditions.

The counterfactual and causal graph approach to causation are not equivalent; counterfactuals provide a finer level of causal detail than directed edges in graphs. Further, stratification is not the only, and perhaps not always the best, technique to get at causal effects. In fact, in longitudinal studies stratification fails to remove confounding and other methods must be used. A powerful and appealing alternative exists in denoting the unobserved counterfactual data for study participants as "missing." This opens the door to modern statistical techniques designed to accommodate missing data with minimal assumptions. In addition to describing, or modeling, causal effects of interest, such methods link extraneous variables to the probability of observing the actual exposure condition of an individual. The appropriate randomization assumption is still required but the method of estimation of a causal effect now relies on "inverse weighting," a technique widely used in estimation from complex surveys (Robins et al., 2000).

Almost all our discussion has focused on a qualitative assessment of confounding. In practice, every observational study suffers from some level of confounding even after controlling for many extraneous factors. Thus, quantitative measures of the amount of confounding are perhaps just as useful as attempts to eradicate it. Recall that the level of distortion due to confounding (how much RR differs from RR_{causal}) depends on the strength of each of the associations in an unblocked backdoor path from E to D. Even one of these links displaying weak association severely limits the amount of confounding. Any relationship determined in an observational study is always vulnerable to the threat that at least part of the observed association may be due to another variable. However, the stronger an observational study association is, the harder it is to explain it away as confounding from a single variable C since such a C would in turn have to be strongly related to both E and D. We return to the quantitative assessment of confounding when we discuss an empirical view of the issue in Chapter 9. Of course, one of the great advantages of a random experiment is that any observed association between a randomized factor E and outcome D cannot be rejected as pure confounding.

When there is more than one causal pathway linking E to D, as in Figure 8.7(b), it is often of interest to disentangle the total causal effect of E in terms of its separate causal pathways. For example, if E represents a measure of fat in the diet, D incidence of breast cancer, and C level of serum cholesterol, it is entirely plausible that an effect of dietary fat on cancer risk is partly due to elevation of cholesterol. With diet studied as a potential target for intervention, the total causal effect is what matters. On the other hand, we may also wish to assess how much of an observed association between diet and breast cancer incidence can be "attributed" to elevated cholesterol, and how much depends on a separate causal path. It is tempting to believe that the direct effect of diet not through cholesterol might be estimated by controlling for cholesterol level, thereby removing the other pathway. However, it is easy for this strategy to give quite misleading results if other uncontrolled factors are involved (Robins and Greenland, 1992; Cole and Hernán, 2002).

As noted in Section 8.1.3, we need measurements on potential confounders in the sample in order to implement stratification as a method of confounding control. There is one situation where this is not the case, that is, where we can achieve some level of control without knowledge of the confounders for study participants. For this to be possible, it is necessary to instead measure individual values of an *instrumental variable*, IV, that has the following properties: (1) IV is independent of the unknown confounders, C; (2) IV is associated with exposure, E; and (3) IV is independent of disease, D, given exposure and confounders. The latter condition simply states that once you know an individual's exposure and confounders, there is no extra information about disease risk contained in the instrumental variable. Figure 8.11 provides a casual graph illustrating a simple situation with an instrumental variable. The key feature of Figure 8.11 that separates it from earlier discussion is that the variables, C, are unobserved. What allows us to still make progress in determining the causal effect of E on D is that both the causal association between IV and D and between IV and E can be obtained without control of C, thereby allowing us to infer properties of the causal association between E and D. Greenland (2000) introduces such use of instrumental variables in this and other epidemiological applications. In many cases, if the variables C are associated directly with E, they will also be with IV, which is not permitted. However, the prototypical study, which fits with the causal graph of Figure 8.11, is a randomized intervention where there is imperfect compliance with assigned "treatment." In this setting, IV measures an individual's assigned intervention group, E the intervention actually experienced (not all participants can or will adhere to their assigned intervention), and D the outcome.

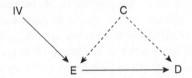

Figure 8.11 *A directed acyclic causal graph with an instrumental variable, IV.*

Sommer et al. (1986) describe such a study of the impact of vitamin A supplementation on childhood mortality in Indonesia. Although children were randomized, by village, to either an intervention group (two oral doses of vitamin A) or to a "no intervention" group, not all children assigned to the treatment group received vitamin A. Although the impact of the intervention can be assessed through the causal effect of intervention *assignment* (the causal association of IV on D in Figure 8.11), a so-called *intent-to-treat* analysis, there is obvious interest on the effect of actual treatment *received* on the outcome (the causal association between E and D in Figure 8.11). However, the latter effect cannot be captured by the observed association between E and D since this is confounded by the presence of C; that is, factors that influence compliance—adhering to the intervention to which one is assigned—and are also associated with the outcome. For example, children from poorer families may be less likely to receive their assigned intervention and, separately, are also at higher risk of death. Instrumental variables allow us to obtain information about the causal effect of E on D, without being able to stratify on C. While a point estimate of this causal effect is usually not available without further assumptions, upper and lower bounds can always be obtained. See Greenland (2000) for further discussion.

The necessary conditions for confounding illustrate that it is possible for C to confound the relationship between E and D, even though E does not confound the C and D association. This happens, for example, with associated factors E and C when E has no direct effect on D. This precludes the possibility of E being a confounder of the C and D relationship, however strong the association between C and E. However, if C is a direct risk factor for both E and D, failure to account for its presence would distort the E and D relationship.

The requirement that a single factor C must be known *a priori* as a causal risk factor for it to be considered a confounder is perhaps overly restrictive, since there are many situations where a factor C, available for measurement, may only be a proxy for an unmeasureable, perhaps unknown, causal factor. Here, we have to be content with treating C as a confounding variable, acknowledging that it is, at best, a stand-in for the true confounder. This is the case in many studies where sex and age are treated as confounders because of prior knowledge of age–sex variations in disease incidence, without specific understanding of the causal mechanism of these demographic factors. This issue also raises concern surrounding the mismeasurement of a confounding factor; if C is measured with error, our abilities to observe and control for its confounding effects are limited, depending on the extent of the measurement error. A related topic is the approximate measurement of an interval-scaled confounder through use of discrete categories. While the adjustment techniques of Chapter 9 can be usefully applied in such cases, the possibility of residual confounding persists. Thus, for example, it is unlikely that a simple dichotomous measure of smoking history (ever or never smoked) will be adequate to control for the confounding effects of smoking in studies of most cancers. Existence of important levels of residual confounding are particular insidious in such cases, as it may appear that the relevant categorized confounder has been successfully accounted for.

The discussion has focused on relatively simple situations with only a limited number of confounding factors, often only one. Considerable effort has been given to linking generalizations of the association criteria (Sections 8.1.2 and 8.4) for several potential confounding variables to the graphical checks for confounding (Sections 8.2.3 and 8.3). Greenland et al. (1999) discuss this as part of a general review of the use of causal diagrams in epidemiologic research. Note that the amount of residual confounding tends to be greater when one categorizes several confounding factors. Stratification by many confounding factors simultaneously with a limited sample size is problematic, and discussed further in Chapters 9, 12, 13, and 14.

As noted earlier in this chapter, the distortion introduced by confounding can be in either direction. That is, an apparent association between E and D can either overstate or understate an underlying causal association. However, design features can influence the direction of confounding. For example, in a case-control study, it is possible, at the design stage, to specify that an equal number of cases and controls be sampled *at each level* of C; essentially, case-control sampling is carried out separately in each subgroup of the population determined by the level of C. With this balance between cases and controls in all C strata, the effect of confounding by C is always toward the null. That is, the observed D and E association in the entire sample, ignoring information on C, will always be closer to the null ($OR = 1$) than when confounding is taken into account. This kind of sampling is known as *frequency matching*, addressed in Chapter 16.

8.6 Problems

Question 8.1

Calculate the chi-square statistic for the three tables in Table 8.8, and comment on the results.

Question 8.2

Suppose variables D, E, and C are all binary, and a case-control study is performed so that interest focuses on the Odds Ratio as a measure of association. If C confounds the relationship between E and D, must E confound the relationship between C and D?

Question 8.3

Smoking increases the risk of giving birth to low birthweight infants. It also causes several respiratory conditions in the mother. Tuberculosis raises both the chances of low birthweight infants and maternal respiratory conditions, but does not alter the probability that an individual smokes. Assuming that the respiratory conditions themselves have no influence on birthweight, draw the causal graph linking smoking, respiratory conditions, tuberculosis, and infant birthweight. With this graph in mind, is the crude association of smoking and birthweight confounded by the other variables? An investigator chooses to perform an analysis of smoking and birthweight, adjusting for the levels of existing respiratory conditions. Is the adjusted association between smoking and birthweight confounded?

Repeat your work but now assuming that the relevant respiratory conditions have a direct effect on birthweight.

Table 8.8 *Three 2 × 2 tables*

I

	B	$\bar{B}$	
A	9	1	10
$\bar{A}$	81	9	90
	90	10	100

II

	B	$\bar{B}$	
A	25	25	50
$\bar{A}$	25	25	50
	50	50	100

Combined I + II

	B	$\bar{B}$	
A	34	26	60
$\bar{A}$	106	34	140
	140	60	200

Question 8.4

Referring to Figure 8.6, assume that *SES* is associated with the childhood health condition by a direct pathway in addition to its association through access to medical care. Add this relationship to the causal graph, and determine which variables you should select to control for confounding of the association between vaccination and the health condition. Are there any other sets of variables that could be controlled to remove confounding effects?

Question 8.5

Referring to Figure 8.6, assume that access to medical care has no influence on vaccination rates or on the risk of the childhood health condition. Draw a new causal graph reflecting these assumptions, and determine whether any confounding of the association between vaccination and the health condition remains. An investigator chooses to adjust for access to medical care in this scenario. Will their analysis be confounded or unconfounded?

Question 8.6

We are interested in the causal relationship between an exposure E and disease outcome D, where there are potential confounding variables A and B. Draw a causal graph so that (1) adjustment for A alone or for B alone is insufficient to remove all confounding of the E–D relationship, and (2) adjustment for both A and B removes all confounding.

Table 8.9 *Hypothetical data on an exposure, E, a proxy for exposure, F, and a disease outcome, D*

			Disease	
Exposure			D	$\bar{D}$
E	Exposure proxy	F	180	600
		$\bar{F}$	200	200
$\bar{E}$	Exposure proxy	F	20	200
		$\bar{F}$	200	600

Question 8.7 (Greenland et al., 1999)

The healthy worker effect refers to the possibility that underlying health conditions affect an individual's choice of employment or length of employment in a specific occupation. Using a simple causal graph, show how this phenomenon confounds the association between employment categories (for example, being an airline pilot) and mortality.

Suppose a study refines its analysis of employment effects on mortality by confining attention to a specific industry, measuring exposure by specific job characteristics, where it is known that underlying health conditions are unrelated to such characteristics. On the other hand, the length of tenure in the industry does vary by job category. Using a causal graph that includes job category, length of job tenure, underlying health conditions, and mortality, show that the unadjusted association between job category and mortality is not confounded by underlying health conditions. On the other hand, use the same graph to illustrate that confounding is introduced to these mortality comparisons by stratification by the length of job tenure.

Question 8.8

Describe a causal graph for the entire population that relates the variables (1) cholecystitis status, (2) diabetes/refractive error, and (3) hospitalization in the example of Chapter 3.5. Show that stratification on hospitalization status induces an apparent association between cholecystitis and diabetes.

Question 8.9 (Robins, 2001)

Table 8.9 provides data on an exposure, E, and a disease outcome, D, where the investigator wishes to assess the causal effect of E on D. For all individuals, there is also information available on a proxy measure of exposure, labeled F. We need to determine which measure of association has a causal interpretation, and ascertain the role of F in our analysis before performing calculations (see Question 9.3). Note that the data reflect that F is related to D, conditional on E.

1. Suppose the data arise from a case-control study of a nonsteroidal anti-inflammatory drug (E) on the incidence of a congenital defect (D) that occurs in the second trimester of pregnancy. Data on E are obtained from comprehensive and accurate medical records of first trimester medications. The proxy measures F on drug use are obtained 1 month postpartum from a maternal interview. Assume all other confounding variables have been controlled, by stratification if necessary (in which case the data in Table 8.9 refer to information in a single stratum). Construct the appropriate causal graph that includes E, F, and D, ensuring that F is related to D, conditional on E; determine whether it is necessary to adjust for F to obtain a causal measure of association between E and D.

2. Now suppose the data arise from a cohort study of the mortality (D) of initially healthy 25-year-old uranium miners who only worked underground for 6 months in 1970. Assume that 30-year follow-up measurement of mortality is complete through 2000. Assume that the factor E measures an above-threshold dose of radon exposure (during a miner's time underground) that is accurately measured by lung dosimetry, while $\bar{E}$ represents a level of exposure known to not increase mortality risk. The variable F represents an estimate of whether a miner exceeds the threshold radon exposure based on the level of radon in the particular mine to which he was assigned. Assume that assignment to a given mine is unrelated to any individual characteristics of the miner, including his mortality risk. Note that a miner's actual exposure will depend not only on the level of radon in his mine, but also on individual characteristics, such as the amount of physical exertion for his job class, that may influence the amount of radon his lungs actually absorb. Note that specific mines may include exposures other than radon that may influence mortality. Again, construct the appropriate causal graph relating E, F, and D, ensuring that F is related to D, conditional on E; determine whether it is necessary to adjust for F to obtain a causal measure of association between E and D.

3. Now suppose the data arise from a randomized trial of a low-fat diet on incidence of breast cancer (D) over 15 years of follow-up. Individuals are assigned to a low-fat and educational group, or to a no intervention group, at random. The variable F measures group assignment, whereas E measures (accurately) whether an individual actually followed the low-fat diet program or not. Again, construct the appropriate causal graph relating E, F, and D, ensuring that F is related to D, conditional on E; determine whether it is necessary to adjust for F to obtain a causal measure of association between E and D.

CHAPTER 9

Control of Extraneous Factors

We can now return to the examples of Chapter 7 with renewed confidence. Let us take a fresh look at the association between coffee drinking and pancreatic cancer. Could this be explained by a confounding variable such as sex? Is some of the effect of behavior type on CHD due to confounding by body weight, say? In the previous chapter, we indicated that, having measured factors D, E, and a potential confounder, C, on individuals sampled through one of the design mechanisms, stratification of the data provides a strategy for the control of confounding by C. In this chapter, we provide a full description of how to extend the ideas of Chapters 6 and 7 to accommodate stratified data. In particular, we wish to both assess the association of D and E, and quantify the extent of the relationship through a measure of association, in both cases having removed or controlled for the confounding effects of one or more extraneous variables. We first turn to testing the association.

9.1 Summary test of association in a series of 2×2 tables

We want to generalize the χ^2 test for association, discussed in Chapter 6, to allow the possibility of a confounding effect from a set of other variables. We assume that the data are stratified into a series of I strata, each of which contains individuals that share common values of all the relevant confounders. So, for example, if sex and age are considered potential confounding variables, and age is divided into six discrete categories (25 to 35 years old, 35 to 45 years old, etc.), then there will be $I = 12$ strata (male and 25 to 35 years old, female and 25 to 35 years old, etc.). The data on D and E are displayed as a 2×2 table for each stratum, with Table 9.1 giving the notation for the data that arises in the ith stratum (where $n_i = a_i + b_i + c_i + d_i$). Illustrating this concretely, Table 9.2 gives the set of 2×2 tables that arise from stratifying the Western Collaborative Group Study data (Table 7.4) on CHD and behavior type by body weight, classified into five groups. Similarly, Table 9.3 displays the data (Table 7.2) on pancreatic cancer and coffee drinking, stratified by sex.

By stratifying we hope to have removed confounding effects. After the data are divided this way, we need a summary test of the association between D and E using the stratified data, and summary estimates and confidence intervals for the relevant measure of association, in all cases combining the information available in each strata. Crudely stated, once we have categorized the data by levels of a confounding variable, how do we put it back together again to answer questions regarding the association between the exposure and disease?

As an aside, it is worth a quick look at the issue of interaction since we have the strata-specific estimates of association in front of us. Recall that this asks whether

Table 9.1 *Symbols for entries in generic ith stratum in stratified analysis*

		Disease		
		D	not D	
Exposure	E	a_i	b_i	$a_i + b_i$
	not E	c_i	d_i	$c_i + d_i$
		$a_i + c_i$	$b_i + d_i$	n_i

Table 9.2 *Coronary heart disease and behavior type, stratified by body weight*

Body Weight (lb)			CHD Event Yes	CHD Event No	$\widehat{OR}$	$\widehat{RR}$
≤150	Behavior type	Type A	22	253	2.652	2.520
		Type B	10	305		
150^+–160	Behavior type	Type A	21	235	2.413	2.297
		Type B	10	270		
160^+–170	Behavior type	Type A	29	297	1.381	1.347
		Type B	21	297		
170^+–180	Behavior type	Type A	47	248	2.524	2.281
		Type B	19	253		
>180	Behavior type	Type A	59	378	2.966	2.700
		Type B	19	361		

Table 9.3 *Pancreatic cancer and coffee drinking, stratified by sex*

Gender			Pancreatic Cancer Cases	Pancreatic Cancer Controls	OR
Females	Coffee drinking (cups per day)	≥1	140	280	2.545
		0	11	56	
Males	Coffee drinking (cups per day)	≥1	207	275	2.676
		0	9	32	

the relevant measure of association is consistent across the I strata. If so, then we can lay aside interaction for the moment. If not, we should determine whether we really want a single measure of association due to the apparent variation in effects. If the variation is extreme, and particularly if in some strata E is a risk factor and in others it is protective (see Chapter 10.4), we will probably seek to separate the data into such distinct groups so we can describe how the effect measure varies across the different levels of the extraneous variables. As a statistical guide to the assessment of interaction, Chapter 10.3 introduces techniques to address whether there is evidence that a measure of association varies across the I strata more than might be expected from random variation.

To illustrate these comments, we examine qualitatively the individual stratum-specific Odds Ratio associated with behavior type at each level of body weight reported in Table 9.2. These estimates show that, at each level of body weight, Type A behavior raises the risk for CHD with estimated Odds Ratios that range from 1.381 to 2.966. Apart from the lower of these values, occurring for individuals with a body weight of 160 to 170 lb, there is little variation in the estimated effects. At first glance, it seems reasonable to assume no interaction with regard to the Odds Ratios, and move on to consider summary measures and tests of the effect of behavior type on CHD, controlling for the potential confounding effects of body weight. Similarly, Table 9.3 shows little variation in the Odds Ratio associating coffee drinking and pancreatic cancer between males and females. In Chapter 10.3.3, we return to further quantitative assessment of the variation in these stratum-specific Odds Ratios and other effect measures.

For now, we focus on the situation where we are confident that there is no important interaction between E and any of the confounding factors, and are thus content with summary tests and estimates. With this assumption, we now discuss such a summary test of association of E and D using the stratified data. In Sections 9.2 to 9.4, we discuss summary estimates and confidence intervals for various measures of association.

9.1.1 The Cochran–Mantel–Haenszel test

We first state a null hypothesis of interest, namely H_0: D and E are independent, controlling for the possible confounding effects of C and assuming no interaction between C and E. We restate this hypothesis in terms of the various measures of association as

$$H_0 \; : \; OR_1 = OR_2 = \cdots OR_I = 1$$
$$\Leftrightarrow RR_1 = RR_2 = \cdots RR_I = 1$$
$$\Leftrightarrow ER_1 = ER_2 = \cdots ER_I = 0$$

where OR_i is the Odds Ratio for the E–D association in the ith stratum etc. Before considering options for assessing this hypothesis, it is important to consider possible alternative hypotheses. The most obvious alternative is just H_{A_1}: D and E are not independent. This is equivalent to claiming that there is at least one Odds Ratio (amongst $OR_1, \ldots, OR_I$) that differs from 1. However, this alternative allows the possibility of arbitrary variation amongst the OR_is; but this would mean interaction is present, which we have excluded by prior examination. A more focused version of the alternative hypothesis is therefore H_{A_2}: $OR_1 = OR_2 = \cdots OR_I \neq 1$, or analogous versions if interest focuses on other measures of association. The value of focusing on specific versions of the alternative hypothesis will soon become apparent.

Each stratum provides a separate piece of evidence regarding the independence of D and E. How do we go about combining these pieces of information into a summary of the evidence "for or against" the null hypothesis H_0? First, it is clear that we cannot simply add the entries in each of the cells of the ith stratum and then do a simple

χ^2 test for independence on the resulting "pooled" table, as this simply ignores the possibility of confounding.

One approach would be to consider each stratum separately, perform a χ^2 test of independence, and reject the null hypothesis H_0 if and only if at least one of these stratum-specific χ^2 tests yields a significant result. An immediate problem with this strategy is that it entails carrying out I separate tests, each with its own risk of a false positive result, so that the overall probability of falsely rejecting H_0 is no longer the nominal significance level α used in each stratum-specific test. This issue of *multiple comparisons* can be addressed by adjusting this significance level, for example, by using the so-called *Bonferroni corrected* level given by α/I. Particularly when I is large, this procedure has little power to detect dependence between E and D, even when more sophisticated alternatives to the Bonferroni corrected significance level are used.

A second possibility is to compute the simple 2×2 table χ^2 test statistic for each stratum separately—call the ith statistic χ_i^2, say—and then add these I test statistics to produce a summary test statistic T. If the sample sizes in each stratum are large, then the sampling distribution of this random variable $T = \sum_{i=1}^{I} \chi_i^2$ is approximated by a χ^2 distribution with I degrees of freedom. This follows from the observation that T is the sum of independent random variables (each χ_i^2 is computed from a separate 2×2 table), each of whose sampling distributions are approximated by a χ^2 distribution with one degree of freedom.

This summary test, based on T, is perfectly reasonable, but it has a significant drawback in that it lacks power to detect deviations from independence in certain scenarios (particularly those covered by H_{A_2}). Recall that the significance level of a test is the probability that the null hypothesis is falsely rejected. Here, the significance level of the test, based on T, has to protect the investigator from an invalid rejection of H_0 (if D and E are in fact independent) over a wide variety of scenarios. For example, all of the Odds Ratios, or only a few, or perhaps only one of the Odds Ratios could be different from 1. Further, the Odds Ratios might all differ from one in the same direction. Or some Odds Ratios could be bigger than 1 and some smaller than 1. In all these scenarios, the test statistic T will ultimately be large as the sample size in each stratum increases, leading to possible rejection of independence.

Figure 9.1 shows schematically the manner in which the stratum Odds Ratios can vary over I degrees of freedom. Notice that the null hypothesis, H_0, has zero degrees of freedom because it completely specifies all the stratum-specific Odds Ratios. The consequence of having a test that must "use" its significance level against incorrectly rejecting the null hypothesis for such a variety of possibilities is that the test has low power to detect departures from H_0 in any specific direction. Note that the test statistic T does not make use of information regarding any pattern in which the OR_is might deviate from 1. In particular, it does not take advantage of an assumption of no interaction between E and C.

We now want to derive a test that is targeted to look only for data that suggest a much more specific alternative to H_0, namely, $H_{A_2} : OR_1 = \cdots OR_I \neq 1$. This is represented in Figure 9.1 and has only one degree of freedom (namely, the value of the unknown common Odds Ratio across the strata). A test statistic designed to detect

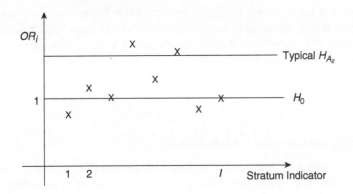

Figure 9.1 *Schematic describing variation of stratum-specific odds ratios.*

this kind of departure from independence will have more power in situations where the data support this kind of alternative, at the cost of having very little, if any, power to detect quite different ways in which the Odds Ratios might reflect dependence of D and E. Note that the assumption of no interaction is now incorporated in both the null (H_0) and alternative hypotheses (H_{A_2}).

The Cochran–Mantel–Haenszel method constructs such a test statistic by considering the observed value in the a cell in the ith stratum, denoted by a_i, and comparing it with its expected value, assuming that D and E are independent. If the marginal totals in the ith stratum are considered fixed, we have from Chapter 6.4.1 the expectation $E(a_i) = A_i = (a_i + b_i)(a_i + c_i)/n_i$, assuming independence. We then add the comparisons $a_i - A_i$ over the I strata, noting that deviations of a_i from A_i will tend to cancel out if they are in different directions but accumulate if they are in the same direction. Under the same assumptions of independence and fixed marginals, the variance of a_i is $V_i = (a_i + b_i)(c_i + d_i)(a_i + c_i)(b_i + d_i)/n_i^2(n_i - 1)$, as also noted in Chapter 6.4.1.

The Cochran–Mantel–Haenszel test statistic is given by the sum of these "deviations," $\sum_{i=1}^{I}(a_i - A_i)$, normalized by the variance of this sum, $\sum_{i=1}^{I} V_i$, since each term in the sum is independent, arising from different strata. Thus, the Cochran–Mantel–Haenszel test statistic is:

$$\chi_{CMH}^2 = \frac{\left(\sum_{i=1}^{I} a_i - \sum_{i=1}^{I} A_I\right)^2}{\sum_{i=1}^{I} V_i}. \tag{9.1}$$

Assuming the null hypothesis, H_0, that D and E are independent, the sampling distribution of χ_{CMH}^2 is approximated by a χ^2 distribution with one degree of freedom. Large values of χ_{CMH}^2, compared with a table of $\chi_{(1)}^2$, thereby suggest that D and E are not independent, allowing for the possible confounding effects of C. Calculation of the Cochran–Mantel–Haenszel test statistic is illustrated in data-based examples in Sections 9.2.3 and 9.2.4.

The Cochran–Mantel–Haenszel test statistic (9.1) is only large, reflecting dependence, when the Odds Ratios in each stratum differ from 1 *consistently*. Conversely, the statistic will not be as big in cases where the Odds Ratios vary from one in an inconsistent manner, particularly those situations where stratum Odds Ratios are on opposite sides of 1, even when they are quite distinct from 1. This stresses the importance of at least a qualitative examination of the stratum Odds Ratios and the possibility of interaction, prior to implementation of the Cochran–Mantel–Haenszel test statistic.

9.1.2 Sample size issues and a historical note

For the naïve summary test statistic T, based on summing individual χ^2 statistics across the I strata, it would be necessary to have a reasonable sample size in each stratum to ensure the accuracy of the separate χ^2 approximations. For the Cochran–Mantel–Haenszel test, this would also be true if we used n_i^3 in the denominator of each V_i calculation instead of $n_i^2(n_i - 1)$. However, with the latter formula, the resulting test statistic, χ^2_{CMH}, has a sampling distribution that is well approximated by the $\chi^2_{(1)}$ distribution as long as $\sum_{i=1}^{I} A_i$ differs, by at least five, from the allowable extremes of $\sum_{i=1}^{I} a_i$, assuming the observed marginal totals in each stratum (note that a set of observed marginals may restrict the minimum and maximum value possible for each a_i). This can be achieved even in situations where each stratum may contain as few as two observations—this is important when we consider matched data in Chapter 16. If small sample size is of concern, an exact test of independence based on hypergeometric distributions is available (Mehta et al., 1985).

Cochran (1954) developed the test statistic given in Equation 9.1, except with the n_i^3 term in the denominator of each V_i. Later, Mantel and Haenszel (1959) introduced the correction by substituting $n_i^2(n_i - 1)$ for n_i^3. Although this change is negligible when each n_i is large, it is particularly important, in terms of validity of the sampling distribution approximation, when each stratum sample size is small. An interesting exchange regarding the failure of the Mantel and Haenszel paper to cite the Cochran work can be found in two letters (Gart, 1976; Mantel, 1977).

9.2 Summary estimates and confidence intervals for the odds ratio, adjusting for confounding factors

Return to the problem of estimating a measure of association while controlling for the possibility of confounding effects due to other important risk factors. We continue to assume that, for the particular association measure under consideration, there is no striking interaction (that is, effect modification) due to the extraneous or strata variables. It makes little sense to produce a summary measure, quantifying the $E–D$ relationship, if substantial effect modification is present because then, by definition, the $E–D$ association differs substantially across at least some of the strata.

In this section we describe two basic strategies for estimation of the Odds Ratio and apply these approaches to both the Relative Risk and the Excess Risk in the following two sections. Regression techniques, introduced in Chapters 12 and 13, provide a further alternative for calculating summary estimates.

9.2.1 Woolf's method on the logarithm scale

The Woolf method uses the simple idea of averaging the individual stratum estimates of the Odds Ratio, taking into account the differing variability associated with each Odds Ratio estimate due not only to varying stratum sample sizes but also changes in the balance of the marginals. Because of the skewness of the sampling distribution of an Odds Ratio estimate, it makes sense to perform the averaging on the logarithmic scale for both the estimate and an associated confidence interval. We can then transform back to the original Odds Ratio scale at the end of our calculations as before.

The summary weighted averaged estimate of the log Odds Ratio is then given by

$$\log \widehat{OR}_W = \frac{\sum_{i=1}^{I} w_i \log \widehat{OR}_i}{\sum_{i=1}^{I} w_i} \tag{9.2}$$

where the w_is are stratum weights and $\log \widehat{OR}_i$ is our previous estimate of the $\log(OR)$ for the ith stratum. Because the sample sizes in some strata may now be moderate or small, we generally use the small sample adjusted estimates given by

$$(\log \widehat{OR}_i)_{SS} = \log \left(\frac{(a + \frac{1}{2})(d + \frac{1}{2})}{(b + \frac{1}{2})(c + \frac{1}{2})} \right).$$

We want the weights to add to one in order to have an appropriate average. This is ensured by normalizing each weight w_i by the sum of the weights, $\sum_{i=1}^{I} w_I$, in Equation 9.2.

The weights account for the fact that the stratum Odds Ratios are estimated with different precision. In averaging quantities that are subject to varying levels of random uncertainty, it is best to use weights that are proportional to the *reciprocal* of the variance of the underlying estimator, so that imprecise components are given low weight. Here, we therefore want to use stratum weights given by $(var(\log(\widehat{OR}_i)))^{-1}$, which we estimate as before, yielding

$$w_i = \left(\frac{1}{a_i + \frac{1}{2}} + \frac{1}{b_i + \frac{1}{2}} + \frac{1}{c_i + \frac{1}{2}} + \frac{1}{d_i + \frac{1}{2}} \right)^{-1}, \tag{9.3}$$

again using the small sample adjustments for safety. A stratum with little information about $\log(OR)$ necessarily has a high $var(\log(\widehat{OR}_i)$ and thus a low w_i. Such a "down-weighted" stratum therefore has less relative influence in the overall estimate $\log \widehat{OR}_W$ than other, more precise, stratum estimates of $\log(OR)$.

If the sample sizes in each stratum are large enough, each $\log(\widehat{OR}_i)$ will have an approximately Normal sampling distribution, the variance of which can be estimated by $V_i = (w_i)^{-1}$. Because the observations in one stratum are independent of those in another, the sampling distribution of $\log \widehat{OR}_W$ will then also be approximately Normal under these same conditions. Since the expectation of each $\log(\widehat{OR}_i)$ is the same population $\log(OR)$, under the assumption of no interaction, the expectation of $\log \widehat{OR}_W$ is just $[\sum_{i=1}^{I} w_i \log(OR)]/[\sum_{i=1}^{I} w_i] = \log(OR)$. In addition, the variance of $\log \widehat{OR}_W$ is approximately $[\sum_{i=1}^{I} w_I{}^2 \widehat{Var}(\log \widehat{OR}_i)/(\sum_{i=1}^{I} w_i)^2] = [\sum_{i=1}^{I} w_i^2(w_i)^{-1}/(\sum_{i=1}^{I} w_i)^2] = (\sum_{i=1}^{I} w_i)^{-1}$. That is,

$$\widehat{Var}(\log \widehat{OR}_W) = \frac{1}{\sum_{i=1}^{I} w_i}.$$

In summary, a $100(1 - \alpha)\%$ confidence interval for $\log(OR)$, based on the Woolf adjusted estimate, is given by

$$\log(\widehat{OR}_W) \pm z_\alpha \sqrt{Var(\log(\widehat{OR}_W))},$$

where z_α is the $(1 - \alpha/2)$th percentile of the standard Normal distribution. The equivalent point estimate and confidence interval for OR is then obtained by exponentiating the analog for $\log(OR)$ in the standard way. These calculations are illustrated in two examples in Sections 9.2.3 and 9.2.4. It is important to stress that the Woolf method is based on approximations that are only effective *when the sample sizes in each stratum are large*. If there are only a few strata with small sample sizes or very poor marginal balance, and the remaining strata possess more substantial information regarding $\log(OR)$, the strata weighting will effectively ignore these few imprecise stratum-specific estimates, $\log(\widehat{OR}_i)$, and the Woolf method will yield valid results. However, the method breaks down when *all* of the strata contain only a few observations.

9.2.2 The Mantel–Haenszel method

Mantel and Haenszel (1959) provided an alternative method for averaging Odds Ratio estimates across strata that works surprisingly well regardless of the sample sizes and marginal balances in the stratum-specific 2×2 tables. Specifically, their estimate is a weighted average of the estimates $\widehat{OR}_i$ themselves and is given by:

$$\widehat{OR}_{MH} = \frac{\sum_{i=1}^{I} w_i^* \widehat{OR}_i}{\sum_{i=1}^{I} w_i^*},$$

where, of course, $\widehat{OR}_i = a_i d_i / b_i c_i$, and the weights are given by $w_i^* = b_i c_i / n_i$. Thus, an equivalent and explicit expression for the Mantel–Haenszel estimate of the Odds Ratio is

$$\widehat{OR}_{MH} = \frac{\sum_{i=1}^{I} (a_i d_i / n_i)}{\sum_{i=1}^{I} (b_i c_i / n_i)}. \tag{9.4}$$

The Cochran–Mantel–Haenszel test statistic is zero ("perfect" independence) if and only if $\sum_{i=1}^{I} a_i - \sum_{i=1}^{I} A_i = \sum_{i=1}^{I} a_i - \sum_{i=1}^{I} [(a_i + b_i)(a_i + c_i)/n_i] = 0$, which is equivalent to $\sum_{i=1}^{I} (a_i d_i / n_i) = \sum_{i=1}^{I} (b_i c_i / n_i)$, that is, $\widehat{OR}_{MH} = 1$. This observation motivates the form of the Mantel–Haenszel estimator given in Equation 9.4.

Even though the Mantel–Haenszel estimator is calculated without using logarithms, we need to move to the log scale in order to calculate a confidence interval. It took almost 30 years from the introduction of the estimator to (1) establish that $\log(\widehat{OR}_{MH})$ has an approximately Normal sampling distribution and (2) find a formula to estimate its sampling variance. The most widely accepted estimator for the variance of

$\log(\widehat{OR}_{MH})$, one that works well if there are either a few strata with substantial data in each or lots of strata with only a few observations in each, was given by Robins et al. (1986). Their formula is as follows:

$$\widehat{Var}(\log \widehat{OR}_{MH}) = \left[\frac{\sum_{i=1}^{I} \left(\frac{a_i+d_i}{n_i} \right)\left(\frac{a_i d_i}{n_i} \right)}{2\left(\sum_{i=1}^{I} \frac{a_i d_i}{n_i} \right)^2} + \frac{\sum_{i=1}^{I} \left(\frac{a_i+d_i}{n_i} \cdot \frac{b_i c_i}{n_i} + \frac{b_i+c_i}{n_i} \cdot \frac{a_i d_i}{n_i} \right)}{2\left(\sum_{i=1}^{I} \frac{a_i d_i}{n_i} \right)\left(\sum_{i=1}^{I} \frac{b_i c_i}{n_i} \right)} \right.$$
$$\left. + \frac{\sum_{i=1}^{I} \left(\frac{b_i+c_i}{n_i} \right)\left(\frac{b_i c_i}{n_i} \right)}{2\left(\sum_{i=1}^{I} \frac{b_i c_i}{n_i} \right)^2} \right].$$

In summary, a $100(1-\alpha)\%$ confidence interval for $\log(OR)$, based on the Mantel–Haenszel summary estimator, is given by

$$\log(\widehat{OR}_{MH}) \pm z_\alpha \sqrt{\widehat{Var}(\log(\widehat{OR}_{MH}))},$$

where z_α is the $(1-\alpha/2)$th percentile of the standard Normal distribution. The associated confidence interval for OR is obtained as usual. Two examples of these computations are given in Sections 9.2.3 and 9.2.4.

9.2.3 Example—the Western Collaborative Group Study: part 2

Return to the data from the Western Collaborative Group Study relating behavior type to the risk of onset of coronary heart disease (CHD), introduced in Section 7.2.1. The data on the 3,154 individuals from Table 7.4, stratified by body weight in five ordered categories, is displayed in Table 9.2. Since body weight is likely to be a risk factor for CHD, and since it is plausible that weight is associated with behavioral characteristics, it is reasonable to consider the possibility that weight confounds the relationship between behavior type and CHD. The causal graph approach of Chapter 8.2 helps us conceptualize this: if body weight (C) causes behavior type (E), then Figure 8.7(a) is applicable and body weight is a potential confounder. On the other hand, if personality type causes body weight, Figure 8.7(b) is relevant and stratification on body weight is inappropriate, since now both pathways, direct and indirect, describe causal effects of behavior type. Perhaps the most likely scenario is that both body weight and personality type have a common unmeasured ancestor, as illustrated in Figure 9.2. With this graph, stratification by body weight is required to remove possible confounding, and we now proceed to the methods derived in Sections 9.1, 9.2.1, and 9.2.2.

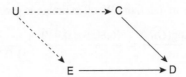

Figure 9.2 *A directed acyclic causal graph linking behavior type (E), body weight (C), and unmeasured variables, U to CHD (D).*

Table 9.4 *Cochran–Mantel–Haenszel test statistic calculations for the data in Table 9.2*

Body Weight (lb)	a_i	A_i	V_i
≤ 150	22	14.915	7.544
150^+-160	21	14.806	7.301
160^+-170	29	25.311	11.546
170^+-180	47	34.339	14.581
>180	59	41.721	17.574
Totals	178	131.091	58.546

Table 9.5 *Calculations for the Woolf and Mantel–Haenszel summary estimates of the odds ratio, based on data from Table 9.2*

Body Weight (lb)	Woolf Method		Mantel–Haenszel Method	
	$\log(\widehat{OR}_i)$	w_i	$a_i d_i / n_i$	$b_i c_i / n_i$
≤ 150	0.949	6.807	11.373	4.288
150^+-160	0.855	6.680	10.578	4.384
160^+-170	0.316	11.477	13.374	9.685
170^+-180	0.910	12.453	20.972	8.310
>180	1.070	13.606	26.070	8.791
Totals		51.023	82.367	35.458

Calculations for the Cochran–Mantel–Haenszel test statistic are displayed in Table 9.4. It immediately follows that $\chi^2_{CMH} = (178 - 131.091)^2/58.546 = 37.6$. Comparing this value to a table of the $\chi^2_{(1)}$ distribution yields a p-value that is less than 10^{-6}. Thus, there continues to be striking evidence that behavior type is strongly related to the incidence of CHD. Recall from Section 7.2.1 that the χ^2 test statistic from the pooled table (Table 7.4) was 39.9. The slight drop in the value of the Cochran–Mantel–Haenszel statistic is due to a slight confounding effect of body weight. Here, confounding is of little concern due to the extremely strong association in play. We now turn to assessment of the impact of this confounding effect on our point and interval estimates of the Odds Ratio.

Table 9.5 shows the intermediate calculations that lead to both the Woolf and Mantel–Haenszel summary estimates of the Odds Ratio. Note that the small sample estimates—adding $1/2$ to all cells—are used in computing both $\log(\widehat{OR}_i)$ and w_i for the Woolf method.

With these calculations in hand, the Woolf estimate is given by

$$\log \widehat{OR}_W = \frac{\sum_{i=1}^{I} w_i \log(\widehat{OR}_i)}{\sum_{i=1}^{I} w_i} = \frac{(6.807 \times 0.949) + \cdots + (13.606 \times 1.070)}{51.023}$$

$$= \frac{41.690}{51.023} = 0.817,$$

leading to $\widehat{OR}_W = 2.264$.

Table 9.6 *Calculations needed to estimate the variance of the Mantel–Haenszel summary estimate of the odds ratio, based on data from Table 9.2*

Body Weight (lb)	$\left(\frac{a_i+d_i}{n_i}\right)\left(\frac{a_i d_i}{n_i}\right)$	$\left(\frac{b_i+c_i}{n_i}\right)\left(\frac{b_i c_i}{n_i}\right)$	$\left(\frac{a_i+d_i}{n_i}\cdot\frac{b_i c_i}{n_i}+\frac{b_i+c_i}{n_i}\cdot\frac{a_i d_i}{n_i}\right)$
≤ 150	6.303	1.911	7.686
150^+–160	5.743	2.004	7.216
160^+–170	6.770	4.782	11.386
170^+–180	11.096	3.913	14.273
>180	13.402	4.272	17.187
Totals	43.315	16.883	57.747

Further, $\widehat{Var}(\log \widehat{OR}_W) = 1/(\sum_{i=1}^{I} w_i) = 1/51.023 = 0.020$, giving a 95% confidence interval for $\log OR$ of $0.817\pm1.96\sqrt{0.020} = (0.543, 1.091)$. The corresponding 95% confidence interval for OR is then $(1.72, 2.98)$.

From Table 9.5, the Mantel–Haenszel estimator is

$$\widehat{OR}_{MH} = \frac{\sum_{i=1}^{I}(a_i d_i/n_i)}{\sum_{i=1}^{I}(b_i c_i/n_i)} = \frac{82.367}{35.458} = 2.323.$$

Additional computations are required to compute the estimate of the variance of $\log \widehat{OR}_{MH}$; these are provided in Table 9.6. These numbers together with those from Table 9.5 give

$$\widehat{Var}(\log \widehat{OR}_{MH}) = \left(\frac{43.315}{2\times 82.367^2} + \frac{57.747}{2\times 82.367\times 35.458} + \frac{16.883}{2\times 35.458^2}\right)$$
$$= 0.020.$$

This yields the 95% confidence interval for $\log OR$ given by $\log 2.323\pm1.96\sqrt{0.020} = (0.567, 1.119)$. The corresponding Mantel–Haenszel 95% confidence interval for OR is then $(1.76, 3.06)$.

In sum, the Woolf and Mantel–Haenszel estimators of the Odds Ratio and their corresponding 95% confidence intervals are given by 2.26 (1.72–2.98) and 2.32 (1.76–3.06), respectively. In comparison, the Odds Ratio estimate and 95% confidence interval, based on the pooled Table 7.4, is 2.34 (1.79–3.11), using small sample computations. We see here, as we did with the Cochran–Mantel–Haenszel test statistic, a slight confounding effect of body weight, with the adjusted Odds Ratio estimates about 4% smaller than the unadjusted. This confounding bias seems insignificant, particularly in light of the much greater level of random variation, and it is quite reasonable in these circumstances to report the unadjusted results without fear of a confounding bias due to body weight.

9.2.4 Example—coffee drinking and pancreatic cancer: part 2

In Section 7.1.3 we examined, using the case-control data of Table 7.3, the association between coffee drinking, dichotomized into abstainers or drinkers, and the risk for pancreatic cancer. The χ^2 test statistic was found to be 16.60, with an estimated Odds

Ratio of 2.75 (95% confidence interval ranging from 1.66 to 4.55). It is previously been established that men experience an elevated risk for pancreatic cancer as compared with women. It is plausible that coffee drinking habits may differ by sex, leading to a possible confounding role for sex in our analysis of the relationship between coffee drinking and pancreatic cancer incidence. In this case, the causal graph in Figure 8.7(a) for sex (C) and coffee drinking (E) seems applicable so that adjustment for sex is appropriate. Table 9.3 abstracts the information from Table 7.2, allowing us to proceed with stratification techniques to accommodate a potential confounding effect.

Without providing full details this time, the Cochran–Mantel–Haenszel test statistic is 14.54, still yielding a p-value smaller than 0.0002. The Woolf estimate of the Odds Ratio is 2.51 with an associated 95% confidence interval of 1.53 to 4.13. For comparison, the Mantel–Haenszel estimate of the Odds Ratio is 2.60 with the 95% confidence interval given by (1.57, 4.32), very similar results to those obtained by the Woolf method. Comparison of the adjusted test statistic and the adjusted Odds Ratio estimates and confidence intervals with those obtained from the pooled data, noted at the beginning of this section, shows a very slight confounding effect of sex on the relationship of coffee drinking to pancreatic cancer incidence, but the decrease in the adjusted Odds Ratio estimate is only around 5 to 9%, a minor adjustment in light of the size of the inherent random error.

9.3 Summary estimates and confidence intervals for the relative risk, adjusting for confounding factors

The two methods used to produce summary estimates and confidence intervals for the Odds Ratio from strata 2×2 tables are easily adapted to cover estimation of the Relative Risk for data arising from either population-based or cohort designs. As for the Odds Ratio, the Woolf method works on the logarithmic scale. With the estimate of $\log RR$ in the ith stratum, $\log \widehat{RR}_i = \log[a_i/(a_i + b_i)/c_i/(c_i + d_i)]$, the summary estimate of $\log RR$ is then a weighted average of these stratum-specific estimates given by

$$\log \widehat{RR}_W = \frac{\sum_{i=1}^I w_i \log \widehat{RR}_i}{\sum_{i=1}^I w_i}.$$

As for the Odds Ratio, the appropriate weights are inversely proportional to the (estimated) variance of the stratum estimates $\log \widehat{RR}_i$; that is,

$$w_i = \frac{1}{\widehat{Var}(\log \widehat{RR}_i)} = \left[\frac{b_i}{a_i(a_i + b_i)} + \frac{d_i}{c_i(c_i + d_i)}\right]^{-1}.$$

An estimate of the sampling variance of $\log(\widehat{RR}_W)$ is again given by $1/(\sum_{i=1}^I w_i)$. A $100(1-\alpha)\%$ confidence interval for $\log(RR)$, based on the Woolf adjusted estimate, is then

$$\log(\widehat{RR}_W) \pm z_\alpha \sqrt{\widehat{Var}(\log(\widehat{RR}_W))},$$

where z_α is the $(1 - \alpha/2)$th percentile of the standard Normal distribution. Exponentiating these confidence limits then gives the analogous confidence interval for the Relative Risk itself.

The Mantel–Haenszel estimate of the Relative Risk is again a weighted average of the stratum-specific Relative Risks; that is, $\widehat{RR}_{MH} = (\sum_{i=1}^{I} w_i^* \widehat{RR}_i)/(\sum_{i=1}^{I} w_i^*)$. Here, $\widehat{RR}_i = [a_i/(a_i + b_i)]/[c_i/(c_i + d_i)]$, with the appropriate weights given by $w_i^* = c_i(a_i + b_i)/n_i$. An alternative equivalent expression for $\widehat{RR}_{MH}$ is then

$$\widehat{RR}_{MH} = \frac{\sum_{i=1}^{I} \frac{a_i(c_i + d_i)}{n_i}}{\sum_{i=1}^{I} \frac{c_i(a_i + b_i)}{n_i}}.$$

To construct the associated confidence interval, we again work on the logarithm scale. An estimate for the sampling variance of $\log(\widehat{RR}_{MH})$ is given by

$$\widehat{Var}(\log(\widehat{RR}_{MH})) = \frac{\sum_{i=1}^{I}[(a_i + b_i)(c_i + d_i)(a_i + c_i) - a_i c_i n_i]/n_i^2}{\left(\sum_{i=1}^{I} a_i(c_i + d_i)/n_i\right)\left(\sum_{i=1}^{I} c_i(a_i + b_i)/n_i\right)}.$$

Confidence intervals for $\log(RR)$ and, subsequently, RR are then obtained as in the Woolf method.

9.3.1 Example—the Western Collaborative Group Study: part 3

The data from the Western Collaborative Group Study are now analyzed, focusing on the Relative Risk for coronary heart disease (CHD) associated with behavior type. Returning to the data in Table 9.2, we estimate this Relative Risk, controlling for the potential confounding effects of body weight.

We again assume that the Relative Risks for CHD associated with behavior type are reasonably constant over the body weight strata. These Relative Risks (see Table 9.2) show a similar pattern to the Odds Ratios and are relatively homogeneous, with perhaps the exception of the stratum with body weight 160^+ to 170 lb. The intermediary calculations for the Woolf and Mantel–Haenszel estimators of the Relative Risk, controlling for body weight, are provided in Table 9.7.

Table 9.7 *Calculations for the Woolf and Mantel–Haenszel summary estimates of the relative risk, based on data from Table 9.2.*

Body Weight (lb)	Woolf Method		Mantel–Haenszel Method	
	$\log(\widehat{RR}_i)$	w_i	$a_i(c_i + d_i)/n_i$	$c_i(a_i + b_i)/n_i$
≤ 150	0.924	7.213	11.746	4.661
150^+–160	0.832	7.136	10.970	4.776
160^+–170	0.298	13.177	14.320	10.630
170^+–180	0.825	14.961	22.547	9.885
> 180	0.993	15.465	27.442	10.163
Totals		57.951	87.024	40.116

Table 9.8 *Calculations needed to estimate the variance of the Mantel–Haenszel summary estimate of the relative risk, based on data from Table 9.2*

Body Weight (lb)	$[(a_i + b_i)(c_i + d_i)(a_i + c_i) - a_i c_i n_i]/n_i^2$
≤ 150	7.590
150^+–160	7.343
160^+–170	11.552
170^+–180	14.898
>180	18.033
Totals	59.416

We then have the Woolf estimate of the adjusted Relative Risk given by

$$\log \widehat{RR}_W = \frac{(7.213 \times 0.924) + \cdots + (15.465 \times 0.993)}{57.951} = \frac{44.224}{57.951} = 0.763.$$

Thus, $\widehat{RR}_W = 2.145$.

Further, $\widehat{Var}(\log \widehat{RR}_W) = 1/\sum_{i=1}^{I} w_i = 0.017$, giving a 95% confidence interval for $\log RR$ of $0.763 \pm 1.96\sqrt{0.017} = (0.506, 1.021)$. The corresponding 95% confidence interval for RR is then $(1.66, 2.77)$.

Further, the Mantel–Haenszel estimator is

$$\widehat{RR}_{MH} = \frac{87.024}{40.116} = 2.169.$$

Table 9.8 provides the additional calculations needed to yield $\widehat{Var}(\widehat{RR}_{MH}) = 59.416/(87.024 \times 40.116) = 0.017$. This gives a 95% confidence interval for $\log RR$ of $(0.519, 1.030)$. The corresponding confidence interval for RR is then $(1.68, 2.80)$. These provide similar results to those based on the Odds Ratio in Section 9.2.3; comparison with the pooled analysis of Section 7.2.1 reaffirms the slight confounding role of body weight.

9.4 Summary estimates and confidence intervals for the excess risk, adjusting for confounding factors

Now we supply the appropriate formulae to construct the Woolf and Mantel–Haenszel estimates of the Excess Risk, adjusting for the influence of potential confounders. Here, we assume that the Excess Risk is consistent across strata defined by constant levels of the confounders.

For the Woolf estimate, we work on the original scale with the Excess Risk. The summary estimate of the Excess Risk is given by

$$\widehat{ER}_W = \frac{\sum_{i=1}^{I} w_i \widehat{ER}_i}{\sum_{i=1}^{I} w_i},$$

where the stratum-specific estimates are just $\widehat{ER}_i = [a_i/a_i + b_i] - [c_i/c_i + d_i]$. The weights are given by

$$w_i = \frac{1}{\widehat{Var}(\widehat{ER}_i)} = \left[\frac{a_i b_i}{(a_i + b_i)^3} + \frac{c_i d_i}{(c_i + d_i)^3} \right]^{-1}.$$

An estimate of the sampling variance of $\widehat{ER}_W$ is then $1/(\sum_{i=1}^{I} w_i)$. The Mantel–Haenszel summary estimate of the Excess Risk is

$$\widehat{ER}_{MH} = \frac{\sum_{i=1}^{I} \left(\frac{a_i(c_i + d_i)}{n_i} - \frac{c_i(a_i + b_i)}{n_i} \right)}{\sum_{i=1}^{I} \frac{(a_i + b_i)(c_i + d_i)}{n_i}}.$$

An associated estimate of the sampling variance of $\widehat{ER}_{MH}$ is given by

$$\widehat{Var}(\widehat{ER}_{MH}) = \frac{\sum_{i=1}^{I} \left(\frac{a_i b_i(c_i + d_i)^3 + c_i d_i(a_i + b_i)^3}{(a_i + b_i)(c_i + d_i)n_i^2} \right)}{\left(\sum_{i=1}^{I} \frac{(a_i + b_i)(c_i + d_i)}{n_i} \right)^2}.$$

9.4.1 Example—the Western Collaborative Group Study: part 4

Table 9.9 provides the necessary components to calculate the Woolf and Mantel–Haenszel estimator of the Excess Risk for CHD associated with behavior type, adjusted for potential confounding by body weight. Before looking at these calculations, note that the five stratum-specific estimates of Excess Risk, displayed in Table 9.9, now show substantial variation beyond the somewhat anomalous stratum of individuals with body weight 160^+ to 170 lb. Thus, there appears to be some evidence of interaction when Excess Risk is used as the measure of association. Chapter 10 gives further detail on the dependence of interaction on the choice of effect measure. Each stratum shows the same *direction* of effect for behavior type, so we can still plausibly consider the summary estimate and confidence interval for the Excess Risk. We thus ignore the possibility of interaction for the time being.

Table 9.9 *Calculations for the Woolf and Mantel–Haenszel summary estimates of the excess risk, based on data from Table 9.2*

	Woolf Method		Mantel–Haenszel Method	
Body Weight (lb)	$\widehat{ER}_i$	w_i	$a_i(c_i + d_i)/n_i - c_i(a_i + b_i)/n_i$	$(a_i + b_i)(c_i + d_i)/n_i$
≤ 150	0.0483	2,738	7.085	146.8
150^+–160	0.0463	2,397	6.194	133.7
160^+–170	0.0229	2,260	3.689	161.0
170^+–180	0.0895	1,443	12.661	141.5
>180	0.0850	2,549	17.279	203.3
Totals		11,388	46.909	786.3

Table 9.10 *Calculations needed to estimate the variance of the Mantel–Haenszel summary estimate of the excess risk, based on data from Table 9.2*

Body Weight (lb)	$\dfrac{a_i b_i (c_i + d_i)^3 + c_i d_i (a_i + b_i)^3}{(a_i + b_i)(c_i + d_i)n_i^2}$
≤ 150	7.873
$150^+\!-160$	7.460
$160^+\!-170$	11.468
$170^+\!-180$	13.877
>180	16.205
Totals	56.882

Using the interim calculations of Table 9.9,

$$\widehat{ER}_W = \frac{(2738 \times 0.0483) + \cdots + (2549 \times 0.0850)}{11{,}388} = 0.0563.$$

The Mantel–Haenszel estimator is

$$\widehat{ER}_{MH} = \frac{46.909}{786.3} = 0.0597.$$

Further, $\widehat{Var}(\widehat{ER}_W) = 1/(\sum_{i=1}^{I} w_i) = 0.000088$, giving a Woolf 95% confidence interval for ER of $0.0563 \pm 1.96\sqrt{0.000088} = (0.0379, 0.0747)$. We need the additional computations given in Table 9.10 to obtain the analogous confidence interval for the Mantel–Haenszel estimator.

These results, plus those of Table 9.9, yield $\widehat{Var}(\widehat{ER}_{MH}) = 56.882/786.3^2 = 0.000092$, leading to a 95% confidence interval for ER of $(0.0409, 0.0785)$. In this example, as before, the results from both the Woolf and Mantel–Haenszel approaches are very similar. These point estimates and confidence intervals are also close to those determined from the pooled table in Chapter 7.3, again indicating only slight confounding.

9.5 Further discussion of confounding

9.5.1 How do adjustments for confounding affect precision?

The main focus of this chapter has been the description of methods to obtain estimates of various measures of association that remove the potential distortion caused by confounding variables. We can ask at this point whether we pay any "price" for constructing these more complex estimators, like the Woolf and Mantel–Haenszel approaches. To provide a context for our discussion, consider again the data from Table 7.3 on the association between coffee consumption and pancreatic cancer. Imagine that the investigators also measured a binary factor C that strongly predicts the incidence of pancreatic cancer (say, a high risk of cancer with C present and a low risk with C absent) and that is not associated with coffee drinking habits (and thus cannot confound the coffee and pancreatic cancer relationship). If we nevertheless stratify on C,

Table 9.11 *Pancreatic cancer and coffee drinking, stratified by a hypothetical strongly predictive factor, C*

Factor			Pancreatic Cancer		
			Cases	Controls	*OR*
C	Coffee drinking (cups per day)	≥ 1	312	113	2.76
		0	18	18	
$\bar{C}$	Coffee drinking (cups per day)	≥ 1	35	442	2.77
		0	2	70	

most of the cases will fall into the C stratum and very few cases will be available for analysis in the $\bar{C}$ stratum. The results of such stratification are shown in Table 9.11.

The techniques of Section 9.2.1 quickly yield 2.76 as the Woolf summary estimate of the Odds Ratio, essentially the same as the pooled sample Odds Ratio estimate of 2.75 discussed in Chapter 7.1.3. However, with regard to precision, the variance of the Woolf summary estimate of the log Odds Ratio is 0.095 (using the data of Table 9.11), whereas the variance of the pooled, or unadjusted, estimate of the log Odds Ratio is 0.065 (using small sample adjustments in both cases). Thus, stratification and adjustment here increase the variance of the log Odds Ratio estimator by 46%, with the consequence that the confidence interval for the Odds Ratio is substantially wider after adjustment. What has happened?

As indicated in Chapters 6 and 7, precision in sample estimates of the Odds Ratio is essentially determined by the balance in the two marginals of the 2×2 table in the sample. After adjustment, it is the "average" balance of these same marginals in the strata that affects the precision of the summary estimate of the Odds Ratio. We use the term "average" loosely, although it is important to recall that strata with larger sample sizes and better balance receive greater weight in summary estimates. In Table 7.3, the balance is about 8:1 on the coffee drinking marginal and a little better than a 2:1 ratio for the case and control marginal totals. In Table 9.11, the coffee drinking marginal shows about a 12:1 ratio of coffee drinkers to abstainers in the C stratum and almost a 7:1 ratio in the $\bar{C}$ stratum. On "average," this does not seem much worse than the pooled table's balance on coffee drinking. However, the case and control marginal totals show a substantial deterioration in balance in comparison to the original pooled table, particularly in the $\bar{C}$ stratum. In essence, most of the controls in the $\bar{C}$ stratum are "wasted," as there are so few cases for comparison. This leads to the considerable increase in variability in the stratification analysis, as reflected in the reported variances of the estimated log Odds Ratio. In this particular situation, since there is no confounding due to C, stratifying on C is unnecessary and even harmful due to the associated loss of precision. This begs the general question: Does stratification always lead to a decline in precision?

Before discussing this further, let us briefly review what we can learn from classical results about the comparison of means of continuous (or interval-scaled) outcome variables, with and without adjustment for covariates of interest (that is, *analysis of variance* compared with *analysis of covariance*). An early and important idea in statistics, originating from Fisher (1932), showed that adjustment for influential covariates is important in the comparison of means of continuous outcome variables, D (contrasting, say, the mean outcome among exposed to the mean among unexposed), not only for the removal of confounding bias, but also for improving precision when estimating the effect of the primary factor (here, exposure E) on the outcome. In particular, in large samples, if the covariate C is an important predictor of the outcome variable, then the variance of the estimate of changes in the mean of D associated with E can be substantially reduced after adjusting for C, whether confounding exists or not. This gain in precision increases as the strength of the C and D relationship grows. Thus, even if there is no need to adjust for C for reasons of confounding (as when E is randomized to individuals), there is substantial advantage in doing so in terms of precision if C is a strong predictor of D. On the other hand, in large samples, if C and D are independent (so that there is no confounding), there is a loss, or at least no gain in precision in estimation of the effect of E on D after adjustment for C, with the loss increasing as the strength of the relationship between E and C grows (this is our first view of the impact of *collinearity*, that is, strongly correlated risk factors). In this case, it is detrimental to adjust for C in terms of precision and unnecessary since there is no confounding.

To what extent are these results, widely used in the analysis of continuous outcome variables, applicable to the case where D is a binary variable? The answer depends on the measure of association under examination. We first consider the Odds Ratio. Robinson and Jewell (1990) showed that somewhat different phenomena occur here with regard to precision, as already illustrated by Table 9.11. The variances of estimated log Odds Ratios depend on the sample distributions of D, E, and C; in comparing the variance of the Woolf adjusted estimate to that of the pooled estimate, we average across the sampling distribution of C (which does not affect the pooled estimate). Robinson and Jewell established that adjustment for any number of discrete covariates *always* leads to an increase in the variance of the Woolf estimate of the log Odds Ratio, in large samples, except when the covariates are independent of both D and E. Further, this result applies equally to the *estimated* variances, used in construction of confidence intervals. In this sense, there is always a price to pay for stratification.

In particular, if there is no confounding because of the absence of a relationship between C and D (see Chapters 8.1 and 8.4), there is a loss of precision in estimating the log Odds Ratio for D associated with E, similar to the loss of precision in comparing means of a continuous outcome. However, in stark contrast to mean comparisons, when C is a risk factor for D but is not related to E (conditional on D; see Chapter 8.4), then adjusting for C still creates a loss of precision in estimating the log Odds Ratio. This loss of precision increases as the strength of the relationship between C and D becomes stronger. This is exactly the scenario of Table 9.11. Either way, there is a cost for unnecessarily adjusting for a nonconfounder when estimating the log Odds Ratio. This will also be true in situations where there is only slight confounding effects. When the relationships of E with C and D are both strong, then the issue of precision is moot. We would usually stratify to remove the bias associated with confounding.

As noted, the variance of the unadjusted and adjusted estimates of the log Odds Ratio depends on other aspects of the population. Specifically, the potential for loss of precision is also dependent on the marginal distribution of the outcome D, *as observed in the sample*, with less increase in variability in the adjusted log Odds Ratio when D is either rare or very common, and greater loss of precision when D is reasonably common (roughly, when the proportion of sample cases in the pooled table is near 0.5). In one sense, the latter situation is when you have the most to lose, in terms of balance, by stratification. Of course, a high frequency of D in the sample often occurs in case-control studies, by design, so that loss of precision due to adjustment generally poses a greater problem here than with the other designs.

As stressed before, variability of the summary estimate of the log Odds Ratio depends on the overall balance of the marginals over the strata. With a pooled analysis, that is, without any stratification, at least one of the marginals can be balanced by design in either a cohort or case-control study. However, such balance can be substantially disturbed by subsequent stratification. One way to think about the fact that adjustment for a potential confounder always leads to loss of precision with the log Odds Ratio is that stratification cannot improve the "average" marginal balance. Controlling the balance in the strata in the process of sample selection can mitigate loss of precision. This is exactly the goal of matched studies, discussed in more detail in Chapter 16.

The effect of stratification on precision of estimates of the Relative Risk and Excess Risk resembles the situation when comparing means of continuous outcome variables. There are no general statements regarding the variance of the estimated log Relative Risk and Excess Risk except when there is no confounding (see Chapters 8.1 and 8.4) and a large sample size. For both measures, if there is no confounding, there is (1) a loss in precision if C is not a risk factor for D and (2) a gain in precision if C is predictive of D but independent of E.

The data in Table 9.12 illustrate issues of precision in considering variability in estimation of the relationship between behavior type and CHD, before and after adjustment for the effects of body weight. The estimated variances of three measures of association, $\log(OR)$, $\log(RR)$, and ER, are given, based on the pooled Table 7.4 and after stratification using Table 9.2. There is a very slight increase in the variance of $\log(OR)$ after adjustment, as body weight is only moderately related to the risk for CHD (as we discuss in later chapters), and since the proportion of CHD cases in the sample is relatively small. On the other hand, the variability of the estimate of ER

Table 9.12 *Comparison of estimated variances of measures of association from both the pooled Table 7.4 and the stratified Table 9.2*

Measure of Association	Pooled Variance Estimate	Adjusted Variance Estimate
$\log(OR)$	0.01956	0.01960
$\log(RR)$	0.01701	0.01726
ER	0.000093	0.000088

decreases after adjustment, as predicted by experience with continuous variables. We might anticipate a similar pattern with $\log(RR)$, but there is, in fact, a slight increase in variability, perhaps because of the presence of some confounding, or the sample distribution of body weights, in addition to factors that mitigated the loss of precision for $\log(OR)$.

We emphasize that observed losses (or gains) in precision are likely to be slight when adjusting for the potential confounding effects of a *single* extraneous factor. However, when the number of potential confounding variables increases and the number of strata thereby grows large, the loss in precision in estimating the Odds Ratio can be substantial. For example, imagine having to subdivide the strata of Table 9.2 to account for age. If age is classified into four groups, we would then face 20 age/body weight strata. If we additionally wish to account for the possible confounding effects of blood pressure history, smoking, alcohol consumption, and so on, we quickly have to accommodate over a hundred strata. At this extreme, many strata may have zeros in the marginals (either, for example, no CHD cases or no Type A individuals); such strata do not contribute to summary estimates. So the information available in all other members of the strata is discarded, effectively reducing the sample size. We tackle this issue in Chapters 12 to 16 on regression models and matching—analysis and design strategies, respectively, for implementing simultaneous adjustment for several extraneous variables.

9.5.2 *An empirical approach to confounding*

In Chapter 8, we introduced several conceptual methods for determining the presence of confounding. However, confounding is a bias and is always present to some degree or other. The key question surrounds the size of the confounding bias or, more directly, the change in the measure of association of interest after adjustment. An empirical assessment of confounding is immediately available by comparing the measure of association *estimates* from the pooled table and from the stratified tables. In and of itself, this numerical comparison only assesses collapsibility of the strata with respect to the effect measure, as discussed in Chapter 8.4, and can be misleading if not accompanied by the appropriate causal graph.

Assuming that the causal graph shows that stratification is needed to remove confounding, we can assess whether the amount of confounding is large enough to warrant the complexity of adjustment. If the difference between the pooled and adjusted estimates is sufficiently great, both in terms of scientific import and in light of the inherent uncertainty, then an adjusted analysis is preferable. If not, then it is appropriate to ignore the limited confounding due to this particular extraneous variable (or set of variables). With the Odds Ratio, we must also take into account any loss of precision due to adjustment as discussed in Section 9.5.1. Occasionally, we will prefer a slightly biased, unadjusted, estimate of the Odds Ratio to a less biased adjusted version that is less precisely estimated. In examples with moderate sample sizes, it is often not valuable to adjust for confounding biases that are less than 10% of the size of the original effect, given the much greater random error in such studies. On the other hand, if there is little or no loss in precision, then it is reasonable to still report an adjusted analysis, particularly if the extraneous variable is generally thought to be a confounder. In both the Western Collaborative Group Study, and for the data relating coffee consumption to pancreatic cancer, we saw, in Sections 9.2.3 and 9.2.4, confounding bias for the Odds Ratio of less than 10%; so in those cases there is no need to adjust for the confounding effects of body weight or sex. We also observed only slightly increased variability in adjusted estimates of the Odds Ratio, so that the stratified analysis can still be used, an advantage if the stratified analysis is likely to be more convincing to the relevant audience. Alternatively, with the hypothetical stratified data of Table 9.11, the substantial loss of precision due to adjustment, coupled with very little confounding, strongly suggests against stratification in this case.

This empirical assessment of confounding, coupled with the concepts provided by causal graphs, is an effective and practical approach. The added value of causal graphs is that they highlight situations (as elucidated in Chapter 8.3.1) where inadvertent stratification by a collider introduces rather than removes confounding.

9.6 Comments and further reading

In principle, the empirical approach to confounding can be used to select a minimal set of confounders for stratification. However, when there are several potential confounders, the order in which they are considered can make a difference. To avoid this possibility, we can stratify on the entire set of confounders and then see if some variables need not be adjusted by removing them from the stratifiers and checking to see if this results in an important change in the effect measure for the exposure of interest. Typically, if the number of confounders is large, this is not possible by pure stratification and alternatives including regression models (Chapters 12 and 13) must be used. Causal graphs can be used to help choose a minimal set of confounders for adjustment, allowing the possible use of stratification on a smaller set of extraneous variables. We discuss the control of many variables simultaneously in regression models in Chapter 15.

Little has been said about the practical definition of strata when the underlying confounder is interval-scaled, as body weight is in the Western Collaborative Group Study. Using too few categories often results in substantial residual confounding in the resulting crude strata. Finer stratification can lead to sparse data in each stratum if taken too far. Again, regression models provide a method to account for a potential confounder using the minimal "degrees of freedom" (see Chapter 14). In a similar vein, stratification may not remove all confounding bias if there is error in measuring the confounder.

The method of *maximum likelihood* is an alternative technique to analyze stratified data. We consider this approach in great detail in Chapters 12 to 14 in the more general setting of regression models. Like the Woolf method, maximum likelihood breaks down when there are few observations in each strata. A variant of the approach, *conditional likelihood*, can be used in such settings; we discuss this approach for matched data sets in Chapter 16.

Stratified analysis and summary estimation of the Relative Risk are also straightforward for case-cohort studies (Greenland, 1986; Sato, 1992b). Similarly, methods for adjusting the estimate of the Attributable Risk to account for potential confounders are available.

As indicated in Section 8.5, there are alternatives to stratification for estimating an adjusted measure of association. These alternatives can be applied generally to more complex data structures. In particular, stratification fails to remove confounding in longitudinal studies where the exposure and confounder vary over time. *Inverse probability weighted* estimators have been recently introduced to deal with time-dependent confounding (Robins et al., 2000). This method and stratification both have difficulty with large numbers of confounders because of the sparseness of the data, in which case they require additional assumptions, often the use of regression models (Chapter 12). Inverse probability weighted estimators have additional appeal in this case because they can be made robust to assumptions regarding (1) the link of exposure and confounders to disease and (2) the way in which potential confounders determine the particular counterfactual observed, and the manner in which these associations evolve over time (van der Laan and Robins, 2002). Robust here means that we can be wrong about either assumption (1) or (2), although not both, and still obtain an appropriate estimator. The use of causal graphs to handle large numbers of confounders, by selecting a minimal set of variables for adjustment (see Chapter 8.3.2), has its own risks, as it can be difficult to ascertain the correct causal graph when there are a large number of variables.

Recall that the association between a randomized exposure, E, and outcome, D, cannot be confounded by any extraneous factor, C. There is no apparent need for adjustment after randomization, as the pooled or unadjusted estimators do not suffer from confounding bias. Nevertheless, in small or moderate samples, the distribution of factors such as C will not be entirely balanced due to the vagaries of randomness, so that some association between C and E will occur in the sample. If C is also a strong risk factor, we will see evidence of empirical confounding, in which case it is still advantageous to use the adjusted estimator. Although not required by confounding bias, the adjusted estimator may be more accurate than the unadjusted estimator. It is similarly important to note that it is the relationships between variables as displayed in the sample that determine the level of empirical confounding, not merely postulated but unobserved associations in the Study or Target Population. Because of this, the use of causal graphs as the sole determinant of whether a stratified analysis is necessary may not, in fact, be the best guide to the most suitable estimator.

9.7 Problems

Question 9.1

In Perez-Padilla et al. (2001) (see Question 6.4) the authors were concerned that the variable, monthly family income (an indicator of economic status), might confound the observed association between indoor air pollution and tuberculosis. The data in Table 6.7, stratified by income, are shown in Table 9.13, with income information coded as "<1000 pesos per month" and "1000 or more pesos per month."

Table 9.13 *Case-control data on biomass fuel exposure and tuberculosis, stratified by monthly income*

Monthly Income			Tuberculosis	
			Cases	Controls
<1000 pesos	Biomass fuel exposure	Yes	38	12
		No	102	141
1000 or more pesos	Biomass fuel exposure	Yes	12	9
		No	136	383

Based on the income strata, (1) what is the Odds Ratio associating biomass fuel exposure, for the low income (<1000 pesos/month) stratum? (2) Similarly, what is the Odds Ratio for the high income (1000^+ pesos/month) stratum? Now estimate the Odds Ratio, associated with biomass fuel exposure, adjusting for income, using the Mantel–Haenszel method. Based on your calculations and those reported from Question 6.4, what is your assessment of confounding by monthly income? Does the income variable fulfill the criteria required for a variable to be a confounder?

In addition to income, the authors considered many other confounding factors: age, sex, urban or rural residence, smoking, crowding, level of education, and socioeconomic status. After controlling for all these confounders, their estimate of the adjusted Odds Ratio between indoor air pollution and tuberculosis was 2.2. Based on the crude and adjusted Odds Ratio, was the association of Question 6.4 confounded?

Question 9.2

Refer again to the data set *oesoph*, found by going to http://www.crcpress.com/e_products/downloads/. The data, associating the binary measure of alcohol consumption (see Question 7.3) with esophageal cancer incidence, can be stratified into two age groups, 25 to 54 years old and 55 years old and above. Use the Cochran–Mantel–Haenszel method to examine the association between alcohol consumption and incidence of esophageal cancer, adjusting for this dichotomous measure of age. Give a summary estimate of the Odds Ratio using both the Woolf and Mantel–Haenszel methods. Provide two 95% confidence intervals based on your summary estimates. Compare these confidence intervals and comment.

Question 9.3

Return to the data in Table 8.9 with your answers regarding confounding and causal effects in situations (1), (2), and (3) of Question 8.9. For each scenario, calculate an appropriate Odds Ratio, with associated 95% confidence interval, that you think best describes the causal effects of exposure on disease.

Question 9.4

> "So they put the poor below, where they'd be the first to go."

The data set, *titanic*, found at http://www.crcpress.com/e_products/downloads/, provides survival data for passengers on the *Titanic* with information on their sex, age, ticket class and fare, and place of embarkation. Stratify the data relating the sex and survival status of the passengers (see Question 4.2) by the three ticket classes. Using the Mantel–Haenszel procedure, estimate the Relative Risk of dying associated with sex, controlling for the potential confounding effects of ticket class; provide an appropriate 95% confidence interval to supplement your point estimate.

CHAPTER 10

Interaction

Epidemiological studies over the past century have revealed many of the common primary risk factors for most major chronic diseases. A fundamental example was the elucidation of cigarette smoking as a risk factor for lung cancer. Nevertheless, for many diseases the mechanism, a biological understanding of how such risk factors lead to disease, remains elusive. Further, in the case of smoking, we are only too aware of individuals who do not develop lung cancer after a lifetime of heavy smoking and those who develop the disease with no apparent exposure to known risks. While these phenomena might be partially explained by the presence of as yet unidentified exposures, the possibility that there exist variables, perhaps genetic, that act synergistically or antagonistically with smoking is especially tantalizing. For example, is there a factor—some form of "immunity"—that protects certain smokers from cancer? Understanding and clarifying the roles of synergistic and antagonistic factors may be of particular value when developing a biological model for disease development or structuring targeted disease screening programs and interventions. For these reasons, questions surrounding synergism and antagonism are of considerable biological as well as epidemiological interest. At first glance, these issues seem to be accessible through the idea of statistical interaction, introduced in Chapter 8. However, in this chapter we discuss that while the ideas of synergism and antagonism appear self-evident, their relationship to statistical interaction is not as straightforward as we might have hoped.

The concept of interaction is focused on the idea that the level of one factor, say, C, influences the action of another factor, E, on the outcome, D. *Webster's Dictionary* defines synergism as the "cooperative action of discrete agencies such that the total effect is *greater* than the sum of the two effects taken independently" (emphasis added). Antagonism has a parallel definition, with "lesser" replacing "greater." Applying these definitions to determine whether two factors of interest, E and C, are synergistic or antagonistic in their association with D, we face two issues that the definition fails to specify:

1. How do we measure the *effect* of a factor or factors?

2. How do we *sum* the effects of individual factors?

The assessment of synergy depends critically on how we address these two questions. Two standard approaches, multiplicative and additive interaction, are often used, each based on different effect measures and different summing tactics.

Before these are described, it is helpful to introduce some additional notation to describe the risks associated at various combinations of the factors C and E. For simplicity, we restrict attention to the situation where both factors C and E are binary.

Now let the risks depend on the levels of C and E according to the following notation:

$$P_{11} = P(D|E\&C) \quad P_{10} = P(D|E\&\bar{C})$$
$$P_{01} = P(D|\bar{E}\&C) \quad P_{00} = P(D|\bar{E}\&\bar{C}).$$

Considering the group of individuals with neither E nor C as a baseline or reference group leads to the definitions of three Relative Risks by dividing the remaining population into three groups, depending on exposure to one or other factor or to both. Specifically, let

$$RR_{11} = \frac{P_{11}}{P_{00}}$$

$$RR_{10} = \frac{P_{10}}{P_{00}}$$

$$RR_{01} = \frac{P_{01}}{P_{00}}.$$

Thus, for example, RR_{10} measures the Relative Risk for those individuals only exposed to E (and not C), against those in the reference group who are exposed to neither factor. We can similarly define OR_{11}, OR_{10}, OR_{01}, and ER_{11}, ER_{10}, ER_{01}. Throughout this chapter, we assume that there is no confounding of the risks at various levels of E and C by other factors, so that all of the noted effect measures have a causal interpretation.

10.1 Multiplicative and additive interaction

In this section the notation above is used, along with our understanding of the measures of association from Chapter 4, to develop two fundamentally different approaches to both defining and combining effects, so we can apply the definitions of synergy and antagonism.

10.1.1 Multiplicative interaction

Relative Risk will first be used as the measure of the effect of a factor, so that RR_{10} describes the effect of E separate from C; RR_{01} describes the effect of C separate from E; and RR_{11} the total effect of both E and C together. With regard to "summing" the effects of individual factors, it is natural to consider multiplication of the separate Relative Risks (equivalent to summing the log Relative Risks). This leads to the definition that E and C *do not interact multiplicatively* if $RR_{11} = RR_{10} \times RR_{01}$.

What does this definition of interaction have to do with the definition in Chapter 8.1.3 in terms of the homogeneity of a measure of association of the E–D relationship across strata of C? To answer this, note that the above definition is equivalent to

$$\frac{P_{11}}{P_{00}} = \frac{P_{10}}{P_{00}} \times \frac{P_{01}}{P_{00}},$$

which, after multiplying both sides by $\frac{P_{00}}{P_{01}}$, yields

$$\frac{P_{11}}{P_{01}} = \frac{P_{10}}{P_{00}}.$$

Note that the left-hand side of this relationship is just the Relative Risk for the $D-E$ relationship among individuals who all have characteristic C, that is, RR for D associated with E, *in the C stratum*. Similarly, the right-hand side is the Relative Risk for the $D-E$ relationship among individuals who do not have characteristic C, that is, RR associated with E in the $\bar{C}$ stratum. The condition of no multiplicative interaction is thus the same as requiring that the Relative Risk associated with E remains constant over levels, or strata, of C.

Analogously the Odds Ratio can be used as the measure of effect, defining the absence of (multiplicative) interaction as $OR_{11} = OR_{10} \times OR_{01}$. Similar algebra shows that this, in turn, is equivalent to the Odds Ratio for D associated with E, being constant over levels of C. The two conditions are, of course, approximately the same in a rare disease setting and we will not further distinguish between these two formulations of multiplicative interaction. Note that for either the RR or OR the definition of multiplicative interaction is symmetric in the roles of C and E, in that C interacts with the relationship between E and D if and only if E interacts with the $C-D$ association.

A classic example regarding the possible presence of interaction concerns the separate and combined effects of smoking and asbestos exposure on the incidence of lung cancer. In approximate terms, it is known that lung cancer incidence is ten times greater for smokers than nonsmokers in a population without exposure to asbestos. On the other hand, asbestos exposure raises the risk of lung cancer in nonsmokers about fivefold. Finally, for individuals who both smoke and have prior asbestos exposure, the risk is roughly 50 times greater than for those who have neither risk factor. Using the notation at the beginning of this chapter, we have $RR_{10} = 10, RR_{01} = 5$, and $RR_{11} = 50$, with E and C representing smoking and asbestos exposure, respectively. Since $RR_{11} = RR_{10} \times RR_{01}$, we conclude that there is no multiplicative interaction between smoking and asbestos exposure with regard to their effects on lung cancer incidence.

10.1.2 Additive interaction

There is, of course, nothing sacrosanct about using the Relative Risk as a measure of effect nor of the notion that separate factor Relative Risks should multiply as a benchmark to compare with the Relative Risk for both factors taken together. We could still use the Relative Risk but, rather than multiplying, add deviations of RR from the null value 1 in order to assess synergism. This leads to the definition that E and C *do not interact additively* if $(RR_{11} - 1) = (RR_{10} - 1) + (RR_{01} - 1)$. This is equivalent to saying that

$$(P_{11} - P_{00}) = (P_{10} - P_{00}) + (P_{01} - P_{00}),$$

that is,

$$ER_{11} = ER_{10} + ER_{01}. \tag{10.1}$$

So, an equivalent approach to additive interaction is the use of Excess Risk as a measure of effect, with summing the Excess Risks the appropriate way to combine individual effects as a reference for considering the joint effect of the factors.

Note that by adding $(P_{00} - P_{01})$ to both sides of Equation 10.1, we see that the condition for no additive interaction is equivalent to

$$P_{11} - P_{01} = P_{10} - P_{00},$$

that is, the Excess Risk associated with E in the C stratum is the same as the Excess Risk from E in the $\bar{C}$ stratum. Hence, the absence of additive interaction is the same as requiring that the Excess Risk arising from E is homogeneous across the C strata. Additive interaction is also symmetric in the roles of C and E.

With the example of Section 10.1.1 regarding smoking and asbestos exposure and their association with lung cancer incidence, we now see quite a different picture with regard to interaction. With $RR_{01} = 5$, $RR_{10} = 10$, and $RR_{11} = 50$, we have $RR_{11} - 1 = 49$, which is considerably larger than $(RR_{10} - 1) + (RR_{01} - 1) = 9 + 4 = 13$. We can conclude that there is substantial additive interaction, synergistically, with regard to the effects of smoking and asbestos exposure, despite the absence of multiplicative interaction.

For two separate risk factors, both with Relative Risks greater than one, it is possible to move from additive or multiplicative antagonism, to no additive interaction and multiplicative antagonism, to additive synergism and multiplicative antagonism, to additive synergism and no multiplicative interaction, and finally to both additive and multiplicative synergism, depending on the sizes of the Relative Risks for individuals exposed to both factors as compared with those exposed to only one. While this is often confusing at first, remember that the definitions of additive and multiplicative interaction refer only to patterns in the Relative Risks for the population subgroups experiencing various combinations of exposures and do not necessarily have any biological meaning. We discuss the implications of the difference between these two definitions of interaction in Sections 10.2 and 10.5.

10.2 Interaction and counterfactuals

We now turn to counterfactuals, introduced in Section 8.1.1, to see if causal ideas can shed light on the appropriate form of interaction that we should look for. We continue with the simplest possible case of two binary risk factors E and C, and we illustrate our discussion in terms of our example where the outcome is CHD and the two variables are behavior type (E) and a dichotomized version of body weight (C). The situation is now more complex than described in Table 8.1, since with two factors there are four possible experimental counterfactuals corresponding to the four possible combinations of the two binary factors. For each of these counterfactual exposure combinations there are two possible outcomes, D or $\bar{D}$, so that in all there are $2^4 = 16$ possible counterfactual outcome patterns. These are listed in Table 10.1,

Table 10.1 *Distribution of possible CHD responses (D) to behavior type (E) and binary measure of body weight (C)*

Group	Type A and High Weight ($E\&C$)	Type A and Low Weight ($E\&\bar{C}$)	Type B and High Weight ($\bar{E}\&C$)	Type B and Low Weight ($\bar{E}\&\bar{C}$)	Number
1	D	D	D	D	Np_1
2	D	D	D	$\bar{D}$	Np_2
3	D	D	$\bar{D}$	D	Np_3
4	D	D	$\bar{D}$	$\bar{D}$	Np_4
5	D	$\bar{D}$	D	D	Np_5
6	D	$\bar{D}$	D	$\bar{D}$	Np_6
7	D	$\bar{D}$	$\bar{D}$	D	Np_7
8	D	$\bar{D}$	$\bar{D}$	$\bar{D}$	Np_8
9	$\bar{D}$	D	D	D	Np_9
10	$\bar{D}$	D	D	$\bar{D}$	Np_{10}
11	$\bar{D}$	D	$\bar{D}$	D	Np_{11}
12	$\bar{D}$	D	$\bar{D}$	$\bar{D}$	Np_{12}
13	$\bar{D}$	$\bar{D}$	D	D	Np_{13}
14	$\bar{D}$	$\bar{D}$	D	$\bar{D}$	Np_{14}
15	$\bar{D}$	$\bar{D}$	$\bar{D}$	D	Np_{15}
16	$\bar{D}$	$\bar{D}$	$\bar{D}$	$\bar{D}$	Np_{16}

together with the population distribution of the 16 groups that share identical patterns. For example, Group 1 individuals develop CHD regardless of their combination of behavior type and body weight, and the population proportion of Group 1 individuals is p_1. Similarly, Group 4 individuals always get CHD when they are Type A but never if they are Type B, regardless of their weight.

Note that some of the counterfactual patterns for a given group exhibit synergistic or antagonistic characteristics. For example, Group 8 individuals only contract CHD when they are *both* Type A and of high weight and not if they have only one or neither risk. For such individuals, each factor is only a risk in the presence of the other. On the other hand, as we already noted, body weight is irrelevant in determining the onset of CHD for Group 4 individuals who do not exhibit synergism or antagonism between factors. Careful consideration of each type reveals that Groups 2, 3, 5, 7–10, 12, and 14–15 show synergistic or antagonistic properties Groups 1, 4, 6, 11, 13, and 16 do not.

We can compute, in terms of the counterfactual proportions, the proportion of Ds in the population if everyone were Type A and high weight, denoted by $P_{11(causal)}$:

$$P_{11(causal)} = p_1 + p_2 + p_3 + p_4 + p_5 + p_6 + p_7 + p_8.$$

Similarly, the probability of D if everyone is Type A and low weight is

$$P_{10(causal)} = p_1 + p_2 + p_3 + p_4 + p_9 + p_{10} + p_{11} + p_{12};$$

if everyone is Type B and high weight,

$$P_{01(causal)} = p_1 + p_2 + p_5 + p_6 + p_9 + p_{10} + p_{13} + p_{14};$$

and, finally, if everyone is Type B and low weight,

$$P_{00(causal)} = p_1 + p_3 + p_5 + p_7 + p_9 + p_{11} + p_{13} + p_{15}.$$

In general, these causal risks can be contrasted using multiplicative or additive interaction, as we did with the observable risks, $P_{11}, P_{10}, P_{01}, P_{00}$, in Section 10.1, although this does not provide much insight. However, one valuable deduction can be gleaned directly. Suppose that there are *no* individuals of any of the groups that display synergism and antagonism as discussed above, that is, $p_2 = p_3 = p_5 = p_7 = p_8 = p_9 = p_{10} = p_{12} = p_{14} = p_{15} = 0$. Then, we can immediately see that

$$\begin{aligned}
ER_{11(causal)} = P_{11(causal)} - P_{00(causal)} &= (p_1 + p_4 + p_6) - (p_1 + p_{11} + p_{13}) \\
&= (p_4 - p_{13}) + (p_6 - p_{11}) \\
&= (P_{10(causal)} - P_{00(causal)}) + (P_{01(causal)} - P_{00(causal)}) \\
&= ER_{10(causal)} + ER_{01(causal)}.
\end{aligned} \tag{10.2}$$

The difference between Equations 10.1 and 10.2 is that the former refers to observed Excess Risks whereas the latter refers to causal Excess Risks. However, assuming the randomization assumption conditional on both E and C (equivalently, that there is no additional confounding after stratification by E and C), the observable and causal measures are the same. We can thus conclude in the absence of confounding by other factors that if we detect additive interaction in a population (Equation 10.1 does not hold) then additive interaction occurs amongst the causal risks (Equation 10.2 does not hold), and therefore at least some members of the population show synergistic or antagonistic behavior with regard to their four counterfactuals. Our back-of-the-envelope assessment of smoking and asbestos exposure as risk factors for lung cancer in the last section thus shows that some fraction of the population possesses antagonistic/synergistic counterfactual patterns, although how many and of which group we cannot say. Despite the weakness of this statement, it suggests that the presence or absence of additive interaction is the right benchmark to claim some form of biological interaction between the two risk factors. We return to this point again in Section 10.5. However, be careful not to equate the absence of additive interaction with a lack of biological synergism or antagonism; it is easy to see that Equation 10.2 can still hold even when some of the synergistic/antagonistic groups exist in the population, that is, some of the proportions $p_2, p_3, p_5, p_7, p_8, p_9, p_{10}, p_{12}, p_{14}, p_{15}$ are nonzero.

10.3 Test of consistency of association across strata

As argued in Chapter 9.1, it is helpful to examine the consistency of effect measures across strata before launching into single summary procedures. Such assessment highlights population subgroups where we believe there to be different impacts of the exposure, E, on disease D. Since we usually deal with population samples, this is a good point to introduce sampling variation into our comparison of various effect measures, in part so that we are not distracted by apparent strata differences in the Relative Risk, say, that are easily explained by mere chance variation. That is, we describe how to use observed data stratified over levels of one or more extraneous variables to assess whether we can plausibly assume that a measure of association associating E with D is consistent across strata. In other words, we assess evidence suggesting that the measure of association of choice may vary across strata, indicating that the stratifying variables modify the effect of E on D. Depending on the particular effect measure used, these techniques help to assess the presence of multiplicative or additive interaction.

As in Chapter 9, we assume that the data on exposure and outcome have been stratified into I strata based on common levels of a set of extraneous variables. We again use the notation of Table 9.1 for the data in the ith stratum. An example of such stratified data was given in Table 9.2 for the Western Collaborative Group Study. In Section 10.3.3, we reexamine this data on behavior type and CHD by body weight to consider whether it is plausible that the observed estimated measures of association, given in Table 9.2, all arise from the same stratum-specific value.

10.3.1 The Woolf method

For the moment, use the Odds Ratio as the measure of association of interest, so that consistency across strata refers to absence of multiplicative interaction. The null hypothesis under investigation is then H_0: $OR_1 = OR_2 = \cdots = OR_I$, where, as before, OR_i is the Odds Ratio for the E–D association in the ith stratum for $i = 1, \ldots, I$. The alternative hypothesis is that there is at least one stratum-specific Odds Ratio that differs from another one. Figure 10.1 illustrates a typical null hypothesis.

Note that the null hypothesis has one degree of freedom since it does not specify the particular constant value of the assumed common Odds Ratio. One approach to testing interaction is to pick a reasonable estimate of a common Odds Ratio, and then look at the variation of the individual stratum Odds Ratio estimates from this common value and determine whether it appears compatible with random variation. Because of skewness in the sampling distribution of the Odds Ratio estimates, we again prefer to work on the logarithm scale, using estimates of $\log OR_i$. We have

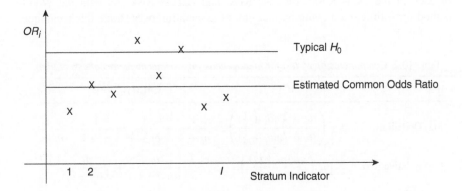

Figure 10.1 *Schematic describing null hypothesis in test for multiplicative interaction.*

already derived an estimate of a plausible "average" of the set of stratum-specific log Odds Ratios, namely, the Woolf estimator (Equation 9.2). We use this as our best guess of a common Odds Ratio. The deviation of the individual stratum-specific Odds Ratio from this "average" value can then be measured by $(\log \widehat{OR}_i - \log \widehat{OR}_W)^2$. These deviations can be added across the strata, each deviation weighted by the reciprocal of the variance of the specific log Odds Ratio estimate, so that we give more precise estimates of $\log OR_i$ a greater role in our assessment of variation. This yields the test statistic

$$\chi_H^2 = \sum_{i=1}^{I} w_i (\log \widehat{OR}_i - \log \widehat{OR}_W)^2,$$

where $\log \widehat{OR}_W$ and w_i are given by Equations 9.2 and 9.3, respectively.

Under the null hypothesis and with sufficiently large samples, χ_H^2 approximately follows a χ^2 sampling distribution with $I - 1$ degrees of freedom. The number of degrees of freedom arises from the fact that the stratum Odds Ratios in Figure 10.1 are all free to vary, in I degrees of freedom, whereas deviations from $\log \widehat{OR}_W$ can only vary with $I - 1$ degrees of freedom, as their weighted average must equal zero (since the weighted average of the $\log \widehat{OR}_i$s equals $\log \widehat{OR}_W$).

This test of the homogeneity of stratum Odds Ratios is easily adapted to cases where the Relative Risk or Excess Risk is being used to describe the E–D relationship. The generic form of the test statistic of homogeneity of a specific measure of association is given by

$$\chi_H^2 = \sum_{i=1}^{I} \frac{[\widehat{MA}_i - Avg(MA)]^2}{Var(\widehat{MA}_i)} = \sum_{i=1}^{I} w_i [\widehat{MA}_i - Avg(MA)]^2, \tag{10.3}$$

where

$$Avg(MA) = \frac{\sum_{i=1}^{I} w_i \widehat{MA}_I}{\sum_{i=1}^{I} w_i}.$$

Table 10.2 provides formulas for calculating $\widehat{MA}_i$ and the associated weights w_i, for each of the Odds Ratio, Relative Risk, and Excess Risk. As with the Woolf method for estimating a common measure of association over strata, this technique

Table 10.2 *Components of χ^2 test for homogeneity for various measures of association*

MA	$\widehat{MA}_i$	$\widehat{Var}(\widehat{MA}_i) = w_i^{-1}$
(log) Odds Ratio	$\log\left(\dfrac{(a_i + \frac{1}{2})(d_i + \frac{1}{2})}{(b_i + \frac{1}{2})(c_i + \frac{1}{2})}\right)$	$\dfrac{1}{a_i + \frac{1}{2}} + \dfrac{1}{b_i + \frac{1}{2}} + \dfrac{1}{c_i + \frac{1}{2}} + \dfrac{1}{d_i + \frac{1}{2}}$
(log) Relative Risk	$\log\left(\dfrac{a_i/(a_i + b_i)}{c_i/(c_i + d_i)}\right)$	$\dfrac{b_i}{a_i(a_i + b_i)} + \dfrac{d_i}{c_i(c_i + d_i)}$
Excess Risk	$\dfrac{a_i}{a_i + b_i} - \dfrac{c_i}{c_i + d_i}$	$\dfrac{a_i b_i}{(a_i + b_i)^3} + \dfrac{c_i d_i}{(c_i + d_i)^3}$

for investigating interaction does not work well when there are many strata with few observations in each stratum. The computation and application of the Woolf test of homogeneity is illustrated for consistency in Section 10.3.3.

10.3.2 Alternative tests of homogeneity

The Woolf test for homogeneity, based on Equation 10.3, focuses directly on a specific measure of association. An alternative approach proposed by Breslow and Day (1980) instead examines variation in the cell counts themselves, assuming a fixed and common association across strata. To illustrate this method, we focus on the Odds Ratio and examine the "a_i" cells, using the notation of Table 9.1 (although we can equivalently use the b, c, or d cells). Based on the data of Table 9.2 from the Western Collaborative Group Study, the observed a_is (namely, 22, 21, 29, 47, and 59) vary, in part because of changes in the sample sizes and marginal totals from stratum to stratum, as well as because the Odds Ratio may also vary by body weight. So first we must evaluate what we expect the values of each of these a_is to be, *assuming that there is a common Odds Ratio* that describes the association between D and E in each stratum. But what is this expectation? For convenience, Table 10.3 revisits the 2×2 table from Table 6.1, with simplified notation.

Assuming that the Odds Ratio underlying this table is OR and that the marginal totals are fixed, then for large n, $A^* = E(a)$ is that value that, when substituted for a in Table 10.3, yields a 2×2 table with exactly these same marginals, $n_E, n_{\bar{E}}, n_D, n_{\bar{D}}$, and the assumed Odds Ratio OR. Table 10.4 gives the large sample expected values, B^*, C^*, D^* for the b, c, and d cells that, along with A^*, yield the observed marginals.

Table 10.3 *Simple notation for general 2×2 table*

		Disease		
		D	not D	
Exposure	E	a	$b = n_E - a$	n_E
	not E	$c = n_D - a$	$d = n_{\bar{E}} - n_D + a$	$n_{\bar{E}}$
		n_D	$n_{\bar{D}}$	n

Table 10.4 *Calculating the expectation of A in a general 2×2 table*

		Disease		
		D	not D	
Exposure	E	A^*	$B^* = n_E - A^*$	n_E
	not E	$C^* = n_D - A^*$	$D^* = n_{\bar{E}} - n_D + A^*$	$n_{\bar{E}}$
		n_D	$n_{\bar{D}}$	n

To calculate $A^* = E(a)$ we simply need to examine the equation

$$\frac{A^* D^*}{B^* C^*} = \frac{A^*(n_{\bar{E}} - n_D + A^*)}{(n_E - A^*)(n_D - A^*)} = OR, \tag{10.4}$$

which gives the required Odds Ratio. This is just a quadratic equation in A^* and easily solved. The values of B^*, C^*, and D^* are then computed by subtracting the value of A^* from the relevant marginals as in Table 10.4. This formulation of the expected value of a when n is large is based on the *noncentral hypergeometric distribution* and extends the (exact) result for $E(a)$ for the special case $OR = 1$ (that is, when E and D are independent), discussed in Chapter 6.4.1 and used in the Cochran–Mantel–Haenszel test.

This then gives the expected value of the a cell, assuming an Odds Ratio fixed at OR. But how big is the variation of a, given the sample size, marginals, and so on? The variance of a, assuming the Odds Ratio is OR, is given by

$$V^* = Var(a|OR) = \left[\frac{1}{A^*} + \frac{1}{B^*} + \frac{1}{C^*} + \frac{1}{D^*} \right]^{-1} \tag{10.5}$$

when n is large and with A^*, B^*, C^*, and D^* given by the calculations above.

We are now in the position to give an alternative test statistic for homogeneity of the Odds Ratio, based on the observed variation of the a_i terms across the strata. Specifically, the test statistic we are aiming for is

$$\chi_H^2(a) = \sum_{i=1}^{I} \frac{(a_i - A_i^*)^2}{V_i^*},$$

where A_i^* and V_i^* denote the expectation and variation of a_i for the ith stratum, assuming a common Odds Ratio, OR, for each stratum. But, of course, A_i^* and V_i^*, given by Equations 10.4 and 10.5, depend on the unknown OR. Instead we substitute an estimate of this assumed common Odds Ratio using, for instance, the Woolf or Mantel–Haenszel estimators described in Chapter 9.2.1 and 9.2.2, and with this estimate compute the A_i^* and V_i^* terms that appear in the formula for $\chi_H^2(a)$. Like χ_H^2, and for the same reasons, $\chi_H^2(a)$ approximately follows a χ^2 sampling distribution with $I - 1$ degrees of freedom, assuming the null hypothesis of a consistent Odds Ratio across strata. Again, this approach is not effective for several strata, all with small sample sizes. In such cases, an exact test (Zelen, 1971) can be used.

10.3.3 Example—the Western Collaborative Group Study: part 5

Return to the Western Collaborative Group Study and the data of Table 9.2, repeated in Table 10.5 for convenience. We first look at evidence of variation of the Odds Ratio for CHD associated with behavior type across the five body weight strata. Here we are checking for multiplicative interaction since the Odds Ratio is the effect measure. Table 9.5 provides the necessary components to calculate the appropriate test statistic; the necessary information has been abstracted in Table 10.6. In particular,

$$\chi_H^2 = 6.807(0.949 - 0.817)^2 + \cdots + 13.606(1.070 - 0.817)^2$$
$$= 3.981,$$

using the fact that the Woolf estimate is given by $\log \widehat{OR}_W = 0.817$.

Table 10.5 *Coronary heart disease and behavior type, stratified by body weight*

Body Weight (lb)			CHD Event		
			Yes	No	$\widehat{OR}$
≤150	Behavior type	Type A	22	253	2.652
		Type B	10	305	
150$^+$–160	Behavior type	Type A	21	235	2.413
		Type B	10	270	
160$^+$–170	Behavior type	Type A	29	297	1.381
		Type B	21	297	
170$^+$–180	Behavior type	Type A	47	248	2.524
		Type B	19	253	
>180	Behavior type	Type A	59	378	2.966
		Type B	19	361	

Table 10.6 *Calculations for the Woolf test of homogeneity of the odds ratio, based on data from Table 10.5*

Body Weight (lb)	$\log(\widehat{OR_i})$	w_i
≤150	0.949	6.807
150$^+$–160	0.855	6.680
160$^+$–170	0.316	11.477
170$^+$–180	0.910	12.453
>180	1.070	13.606

In this case, there are five body weight strata; so under the null hypothesis that the Odds Ratios associated with behavior type are constant across these strata, the test statistic χ_H^2 should have a χ^2 sampling distribution with 4 degrees of freedom. With this as a benchmark, the observed test statistic χ_H^2 yields a p-value of 0.41. Thus there is little convincing evidence that the Odds Ratios for CHD associated with behavior type are modified by body weight.

Analogous calculations can be carried out to examine homogeneity of both the Relative Risk and Excess Risk. Specifically, for the Relative Risk the computation of χ_H^2 follows from the calculations of Table 9.7 and is given by

$$\chi_H^2 = 7.213(0.924 - 0.763)^2 + \cdots + 15.465(0.993 - 0.763)^2$$
$$= 3.948,$$

also yielding a p-value of 0.41 in comparison with a $\chi_{(4)}^2$ distribution. For the Excess Risk, we have, using the results of Table 9.9,

$$\chi_H^2 = 2738(0.0483 - 0.0563)^2 + \cdots + 2549(0.0850 - 0.0563)^2$$
$$= 6.623.$$

Table 10.7 *Breslow–Day test statistic calculations for the data in Table 10.5, assuming the common odds ratio =* $\widehat{OR}_W = 2.264$

Body Weight (lb)	a_i	A_i^*	B_i^*	C_i^*	D_i^*	V_i^*
≤ 150	22	20.937	254.063	11.063	303.937	6.879
150^+–160	21	20.587	235.413	10.413	269.587	6.555
160^+–170	29	34.300	291.701	15.700	302.300	10.042
170^+–180	47	45.650	249.350	20.350	251.650	12.653
> 180	59	55.193	381.807	22.807	357.193	14.840

Here the associated p-value is 0.16, suggesting some evidence that the variation in Excess Risks across the body weight strata may not be compatible with a common Excess Risk for behavior type at each body weight. We raised this possibility earlier in Chapter 9.4.1 following a qualitative examination of the stratum Excess Risks.

Finally, we compute the Breslow–Day test statistic for homogeneity of the Odds Ratio, described in Section 10.3.2. We first need to compute the expected values, A_i^*, for the a_i cells in each stratum, as given by Equation 10.4. For example, suppose we use the Woolf estimate, $\widehat{OR} = 2.264$, of an assumed common Odds Ratio, calculated in Chapter 9.2.3; for the stratum with body weight ≤ 150 lb of Table 10.5, Equation 10.4 then becomes $A^*(283 + A^*)/(275 - A^*)(32 - A^*) = 2.264$. The solution of this quadratic equation that gives positive values for each of A^*, B^*, C^*, and D^* in Table 10.4 is $A^* = 20.937$, which then yields the values $B^* = 254.063$, $C^* = 11.063$, and $D^* = 303.937$. In turn, this gives $V^* = [20.937^{-1} + \cdots + 303.937^{-1}]^{-1} = 6.879$, from Equation 10.5. Solutions for A_i^*, B_i^*, C_i^*, D_i^* and the associated values for V_i^* for each stratum are given in Table 10.7.

Thus,

$$\chi_H^2(a) = \frac{(22 - 20.937)^2}{6.879} + \cdots + \frac{(59 - 55.193)^2}{14.840}$$
$$= 4.108,$$

yielding a p-value of 0.39 from a table of the $\chi_{(4)}^2$ distribution. Here, the Breslow–Day test gives almost equivalent results to the Woolf test for consistency of the Odds Ratio, calculated at the beginning of this section.

10.3.4 The power of the test for homogeneity

Suppose for a moment that we reassign the strata in Table 10.5 to a different hypothetical covariate, labeled X for convenience, as in Table 10.8. Note that we have kept the data exactly as it was in the body weight strata, just changed the labels of the strata. If we now carried out the χ^2 test for homogeneity of the Odds Ratio across these strata of X we would obtain exactly the same result, $\chi_H^2 = 3.981$ and p-value $= 0.41$, as calculated in the previous subsection. This is because the test of homogeneity pays no attention to any underlying structure in the definition of the

Table 10.8 *Coronary heart disease and behavior type, stratified by hypothetical variable X*

X				CHD event		$\widehat{OR}$	$\widehat{RR}$
				Yes	No		
X = 1	Behavior type		Type A	29	297	1.381	1.347
			Type B	21	297		
X = 2	Behavior type		Type A	21	235	2.413	2.297
			Type B	10	270		
X = 3	Behavior type		Type A	47	248	2.524	2.281
			Type B	19	253		
X = 4	Behavior type		Type A	22	253	2.652	2.520
			Type B	10	305		
X = 5	Behavior type		Type A	59	378	2.966	2.700
			Type B	19	361		

strata. On the other hand, with the data of Table 10.8, we might be considerably more reluctant than for body weight to say that there is no evidence of effect modification by X, due to the obvious pattern of an increasing Odds Ratio for behavior type as X increases.

It is important to note that the χ^2 test for homogeneity looks for all possible departures from the null hypothesis. As discussed in our treatment of the Cochran–Mantel–Haenszel test, the consequence of extremely broad alternative hypotheses is a lack of power in the resulting test, since a fixed significance level is "used up" in protecting the procedure from falsely rejecting the null in comparison to such a wide variety of alternatives. There are two immediate ways around this difficulty. First, we can increase power by simply raising the nominal significance level from the arbitrary level, 0.05, to 0.2, say, below which point we consider there to be signs of nonconsistency. While this appears to be an artificial adjustment, it often produces the desired effect of drawing attention to important variations that might be missed by inappropriately fixating on the standard 0.05 level of significance.

Second, as in the Cochran–Mantel–Haenszel situation, we can develop a more targeted test statistic by restricting the alternatives of interest. This can be achieved, for example, by designing a test of homogeneity where the alternative hypothesis is that the measures of association increase (or decrease) corresponding to a natural order in the strata labels. With the data of Table 10.5, this alternative would focus on evidence that the Odds Ratio for CHD associated with behavior type increases or decreases as body weight increases. We will defer the development of such targeted tests for interaction until Chapter 14, where they arise naturally in the context of regression models. Note that the gain in such an approach is the increase in power in detecting a specific kind of departure from the null hypothesis of homogeneity (such as a trend in the measures of association); the disadvantage is that such a targeted test will have very little, if any, power against other kinds of alternatives.

10.4 Example of extreme interaction

We end this chapter by giving a practical example of extreme interaction, a case where the $E-D$ association is in one direction at one level of C and in the other direction at the other level. While this was illustrated with hypothetical data in Table 8.6, it is valuable to look at some real data.

Infection with human cytomegalovirus (CMV) is a primary concern in renal transplants. The need for immunosuppression to prevent organ rejection leaves a transplant recipient vulnerable to reactivation of a prior asymptomatic infection or to a new infection from a CMV-positive but asymptomatic donor. (In the general U.S. population, CMV infection is extremely common but rarely causes symptoms; approximately 80% of Americans test positive for CMV by the age of 60.) On the other hand, prior exposure to infection in the recipient may lead to a partial immunity that will be of value in resisting CMV after a transplant. Thus, the nature of the risk associated with either a recipient testing CMV-positive or the organ donor testing CMV-positive, prior to transplant, is unclear. In unpublished work, Stafford (1988) pooled data from five studies and looked at the Relative Risk for a CMV infection after transplant associated with these two risk factors.

Table 10.9 gives the Relative Risks for posttransplant CMV disease, associated with receiving a kidney from a CMV-positive donor, first for the stratum where the recipient patient is already CMV-positive ($RR = 1.3$) and then for the stratum where the recipient is CMV-negative ($RR = 15.1$). A CMV-negative patient therefore experiences a huge increase in risk when receiving the organ from a CMV-positive donor as against a CMV-negative donor, presumably in large part due to the effects of immunosuppressant drugs. On the other hand, there is little elevation in risk when the patient is already CMV-positive prior to the transplant, perhaps due to some form of developed immunity. Similarly, the Relative Risk associated with being CMV-positive prior to transplant is very different depending on whether the donor is CMV-positive ($RR = 0.5$) or CMV-negative ($RR = 6.1$). The latter high Relative Risk is again perhaps the result of immune suppression with resulting reactivation of CMV. By either consideration of the roles of the two risk factors, the donor's and recipient's prior CMV status, the data present a striking interactive effect.

This discussion is not necessarily advocating stratification on a donor's CMV status in assessing the causal effect of a recipient's CMV status on posttransplant disease. In fact, a possible causal graph relating the three variables is illustrated in Figure 10.2.

Table 10.9 *Relative risks for CMV disease associated with organ donor and recipient's prior CMV status*

Risk Factor is CMV+ Donor		Risk Factor is CMV+ Recipient	
Stratum	RR	Stratum	RR
Recipient CMV+	1.3	Donor CMV+	0.5
Recipient CMV−	15.1	Donor CMV−	6.1

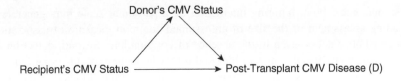

Figure 10.2 *A simple directed causal graph linking a donor and recipient's predisease CMV-status to posttransplant CMV disease in renal transplants.*

This figure assumes that the selected donor organ is influenced by the characteristics of the recipient, rather than the other way around. In this case, both pathways from the recipient's CMV status to posttransplant disease represent causal effects, so that stratification is unnecessary to remove confounding. On the other hand, the data of Table 10.9 show that a single measure of the effect of the recipient's CMV status conceals huge variation across the donor's status, with important practical implications.

10.5 Comments and further reading

We already know that in a given population it is possible for two risk factors to interact multiplicatively but not additively, and vice versa. Further, Siemiatycki and Thomas (1981) describe a range of multistage models for carcinogenesis, all leading to the same population risk patterns for exposure combinations, that have very different interpretations regarding the joint action of risk factors. Thompson (1991) makes a similar point. As a result, it is difficult to definitively conclude from epidemiological data that a specific form of biological synergism (or antagonism) exists. Without further understanding of a true biological model or mechanism describing in detail how factors act, together and alone, to produce the disease outcome, it is misleading to focus on a specified "interaction scale," additive, multiplicative, or any other alternative.

By using counterfactuals, we have seen that additive interaction points to synergistic/antagonistic behavior in at least some fraction of the population. A similar conclusion is reached by Rothman (1976), based on the conceptual idea of sets of "sufficient" causes or pathways for the disease outcome, with the subsequent interpretation that two factors do not biologically interact if they do not appear together in at least one of these pathways. Further, the additive scale is usually the scale of choice when either contemplating the contribution of risk factors to the total disease burden or designing effective interventions.

While counterfactuals provide the basis of causal inference when examining the total effects of one or more risk factors, we have seen that they only slightly illuminate subtleties of joint actions. This inability to definitively identify specific forms of joint actions of risk factors is an additional weakness of nonexperimental studies in determining causal effects.

On a positive note, we stress that statistical modeling of interactive effects is still a key component in exploring the contribution of two or more risk factors to explaining disease outcomes. First, ignoring interaction on a particular scale may generate a misleading assessment of the size of an assumed common measure of association for one or both factors, even in the absence of confounding. Second, detection of interaction may give insight into specific conditions where one exposure is particularly strongly related to disease. Careful consideration of the various kinds of interaction may also lead to a simple or parsimonious description of the association of a series of factors with disease. Finally, highlighting the nature of observed interactions can suggest targeted screening programs and interventions.

All of the above points are particularly important in cases of extreme interaction, where the direction of the effect of one factor changes over levels of the other factor. For example, the data in Table 10.9 indicate that in renal transplants, a CMV-positive donor raises the risk of a posttransplant CMV infection only if the recipient is CMV-negative. This strongly suggests that CMV-positive donors, if used at all, be matched with CMV-positive recipients only. In another setting, Colditz et al. (1996) examine the impact of bearing children on the risk of breast cancer and how this association is modified by a family history of breast cancer in close female relatives. They report a decrease in the risk for breast cancer of about 20% in women who have ever given birth, as compared to nulliparous women, absent any family history. On the other hand, they observed an increase of risk of about 40% for the same comparison when there is family history. These findings suggest that breast cancer screening assessments should occur more frequently amongst parous women with a family history of breast cancer (McKnight, 1998).

10.6 Problems

Question 10.1

Determine if the following statements are true or false:

1. For C to interact multiplicatively with the association between E and D, it is required that C and E are not independent.

2. It is impossible to have data reflecting both additive and multiplicative interaction between two factors at the same time.

Question 10.2

Suppose a moderately sized case-control study of the relationship between a binary risk factor, E, and a disease, D, provides the following results:

- Pooled Odds Ratio estimate is 2.02 with associated 95% confidence interval of (1.25, 3.15).

- After stratification on another factor C, the Odds Ratio estimate when C is present is 1.10 with associated 95% confidence interval of (0.55, 2.70).

- After stratification on another factor C, the Odds Ratio estimate when C is absent is 1.01 with associated 95% confidence interval of (0.72, 1.65).

Discuss whether the following statements are likely to be true or false and give a brief reason:

1. The χ^2 test for independence of E and D in the pooled table yields a p-value < 0.05.

2. The χ^2 test for independence of E and D among those individuals with C yields a p-value < 0.05.

3. The χ^2 test for homogeneity of the two Odds Ratios in the C and $\bar{C}$ strata yields a p-value < 0.05.

4. The Cochran–Mantel–Haenszel χ^2 test for independence of E and D yields a p-value < 0.05.

Question 10.3

Refer to the data of Perez-Padilla et al. (2001) in Question 9.1, given in Table 9.13. Using both the Woolf and Breslow–Day test for interaction, examine the empirical evidence of multiplicative interaction of income and indoor air pollution. Given your results and interpretation, which Odds Ratio would you present for the data of Table 9.13: (1) the pooled Odds Ratio, (2) the Odds Ratio, adjusted for income, or (3) the stratum-specific Odds Ratios?

Question 10.4

In Perez-Padilla et al. (2001), the authors also stratified by smoking the data of Table 6.7 on association between indoor air pollution and tuberculosis. The stratified data are shown in Table 10.10, with smoking information coded as "never" and "past or present." The authors were particularly concerned that smoking might modify the effect of indoor air pollution on tuberculosis. In other words, they were looking for (multiplicative) interaction between smoking and indoor air pollution.

Based on the stratified data, what is the Odds Ratio, associated with biomass fuel exposure, for the never smokers stratum? What is the Odds Ratio for the past or present smokers stratum? Using the Mantel–Haenszel method, estimate the Odds Ratio associated with biomass fuel exposure after adjusting for smoking. Provide your assessment of the role of smoking as a confounding variable.

Table 10.10 *Case-control data on biomass fuel exposure and tuberculosis, stratified by smoking*

| Smoking Status | | | Tuberculosis | |
			Cases	Controls
Never smokers	Biomass fuel exposure	Yes	33	17
		No	186	411
Past or present smokers	Biomass fuel exposure	Yes	17	4
		No	52	113

Using the Breslow–Day method, now examine the evidence for multiplicative interaction between smoking and indoor pollution. Given all your computations, which Odds Ratio would you report for the data of Table 10.10: (1) the pooled Odds Ratio, (2) the Odds Ratio, adjusting for smoking, or (3) the stratum-specific Odds Ratios?

Question 10.5

Refer again to the data set *oesoph*, found by going to http://www.crcpress. com/e_products/downloads/. Using both a binary measure of alcohol consumption (Question 7.3) and a binary measure of age (Question 9.2), examine the evidence for multiplicative interaction of age on the relationship between alcohol consumption and the incidence of esophageal cancer.

Question 10.6

Using the stratified data on the *Titanic* passengers of Question 9.4, examine the evidence for multiplicative interaction between sex and ticket class, using the Woolf method, with the Relative Risk as the basic measure of association.

CHAPTER 11

Exposures at Several Discrete Levels

In the previous chapters we have confined our attention to the simplified situation where the primary exposure variable of interest is limited to two levels: exposed (E) or unexposed ($\bar{E}$). Such a crude assessment is rarely an effective measure and does not allow us to develop a detailed understanding of how disease risk changes over subtle shifts in exposure. Fortunately, even the most basic exposure measurements allow a finer level of gradation; for example, in capturing coffee drinking, the data of Table 7.2 have exposure measured by average daily consumption in cups per day with four distinct categories. We now want to expand the methods to look at more complex risk factors that allow for several differing levels of exposure. For the moment we do not draw a distinction between exposure variables where these levels may be ordered and those for which there is no natural ordering. This issue will be of considerable relevance, however, in Section 11.3.

11.1 Overall test of association

Suppose that, in the population of interest, the exposure variable E now has K natural levels, labeled for convenience by $1, 2, \ldots, K$. We first wish to extend the simple χ^2 test for association between the outcome, D, and E to cover this situation. Arbitrarily, we pick reference level $E = 1$ as a baseline or reference level of exposure; note that we now have $K - 1$ measures of association if we compare the remaining $K - 1$ exposure levels with the reference level. For example, for the Relative Risk, we can define RR_2 as the Relative Risk that compares risk at level 2 of E with the baseline level $E = 1$; that is, $RR_2 = P(D|E = 2)/P(D|E = 1)$. We define $RR_3, \ldots, RR_K$ similarly. The null hypothesis that D and E are independent can then be specified by

$$H_0 : D \text{ and } E \text{ are independent } \Leftrightarrow RR_2 = RR_3 = \cdots = RR_K = 1.$$

If we use alternative measures of association, then H_0 can be written as $OR_2 = \cdots = OR_K = 1$ or $ER_2 = \cdots = ER_K = 0$, where OR_k and ER_k are defined by comparing the risk at level $E = k$ to the baseline level $E = 1$, respectively, for each k with $2 \leq k \leq K$.

The alternative hypothesis that immediately comes to mind is $H_A : D$ and E are not independent. This can be written, for example, as

$$H_A : RR_k \neq 1 \text{ for some } k \text{ with } 2 \leq k \leq K.$$

Table 11.1 provides the notation that we use to describe the generic $K \times 2$ table that cross-classifies the data according to disease status and exposure level. Note that,

Table 11.1 *Symbols for entries in generic $2 \times K$ table*

		Disease		
		D	not D	
Exposure level	1	a_1	b_1	m_1
	2	a_2	b_2	m_2
	...	...	...	...
	K	a_K	b_K	m_K
		n_D	$n_{\bar{D}}$	n

in this context, a cohort design involves the selection of K random samples, one for each level of exposure. On the other hand, a case-control design still requires two random samples, one of cases and one of controls.

The natural extension of the χ^2 statistic that allows for K levels of the risk factor is given by

$$\chi^2_{overall} = \frac{n^2}{n_D n_{\bar{D}}} \sum_{k=1}^{K} \frac{\left(a_k - \frac{n_D m_k}{n}\right)^2}{m_k}. \tag{11.1}$$

If H_0 is true, the sampling distribution of $\chi^2_{overall}$ approximately follows a χ^2 distribution, as we saw for the simple 2×2 table. The degrees of freedom of this null sampling distribution are now $K - 1$ in the general case. As was true for the 2×2 table, this result applies for data generated by either a population-based, cohort, or case-control design. The derivation of the statistic differs across the three study designs, although the result is the same in all cases.

A heuristic for figuring out the correct number of degrees of freedom is most easily seen for a cohort study. Here, there are K separate proportions or risks, $P(D|E = k)$, for $k = 1, \dots, K$ of interest. Under the alternative hypothesis, H_A, these proportions can assume any values between 0 and 1. That is, they have K "degrees of freedom." However, under the null hypothesis, H_0, all these proportions are constrained to be equal and thus there is only one degree of freedom (the unspecified common value of $P(D|E = k)$). If H_0 is true, then, by chance, the value of the $\chi^2_{overall}$ statistic has $K - 1$ degrees of freedom to "use" for random variation between the null and alternative hypotheses. A similar heuristic can be used for population-based and case-control designs. Alternatively, one can think of the null hypothesis as completely specifying the Relative Risks, $RR_2, \dots, RR_K$ (thus they have zero degrees of freedom), whereas under the general alternative hypothesis, these Relative Risks are free to move over $K - 1$ degrees of freedom (as there are $K - 1$ "free" Relative Risks).

When there are only two levels of E (that is, $K = 2$), the test statistic, Equation 11.1, reduces to the familiar χ^2 statistic for testing association in a 2×2 table, described at length in Chapter 6.

Table 11.2 *Pancreatic cancer data with multiple levels of coffee consumption*

		Disease Status		
		D	not D	
Coffee drinking (cups per day)	0	20	88	108
	1–2	153	271	424
	3–4	106	154	260
	≥5	88	130	218
		367	643	1010

11.2 Example—coffee drinking and pancreatic cancer: part 3

We return to our analysis of the case-control data given in Table 7.2, relating the incidence of pancreatic cancer to coffee drinking. Up to this point, we have simply dichotomized exposure into abstainers (no cups per day) or drinkers (one or more cups per day). With the ideas of Section 11.1 at hand, we can make use of the data that gives four levels of coffee consumption.

Table 11.2 reproduces the data from Table 7.2 where we have, for the time being, combined the information across sex strata. We use this data to take a more refined look at the putative association between coffee drinking and pancreatic cancer. The overall χ^2 test statistic is given by

$$\chi^2_{overall} = \frac{1010^2}{367 \times 643} \left[\frac{\left(20 - \frac{367 \times 108}{1010}\right)^2}{108} + \cdots + \frac{\left(88 - \frac{367 \times 218}{1010}\right)^2}{218} \right]$$

$$= \frac{1010^2}{367 \times 643} \times 4.296$$

$$= 18.6.$$

The value of the statistic now can be compared with a χ^2 distribution with 3 degrees of freedom, since there are 4 levels of coffee consumption, yielding a p-value of 0.0003. We thus see a continued strong association of coffee drinking with the incidence of pancreatic cancer when we use a more refined measure of consumption.

11.3 A test for trend in risk

In examining the possible association between D and E, the methods of Section 11.1 have made no use of the underlying meaning of the various exposure levels, particularly whether there is any apparent ordering among these levels. This is certainly the case in the pancreatic cancer case-control study, where coffee consumption levels are ordered in terms of cups per day. Further, as we have now seen several times, the overall test of association has such a broad set of alternatives to the null hypothesis of independence that it will have low power against a specific alternative of interest. As we saw in the discussion of χ^2 tests for homogeneity in Section 10.3.4, one approach is to narrow our set of alternative hypotheses substantially. For an exposure with several levels that have a *natural order*, it makes sense to consider alternatives—to the null hypothesis of independence—that focus on whether the risk of D increases (or decreases) as the level of exposure increases. Symbolically, the alternative hypothesis is now

$$H_A : 1 < RR_2 < RR_3 < \cdots < RR_K \text{ or } 1 > RR_2 > RR_3 > \cdots > RR_K.$$

This alternative, if supported by the data, suggests a possible causal link between exposure and disease, since it is plausible to expect that if an exposure is causally linked to D, the higher the exposure the higher the risk. On the other hand, if we detect some association for an exposure E with ordered levels but observe no trend to the association, we may suspect that the apparent association is not causal, but is possibly reflecting the risk from a hidden causal factor to which E is only loosely correlated.

Cochran (1954) and Armitage (1955) developed a test for trend in the risk for D associated with increasing levels for E when the exposure levels can be *quantified*. In other words, we assume that levels of exposure can be linked to a graded numerical scale. For many risk factors, the scale not only possesses a natural ordering but also an associated numerical scale. This is certainly true for age, body weight, and even cups of coffee as described in the pancreatic cancer study data of Section 11.2. In the latter case, however, it is hard to measure participants' exact daily consumption of coffee; a more crude ordered numerical scale is necessary. We discuss this further in our analysis of Section 11.5.

We therefore assume an ordered scale for E such that for each level k of E, there is a numerical measure of exposure given by x_k. The test for trend is based on the plot of the risk for D at level k of E, $P(D|E = x_k)$, against the scaled exposure value x_k. Of course, we are unable to observe $P(D|E = x_k)$ exactly, but at least in population-based and cohort studies these risks can be estimated and plotted. Figure 11.1 illustrates the generic version of such a plot.

Note that Figure 11.1 illustrates a typical set of risks under the null hypothesis, namely, risks that stay constant (at an unspecified value) as you change levels

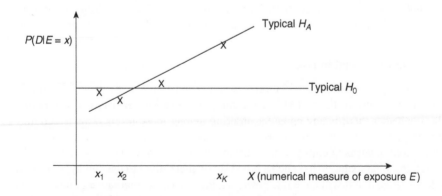

Figure 11.1 *Plot of estimated risks against exposure levels.*

of exposure. Similarly, a typical alternative hypothesis is shown here, allowing the risks to grow linearly with exposure level.

Using simple linear regression techniques, we can examine the evidence for or against a constant level of risk in comparison with a (linear) trend in the risks as exposure level increases. In applying these ideas, it is important to weight the separate plotted points in Figure 11.1 by some measure of precision in the estimate of $P(D|E = x)$ associated with that point. It is simplest to just use the number of sample observations at exposure level $E = x_k$ as a (relative) weight for the estimate of $P(D|E = x_k)$ for each k. This leads to the following test statistic to assess trend:

$$\chi_{trend}^2 = \frac{n^3}{n_D n_{\bar{D}}} \frac{\left[\sum_{k=1}^{K} x_k \left(a_k - \frac{n_D m_k}{n}\right)\right]^2}{\left[n \sum_{k=1}^{K} x_k^2 m_k - \left(\sum_{k=1}^{K} x_k m_k\right)^2\right]}. \tag{11.2}$$

This is derived from a regression test of slope; the test statistic is thus compared to a χ^2 distribution with one degree of freedom for the purpose of calculating a p-value. As intended, the test statistic quantifies evidence suggesting an increase (or decrease) in values of $P(D|E)$ as exposure rises.

We can most simply justify the use of the test statistic (Equation 11.2) with case-control data by considering the marginal totals of Table 11.1 as fixed (of course, in case-control studies the D and $\bar{D}$ marginals are already fixed by design), as discussed briefly in Chapter 6.4.1. We then make use of properties of the K-dimensional hypergeometric distribution as the basis for the sampling distribution of the test statistic (Equation 11.2) under the null hypothesis of independence (although technically this replaces the n^3 term with $n^2(n-1)$ in Equation 11.2). For case-control studies, naïve sample estimates of $P(D|E)$ have no direct population interpretation because of the sampling, but their relative size still indicates whether the risk of D possesses a trend as you increase the level of exposure. Because of the property of the Odds Ratio under case-control sampling (Chapter 5.3), it makes more sense to plot the estimated log Odds when $E = x_k$, against x_k, rather than a plot akin to Figure 11.1 (or plot the Odds Ratio or log Odds Ratio comparing the exposure levels, $E = x_k$, to the baseline level $E = x_1$, against x_k). Although linearity of these plots does not exactly correspond with the linearity underlying Figure 11.1 and Equation 11.2, such a plot still provides insight into the existence of an increasing or decreasing risk as exposure increases. As we see in Chapters 12 and 13, linearity of the log Odds Ratio, when plotted against exposure level, is the basis for the ubiquitous logistic regression model. We illustrate plots of this kind in Sections 11.4 and 11.5, supplemented with application of the test statistic (Equation 11.2).

11.3.1 Qualitatively ordered exposure variables

The application of the test for trend statistic (Equation 11.2) requires a numerical score for each level of exposure. In some cases, the exposure scale may only possess a qualitative ordering; for example, when measuring the use of barrier contraceptives in assessing the risk for HIV infection, individuals may be classified simply by whether they always use, sometimes use, or never use condoms. In other situations, initial measurements of exposure may be based on an interval scale, but are subsequently grouped for convenience. The variable age is often reported in this manner; coffee consumption, introduced in the example of Chapter 7.1.3, is grouped in a similar fashion. There are a variety of ad hoc techniques used to assign numerical values to exposure groups that possess either of these types of qualitative ordering.

For purely qualitative variables, the simplest option is merely to assign the values $0, 1, 2, \ldots$ to the ordered categories of exposure, and then apply the test statistic (Equation 11.2). With grouped exposure levels, one possibility is to use the midpoint of the interval of exposure that defines a particular exposure category. For example, if ages are grouped by the intervals, 20 to 30, 30 to 40 years old, etc., we might use the quantitative values 25, 35, and so on for the various age categories. If the age group has no upper or lower bound, that is, one category is defined, say, by age >70, then an ad hoc value has to be chosen using common sense. If the original values for grouped exposures are known, then an alternative option is to use the median of all sample exposure values in a particular category. For example, if the actual age of all study participants is available, a suitable summary age measure for the group 20 to 30 years old is the median age of all study participants of ages between 20 and 30 years. This approach also applies directly to open-ended categories.

Fortunately, the test for trend, although designed for a linear trend in risk as exposure increases, is not particularly sensitive to the choice of scores. This is related to our discussion in the next section on nonlinear trends. The power of the test will decrease if "incorrect" scores are used, but only slightly. Here, "incorrect" supposes that there is a true set of scores that linearly predicts the trend in risk, but that a proxy or guessed exposure measure is used instead, the approximate measure maintaining a reasonable level of correlation with the unknown true exposure score. This is not to be confused with the potential loss of power that can arise from excessive grouping, that is, placing individuals who possess quite different levels of risk into a common group with a single score (Lagakos, 1988).

11.3.2 Goodness of fit and nonlinear trends in risk

The test for trend, with the test statistic (Equation 11.2), is predicated on a linear trend in risk as exposure increases. This raises the question of how well the variation in risk over the exposure categories is captured by such a linear assumption. A *goodness of fit* test, based on the variation in risk not explained by a linear pattern, can help us address this question. A suitable test statistic is given by the size of the overall χ^2 statistic, Equation 11.1, reduced by the component of this χ^2 statistic that is attributable to a linear trend. Specifically, we let

$$\chi^2_{gof} = \chi^2_{overall} - \chi^2_{trend}. \tag{11.3}$$

Assuming that the change in risk is captured by a linear trend, the test statistic (11.3) approximately follows a χ^2 sampling distribution with $K - 2$ degrees of freedom. Large values of the statistic reflect variation in the risk of D that is not adequately described by a linear trend.

It is unusual, *a priori*, to anticipate complex, highly nonlinear descriptions of the changes in risk as exposure increases. Nevertheless, it is plausible that some nonlinearity is reflected in the data. It is possible to derive a test statistic designed to detect not just linear trends but any *monotonic* change in risk as exposure levels increase. However, Collings et al. (1981) showed that there is little, if any, gain in power by using this approach in lieu of the test for trend based on Equation 11.2. In large part, this finding reflects that the linear component of any nonlinear monotonic function is the easiest component to detect. Indirectly, this also shows that, as discussed in Section 11.3.1, minor changes in the choice of scores for exposure—which may change a linear trend in the risk of D against some unknown "true" scores into a nonlinear association with the chosen scores—are unlikely to make a substantial difference in the power of the test for trend.

11.4 Example—the Western Collaborative Group Study: part 6

The techniques of this chapter are used to examine the association between body weight and incidence of CHD. For the time being we ignore the role of behavior type. Table 11.3 provides the relevant information abstracted from Table 9.2 or Table 10.5. For the data in this table, $\chi^2_{overall} = 21.4$, yielding a p-value of 0.0003 from tables of a χ^2 distribution with 4 degrees of freedom, strong evidence of an association between levels of body weight and incidence of CHD. We now use the test for trend to examine whether this association reflects increasing (or decreasing) risk as body weight increases.

Examined first are some plots of estimated risk of D against body weight. Here we use the codes $x = 0$ for the stratum with body weight less than or equal to 150 lb, $x = 1$ for body weights between 150 and 160 lb, and so on, up to $x = 4$ for the group with body weight greater than 180 lb. With regard to trends, these scores are, of course, equivalent to the choices $x = 145, 155, 165, 175$, and 185, which roughly correspond to the midpoints of the body weight intervals. Figure 11.2 shows plots of the estimated risk, odds, and log odds of CHD for each body weight category against x, the relevant code. It is often helpful to add confidence interval bars to each of these estimated risks to reflect the amount of sampling variation. The pattern of risk change is extremely similar in each plot, reflecting that with the low risk values observed in

Table 11.3 *Body weight and coronary heart disease*

		CHD Event		
		D	not D	
Body weight (lb)	≤150	32	558	590
	150+–160	31	505	536
	160+–170	50	594	644
	170+–180	66	501	567
	>180	78	739	817
		257	2897	3154

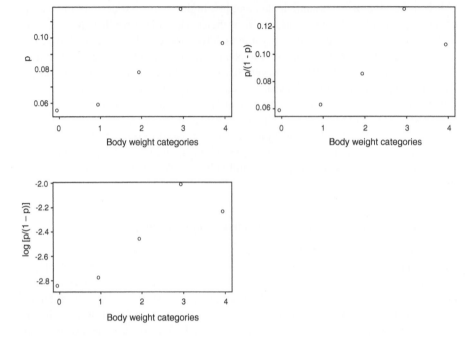

Figure 11.2 *Plots of the estimated risk ($p = \hat{P}(D|X = x)$), odds ($p/(1 - p)$), and log odds ($\log(p/(1 - p))$) for CHD for various body weight categories.*

the data, there is little difference between relative differences in p, $p/(1 - p)$ and $\log(p/(1 - p))$. Thus, although the test for trend is designed to detect linear changes in the risk $P(D|X = x)$, it will be just as effective in highlighting linear trends in the odds or log odds.

The plot of $\hat{P}(D|X = x)$ against x, while not monotonic, suggests a strong linear component in the change in risk as x, body weight, increases, using the simple scale chosen. We examine this formally using the test for trend. The test statistic, Equation 11.2, is then

$$\chi^2_{trend} = \frac{3154^3}{257 \times 2897}$$

$$\times \frac{\left[0 + 1\left(31 - \frac{257 \times 536}{3154}\right) + \cdots + 4\left(78 - \frac{257 \times 817}{3154}\right)\right]^2}{[3154(0 + (1^2 \times 536) + \cdots + (4^2 \times 817)) - (0 + (1 \times 536) + \cdots + (4 \times 817))^2]}$$

$$= \frac{3154^3}{257 \times 2897} \times \frac{7652.8}{20,994,349}$$

$$= 15.4.$$

Under the null hypothesis of independence, this statistic approximately follows a χ^2 distribution with one degree of freedom, yielding the associated p-value of 0.00009.

There is thus striking evidence of an increasing trend in risk of CHD as body weight increases. (Note that the smaller p-value here, as compared with the overall test, is explained by the clear presence of a strong trend, as illustrated in Figure 11.2.) Finally, the goodness of fit test statistic $\chi^2_{gof} = 21.4 - 15.4 = 6.0$, which when compared with a χ^2 distribution with 3 degrees of freedom gives a p-value of 0.11. There is thus no major evidence that the linear trend gives an inadequate description of the pattern of increasing risk for CHD as body weight increases (see Figure 11.2).

11.5 Example—coffee drinking and pancreatic cancer: part 4

We now return to the data from Table 11.2 for further examination of the relationship between coffee consumption and pancreatic cancer. In particular, we examine evidence of a trend in the apparent association observed in Section 11.2. Before performing the test for trend in Section 11.3, we look at the estimated Odds Ratios that measure changes in risk of pancreatic cancer at various levels of coffee consumption against the baseline group of coffee abstainers. From Table 11.2, we see that $\widehat{OR}_2 = (153 \times 88)/(271 \times 20) = 2.5$, suggesting that individuals who regularly consume 1 to 2 cups of coffee per day have more than a twofold higher risk of pancreatic cancer than those who never drink coffee. Similarly, $\widehat{OR}_3 = 3.0$ and $\widehat{OR}_4 = 3.0$ if we compare the groups who drink 3 to 4 and more than 5 cups per day, respectively, to the baseline group. Thus, there is an immediate increase in risk as coffee consumption increases from abstinence, but only slight further risk increases are observed after the first jump from nondrinkers to the 1 to 2 cups-per-day group. After this initial increase, the risk seems surprisingly flat as coffee consumption increases.

We can display this graphically by plotting the naïvely estimated odds for pancreatic cancer, from Table 11.2, against the level of coffee consumption, as shown in Figure 11.3. It would be natural to try to mimic the actual amount of coffee consumption in each group by choosing $x_1 = 0$ for the nondrinkers, $x_2 = 1.5$ for the 1 to 2 cups-per-day group, and so on. Some form of reasonable but arbitrary level needs to be chosen for the group defined by more than 5 cups per day. It is easier and just as plausible to simply use the values $x_1 = 0$ (0 cups per day), $x_2 = 1$ (1 to 2 cups per day), $x_3 = 2$ (3 to 4 cups per day), and $x_4 = 3$ (≥ 5 cups per day), as we do in Figure 11.3. Further, these codes should make very little difference to the test for trend as compared to alternatives such as $x_1 = 0$, $x_2 = 1.5$, $x_3 = 3.5$, and $x_4 = 5.5$.

Note that the scale on the Y-axis in Figure 11.3 cannot be interpreted in terms of the population log odds of disease due to case-control sampling. However, the vertical distances between the plotted points at differing levels of coffee consumption do reflect the analogous population quantities, that is, log Odds Ratios, as discussed in Chapter 5.3. Thus, the *shape* of the plot is meaningful in a population sense even though the values on the Y-axis are not. Further, as for Figure 11.2, given the low risk of pancreatic cancer in the population, this shape is similar to what would be observed in a plot of the estimated risk, $\hat{P}(D|X = x)$, against x.

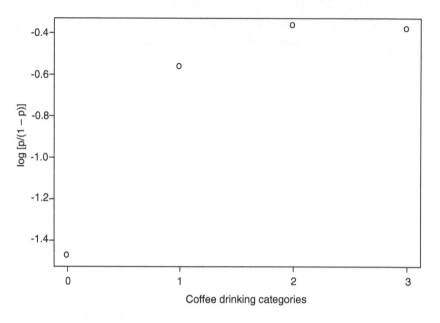

Figure 11.3 *Plots of the observed log odds* ($\log(p/(1-p))$) *for incidence of pancreatic cancer for various coffee drinking categories.*

With $x_1 = 0$, $x_2 = 1$, $x_3 = 2$, and $x_4 = 3$, the test for trend calculation is

$$\chi^2_{trend} = \frac{1010^3}{367 \times 643}$$

$$\times \frac{\left[0 + 1\left(153 - \frac{367 \times 424}{1010}\right) + \cdots + 3\left(88 - \frac{367 \times 218}{1010}\right)\right]^2}{[1010(0 + (1^2 \times 424) + \cdots + (3^2 \times 218)) - (0 + (1 \times 424) + \cdots + (3 \times 218))^2]}$$

$$= \frac{1010^3}{367 \times 643} \times \frac{2336.8}{906,656}$$

$$= 11.3.$$

Under the null hypothesis of independence, this statistic follows approximately a χ^2 distribution with one degree of freedom; the value 11.3 yields a p-value of 0.0008 for the χ^2 test for trend. There is thus strong evidence of an increasing trend in incidence of pancreatic cancer as coffee consumption increases, as reflected in Figure 11.3. Here, however, the goodness of fit statistic is $\chi^2_{gof} = 18.6 - 11.3 = 7.3$, which, when compared to a χ^2 distribution with 2 degrees of freedom, yields a p-value of 0.026. This suggests that a linear trend is insufficient to describe the pattern of increasing risk with greater coffee consumption. As in our examination of the Odds Ratios at each level of coffee drinking, as compared to nondrinkers, in Figure 11.3, there appears to be a (nonlinear) threshold relationship. The risk increases immediately with some coffee drinking (1 to 2 cups per day) and then stays flat for the groups with even greater consumption. This observation undermines the plausibility of a causal relation between coffee drinking and pancreatic cancer, although we acknowledge that the quantitative assessment of consumption is crude and therefore some mismeasurement of exposure may have occurred among the coffee drinkers.

11.6 Adjustment for confounding, exact tests, and interaction

Just as we adjusted the χ^2 test for independence for a single 2×2 table, all of the tests in this chapter can be modified to allow for the potential confounding effects of extraneous variables using the Cochran–Mantel–Haenszel procedure of Chapter 9.1. In particular, we describe the extension of the test for trend (see Equation 11.2) to allow stratification on one or more possible confounders. We use notation akin to that of Chapter 9, in that the subscript i denotes the data from Table 11.1 that are assigned to the ith stratum; the index i ranges over the I strata, defined by common levels of the confounding variables. To describe the adjusted test statistic concisely, we set

$$\bar{a}_k = \sum_{i=1}^{I} a_{ki}$$

$$\bar{A}_k = \sum_{i=1}^{I} A_{ki} = \sum_{i=1}^{I} \frac{n_{Di} m_{ki}}{n_i}$$

$$\bar{m}_k = \sum_{i=1}^{I} m_{ki}$$

$$\bar{n}_D = \sum_{i=1}^{I} n_{Di}, \qquad \bar{n}_{\bar{D}} = \sum_{i=1}^{I} n_{\bar{D}i}.$$

We can now calculate a test statistic for trend, controlling for the effects of the stratifying variables (and assuming no interaction between these variables and the exposure of interest) as

$$\chi^2_{trend(adjusted)} = \frac{\left[\sum_{k=1}^{K} x_k (\bar{a}_k - \bar{A}_k) \right]^2}{\sum_{i=1}^{I} \frac{n_{Di} n_{\bar{D}i}}{n_i - 1} \left[\sum_{k=1}^{K} x_k^2 \left(\frac{m_{ki}}{n_i} \right) - \left(\sum_{k=1}^{K} x_k \left(\frac{m_{ki}}{n_i} \right) \right)^2 \right]},$$

which again approximately follows a χ^2 distribution with one degree of freedom under independence of D and E. Here, the assumption of no interaction indicates that the trend in risk, if it exists, is considered to be consistent across all strata. Note that this adjusted test statistic simplifies to the Cochran–Mantel–Haenszel statistic (Equation 9.1) with only two levels of exposure. Further, if there is only one stratum, the statistic is the same as Equation 11.2, with the term $n^2(n-1)$ replacing n^3.

The value of $\chi^2_{trend(adjusted)}$ for the data in Table 11.2, now stratified by sex (see Table 7.2), is 8.6. Tables of a χ^2 distribution with one degree of freedom yield a p-value of 0.003. Note that the adjusted test for trend statistic is somewhat less than the unadjusted value, 11.3 (see Section 11.5). This reflects a moderate amount of confounding (due to sex), compatible with what we have previously noted in other analyses of this data.

Various interactive effects between the stratifying variables and the exposure of interest may be studied. In the context of an overall test of association, interaction usually reflects differences in the pattern of association between D and E over strata. When examining trend, it may be most useful to consider interaction in terms of whether any trend in risk, as exposure increases, is consistent from stratum to stratum. We defer further discussion of assessment of these varying forms of interaction to the following chapters on regression models, where such issues are most naturally addressed.

For small samples, exact tests are available for each of the testing scenarios considered in this chapter; see Mehta and Patel (1998) for a summary with relevant references.

11.7 Comments and further reading

In light of our comments in Chapter 6.1.1 regarding focus on estimation, it is odd to stop this chapter when all we have discussed relates to hypothesis tests. Figures 11.2 and 11.3 beg for a quantitative description of how the risks for CHD and pancreatic cancer change as exposures are modified. Statistical approaches to this question fall under the rubric of *regression models*, which are covered in the next chapters. Chapters 12 to 15 introduce highly structured regression models where risk changes are assumed to follow prescribed patterns such as linearity. In Chapter 17, we briefly discuss more flexible approaches that allow the data to suggest the way in which exposure levels influence risk.

It is possible for nondifferential misclassification of exposures with several categories to lead to an apparent trend that is the reverse of the true pattern (Dosemeci et al., 1990). However, such behavior is unusual. Nondifferential misclassification typically "weakens" the association, for example, by decreasing the slope of the linear pattern of Figure 11.1. Weinberg et al. (1995) discuss situations that guarantee, modulo sampling variation, that misclassification cannot change the direction of a trend.

We have said little about the choice of exposure categories or the singling out of one particular level as the baseline or reference group, although we return to the topic briefly in Chapter 12.6.1. The choice of baseline group can affect the appearance of plots of Odds Ratios or log Odds Ratios when there are few observations in the reference category. This is because the variability of all comparative measures is necessarily high due to the lack of information in the baseline group. This is why we prefer to plot risks, odds, or log odds directly as we do in Figures 11.2 and 11.3. More sophisticated approaches to plotting effect measures against risk levels are described in Easton et al (1991).

11.8 Problems

Question 11.1

Suppose you are investigating the pattern of how the risk of a disease, D, changes over four ordered levels of beef consumption (e.g., eats no beef, eats beef less than once a week, eats beef about once a week, eats beef more than once a week):

Table 11.4 *Case-control data on biomass fuel exposure and tuberculosis, stratified by age*

		Exposure and Tuberculosis Distribution	
		Exposure among Cases	Exposure among Controls
	<25	8/59	7/133
	26–35	7/54	6/150
Age group (in years)	36–45	12/53	3/120
	46–55	8/61	3/120
	>55	15/61	1/57

1. Describe a scenario where a χ^2 test for trend will have less power to detect an association between beef consumption and the disease than the overall χ^2 test of association.

2. Suppose you calculate both χ^2_{trend} and $\chi^2_{overall}$. The goodness of fit statistic $\chi^2_{gof} = \chi^2_{overall} - \chi^2_{trend}$ is calculated to be 13.8. How many degrees of freedom should be used for the reference χ^2 distribution? What is your interpretation of the observed χ^2_{gof}?

Question 11.2

The data on biomass cooking fuel exposure and tuberculosis (Perez-Padilla et al., 2001) (see Question 6.4) included additional information on age of the respondent. Table 11.4 provides the data on exposure and tuberculosis across various age subgroups. For example, among respondents less than 25 years old, there were 59 tuberculosis cases, of whom 8 were exposed, and 133 controls, of whom 7 were exposed.

Ignoring biomass fuel exposure for the moment, perform an overall test for the association between age and tuberculosis and report a p-value. Now perform a test for trend to evaluate the evidence for increasing risk of tuberculosis with age.

Estimate the Odds Ratio for tuberculosis associated with indoor pollution for each age stratum separately. Qualitatively describe your assessment of how age modifies the effect of biomass fuel exposure on tuberculosis.

Question 11.3

The data set *oesoph*, found by going to http://www.crcpress.com/e_products/downloads/, contains more detailed information on alcohol consumption; see Question 7.3. Using the full data on four levels of alcohol consumption, perform an overall test for the association between alcohol consumption and incidence of esophageal cancer. Also assess the evidence for increasing risk over the four increasing levels of alcohol consumption, with an appropriate choice of ordered code, k, say, for each of the consumption groups. Make two plots with (1) $\hat{p}_k = \hat{P}(\text{case}|\text{alcohol level } k)$ and (2) OR_k (Odds Ratio for kth level vs. baseline level of 0 to 39 g/day alcohol consumption) on the Y-axis, both against k on the X-axis. Interpret the results of the two tests in light of these plots.

Question 11.4

Using the data set, *titanic*, found by going to http://www.crcpress.com/e_products/ downloads/, examine the existence of a trend in the risk of dying as a passenger's ticket class changes from 1st to 2nd to 3rd. Plot the Relative Risk of dying for each ticket class using the 1st class passengers as the reference group, and plot the three Relative Risks against the ticket class.

CHAPTER 12

Regression Models Relating Exposure to Disease

The stratification methods discussed in Chapters 9 and 10 are effective for addressing the issues of confounding and interaction in studies with large sample sizes. In addition, if availability of data is not a concern, the techniques of Chapter 11 work well in considering the role of an exposure level that has many levels, possibly ordered. Although these techniques work well in a wide variety of situations, there are substantial challenges still to face.

As noted in Chapter 2, we are keenly interested in effective and refined measurement of exposure when identifying an association with a disease outcome. The methods of Chapter 11 allow analysis of exposures at several discrete levels; nevertheless, both the need to (1) accommodate more refined exposure measurements and to (2) elucidate the pattern of disease risks over a variety of exposure levels, as illustrated in our discussion of linear and nonlinear trends in risks, suggest consideration of succinct models that relate exposure to disease risk. *Regression models* provide exactly such a tool. Now that we have entered the real world, where coffee drinking can be measured by more than just "yes" or "no," we are chomping at the bit for methods that allow us to describe changes in risk invoked by incremental changes in exposure. If drinking one cup of coffee per day increases your risk, is two cups per day twice as bad? If an increase of 50 lb over an ideal weight doubles your risk of a disease, does 100 lb double the risk again, or have an even worse effect? Regression models can also be an effective tool in describing interactive effects as hinted at in Chapter 10.3.4.

There is a more fundamental statistical argument behind the value of regression models. In Chapter 9.5.1, we noted that estimation of the association between a primary exposure and a disease is usually less precise when it is necessary to stratify on many potential confounding variables simultaneously. This is because the balance on the marginals at the stratum level tends to deteriorate as an increasing level of stratification is used to remove confounding bias. In the pooled table balance can be controlled, at least on one marginal, in either cohort or case-control studies. However, there is no guarantee that even this balance can be maintained as the sample is divided into a large number of strata. Stratifying on even a moderate number of potential confounders leads to a very large number of strata, accompanied by an ever increasing loss of marginal balance, with the consequence of imprecise estimates of adjusted measures of association. For example, in the analysis of the Western Collaborative Group Study data of Table 9.2, we considered just five body weight strata; however, if we now wish to further adjust the analysis for the potential confounding effects of smoking history (say, three levels), initial serum cholesterol (say, four levels), initial blood pressure (say, three levels), we would then have to juggle 180 ($= 5 \times 3 \times 4 \times 3$) strata to ensure common levels of each confounder in a given stratum. And this level of complexity is required to control merely four confounders in a situation where there are plausibly several others of importance. At this fine level of stratification, the methods of Chapters 9, 10, and 11 simply break down with regard to maintaining reasonable levels of precision. Further, classifying exposures in smaller number of categories is a false economy because this strategy increases residual confounding and measurement error, which may more than offset apparent precision gains from fewer strata.

What then can we do in such situations, which are common to most if not all studies? Increasing the sample size in the design is one approach, but clearly raises the cost of studies substantially and is not an option *post facto*. The next obvious alternative would be to ensure against any loss of balance, on at least some marginals, through a *design strategy* known as *matching*. For example, in the case-control study of pancreatic cancer, we might choose a similar ratio of cases and controls for both sexes in our sample design, effectively carrying out a mini case-control study for each sex separately and then combining the information. Matching has a long history in observational studies, discussed at greater length in Chapter 16.

Absent a design strategy, how can we accommodate the role of many explanatory factors in our analysis without the concomitant loss of precision? A natural way to increase information in one stratum, that in itself is not particularly informative, is to "borrow" information from other strata where there may be more data on the relationship of interest. One way to achieve a link between strata is through the use of "smoothing," or, in more familiar terminology, a *regression model*. Figure 12.1 illustrates this idea schematically for a single exposure variable X.

Notice here that we wish to understand the relationship between risk of D and E at two disparate levels of exposure, one around the values $E = x_1 - x_2$, the other containing $E = x_3 - x_4$. We may be faced with a limited sample size in one or both of these regions of exposure. A smooth regression model allows us to

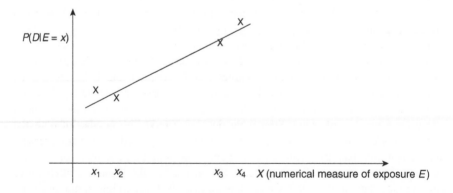

Figure 12.1 *Schematic linking effects at disparate levels of a risk factor.*

link the behavior of $P(D|E = x)$ in one region of exposure to another, thereby making effective use of the sample information in both exposure regions. Figure 12.1 illustrates this idea for a linear model that is, by nature, extremely smooth. The disadvantage of such models is that the smooth link—in Figure 12.1 a straight line in the scale of $P(D|E = x)$—may not be an accurate description of population risk, and taking advantage of such a regression model can thereby lead to distorted or biased estimates of population effects. The gain, as discussed, is an efficient use of sample information when simultaneously adjusting for many possible risk or confounding factors, mitigating a degradation in precision as occurs with fine levels of stratification. Note that in comparison, stratification approaches make no use of the definition of the strata; for example, the methods ignore the fact that a stratum of individuals whose body weight is <150 lb is "closer" to the stratum with body weights between 150 and 160 lb than to the stratum of weights >180 lb. Regression techniques take advantage of such information through model assumptions. Further, regression models often provide a simple and parsimonious description of the joint effects of risk factors on the risk of D, thereby allowing targeted examination of such effects and their possible interaction. In the remainder of this chapter we introduce some basic regression models, all of which use the concept of linearity, their chief difference being the chosen scale for $P(D|E = x)$.

12.1 Some introductory regression models

For convenience, and for consistency with standard treatments of regression models, we now label our exposure variable of interest with X instead of E. This reinforces the possibility that exposure may now be measured on a continuous scale, while not ruling out discrete risk factors. For an exposure variable X, we are interested in how the risk for D changes as the amount of exposure changes; that is, how does $P(D|X = x)$ depend on x? For simplicity, write $p_x = P(D|X = x)$.

In an ideal world we would like to see the plot of p_x against x, since this graph would tell us everything about the risk for disease at all possible exposure levels. In fact, for discrete or grouped exposure variables, such plots were extremely useful in examining the possibility of risk trends; see Figures 11.2 and 11.3. However, we also want to allow for the possibility of continuously scaled exposure variables where there may only be a single sampled individual that exhibits a specific exposure level. In such cases, we do not have sufficient data to tackle direct estimation of risk plots, in general. Regression models provide the simplifying assumptions necessary to allow description, and plots, of risk and exposure relationships.

12.1.1 The linear model

The simplest model that comes to mind is the *linear model*, ubiquitous in other applications. In this context, the linear model can be described by

$$p_x = P(D|X = x) = a + bx. \tag{12.1}$$

This model assumes that as the exposure level $X = x$ changes, the risk changes *linearly in x*. The two numbers a and b are *model parameters* and particular values of these parameters determine the specific linear model that applies to a given population. That is, as you modify either a or b or both, a new linear model is determined. In this sense, the linear model is a family of models indexed by the values of a and b. The parameters a and b are often referred to as the *intercept* and *slope* parameters, respectively.

In using any regression model effectively, our first responsibility is to understand the explicit meaning of the various parameters of the model, here a and b. First, note that when $X = 0$, the linear model yields $p_0 = a$. Therefore, a is simply the risk of D when $X = 0$, often referred to as the baseline or reference value of X.

Now, consider two levels of exposure that differ by *one unit on the scale of X*, say, $X = x + 1$ and $X = x$. If X denotes coffee consumption in cups per day, then a unit increase in exposure refers to an additional cup of coffee per day; if X denotes body weight, measured in pounds, then a unit change in X is simply one pound difference in weight. Note the dependence of a "unit change" on the scale in which X is quantified. The linear model tells us that the difference in the risks of D at the levels, $X = x + 1$ and $X = x$, is just

$$p_{x+1} - p_x = P(D|X = x + 1) - P(D|X = x) = [a + b(x + 1)] - [a + bx] = b.$$

So, the slope parameter b is simply the Excess Risk associated with a unit increase (in the scale of X) of exposure. In general, when comparing two levels of exposure, the model (Equation 12.1) assumes that the Excess Risk in going from, say, a group with exposure $X = x$ to a group with $X = x^*$ is given by $ER = b(x^* - x)$. Note that the Excess Risk associated with a unit increase in X does not depend on what level of X you start from. For example, suppose the linear model (Equation 12.1) with parameters a and b describes the relationship between the risk of infant mortality and birthweight, measured in grams (X). The model has the following interpretation and consequences: first, the intercept a refers to the risk of infant mortality for a baby with zero birthweight $(X = 0)$! This is, of course, an extrapolation beyond the range of values of X in the population. Second, the Excess Risk comparing babies with birthweights of 2001 g to those with birthweight 2000 g is given by b; similarly, the Excess Risk comparing babies with birthweights of 2501 g to those with birthweight 2500 g is also b. The fact that the Excess Risk associated with a unit increase in X does not depend on which level of X the increase is measured from is, of course, the heart of the linear assumption—risk goes up in a straight line.

In this example, neither of the parameters has a particularly useful interpretation: zero birthweight is not possible, and an increase in birthweight of 1 g is too small to expect any meaningful increase in mortality risk. Recentering the scale of birthweight to be, say, $X = $ birthweight $- 2500$ g gives an intercept with a more useful interpretation. With regard to the slope parameter, it is possible immediately to obtain the Excess Risk associated with an increase of 100 g in birthweight, since this is just $100b$. More directly, one can simply rescale birthweight in terms of 100 g, for instance. Both of these changes would lead to a new scale given by $X^* = (X - 2500)/100 = $ (birthweight $- 2500)/100$. Of course, a linear model applies in this scale if and only if it applies in the original scale in grams; the advantage of the new scale, with the resulting linear model $p_{x^*} = a + bx^*$, is a more simple and direct interpretation of the intercept (risk of infant mortality at 2500 g) and slope (Excess Risk for infant mortality associated with an increase of 100 g in birthweight) parameters. These brief remarks also show that while a linear change in scale for an exposure does not change the basic assumption of linearity underlying Equation 12.1, the interpretation of the parameters a and b are tied to the particular scale chosen. Nonlinear changes in exposure scales require a quite different linear model since unit increases at various levels now carry different meaning.

12.1.2 Pros and cons of the linear model

As the interpretation of b reveals, the linear model is most useful for modeling Excess Risk. It is difficult to translate the parameters directly into a Relative Risk or Odds Ratio. A further consequence is that the linear model cannot be directly applied to case-control data since Excess Risks cannot be estimated from such designs without additional information.

There is an additional structural drawback to use of the linear model with binary outcome data. Whatever the value of the parameters a and b ($\neq 0$), at some values in the range of X, either low values or high values, the model (Equation 12.1) predicts values of $p_x < 0$ or $p_x > 1$, not permissible for risks. This may not be a practical concern when this occurs for X values that are far from those observed in the population; for example, if the risk of infant mortality is predicted to become negative for birthweights less than 10 g. However, in cases where the risks are either very low or very high, the true values of risk are already close to these boundaries, and it may be safer to use a model that does not allow for negative risks or risks greater than one. Section 12.5 gives a simple example of the linear model at the population level.

12.2 The log linear model

An alternative specification to the linear model that has been used extensively is the *log linear model*, which invokes linearity in the relationship between the log risk and exposure. That is, we have

$$\log(p_x) = \log(P(D|X = x)) = a + bx, \qquad (12.2)$$

or equivalently,

$$p_x = P(D|X = x) = e^{a+bx}.$$

Using the same approach as for the linear model, we can easily interpret the two parameters a and b. Specifically, a is the log of the risk at the baseline level $X = 0$. Equivalently, this risk, $P(D|X = 0)$, is given by e^a. Comparing two groups, one unit apart in their exposure levels, Equation 12.2 yields

$$\log(p_{x+1}) - \log(p_x) = [a + b(x + 1)] - [a + bx] = b.$$

But $\log(p_{x+1}) - \log(p_x) = \log(p_{x+1}/p_x) = \log[P(D|X = x + 1)/P(D|X = x)]$, so that b is just the log Relative Risk associated with a unit increase in exposure.

Equivalently, e^b is the Relative Risk associated with a unit increase in the level of X. Again, note that this Relative Risk does not change whether you raise exposure starting from $X = 1$, $X = 5$, $X = 100$, or any other value, reflecting the core of the linear assumption in Equation 12.2. As with the linear model, simple translation or constant rescaling can be used on the original scale of X to make the parameters more immediately relevant to an application.

The log linear model is useful when the Relative Risk is the primary measure of association. Since e^{a+bx} can never be negative, this model avoids one of the structural issues of the linear model; however, the risk e^{a+bx} can still exceed one for any nonzero value of b with large (or small, depending on the sign of b) values of X. Given the role of the Relative Risk within the log linear model, it is not surprising that this model cannot be applied directly to traditional case-control data.

12.3 The probit model

The probit model is one model designed to avoid the possibility of negative risks or risks greater than 1, by choosing a relationship between x and p_x that cannot take values outside the range 0 to 1. Specifically, the probit model is given by

$$p_x = P(D|X = x) = \Phi(a + bx),$$

where $\Phi(u)$ is the area under the standard Normal curve to the left of u, as illustrated in Figure 12.2. Note that as $u = a + bx$ increases from very large negative to large

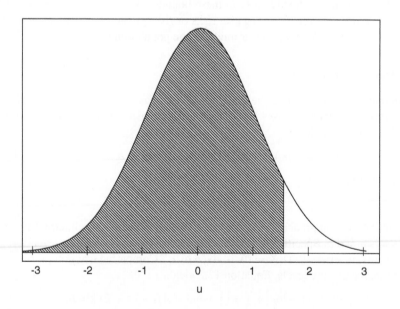

Figure 12.2 *Plot of the standard normal density, N(0, 1): shaded area to the left of a value, e.g., u = 1.5, = $\Phi(u)$, the cumulative normal distribution.*

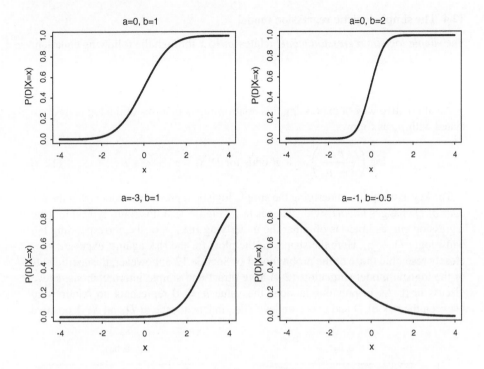

Figure 12.3 *Plot of the probit relationship for various choices of parameters a, b.*

positive, $p_x = \Phi(a + bx)$, the area to the left of $a + bx$, grows from 0 to 1, but can never be negative or larger than 1.

The probit model reflects a monotonic dose-response since, if $b > 0$, the risk of D increases as the exposure level x increases, while the risk decreases as x increases if $b < 0$. Typical probit curves are shown in Figure 12.3. These plots illustrate the pattern of change in risk as exposure increases or decreases. Note that this model is appropriate if the binary outcome D is believed to represent whether an underlying— and unobserved—continuous measure of disease, say, Y, exceeds a fixed threshold Y_0 or not (that is, $D = 1$ if $Y > Y_0$ and $D = 0$ if $Y \leq Y_0$), where the population mean of this continuous measure Y varies linearly with X, as in standard linear regression. As in the linear model, the null value of the parameter b is $b = 0$ since then the exposure level x has no effect on the risk of D. However, there is no natural interpretation of the parameter b in terms of the measures of association introduced so far. Qualitatively, the larger the (positive) value of b, the faster risk grows with increasing exposure, and vice versa.

As with the other regression models, the parameter a is a measure of the risk when the exposure $X = 0$; in this case, $P(D|X = 0) = p_0 = \Phi(a)$. As a consequence, we cannot hope to estimate a from case-control data; in addition, it is impossible to estimate b from this study design without additional information.

12.4 The simple logistic regression model

The *simple logistic regression model* relates p_x to x through the following equation:

$$p_x = P(D|X = x) = \frac{1}{1 + e^{-(a+bx)}}. \tag{12.3}$$

An alternative way of expressing this relationship is in terms of the log odds associated with p_x as follows:

$$\log\left(\frac{p_x}{1 - p_x}\right) = \log(\text{ odds for } D|X = x) = a + bx. \tag{12.4}$$

The key assumption underlying the simple logistic regression model is that the *log odds of D* changes *linearly* with changes in X. Figure 12.4 illustrates typical logistic regression curves in terms of either the underlying risk, p, or the corresponding log odds, $\log(p/1 - p)$. Here the shapes of the plots for the risk against exposure very closely resemble those of the probit model of Section 12.3; however, the coefficients of the logistic model (Equation 12.4) have direct and simple interpretations, as we discuss next. As in previous models, the value $b = 0$ represents no relationship between the risk of D and exposure level, i.e., independence of D and X. A positive

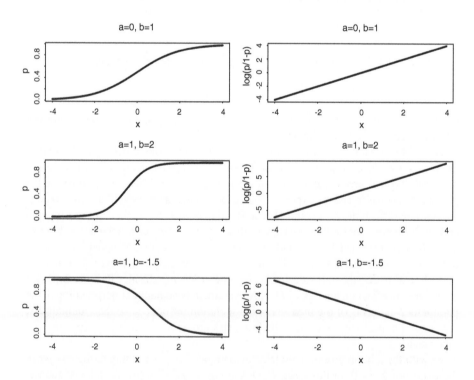

Figure 12.4 *Plot of the logistic relationship (Equation 12.3 or 12.4) for various choices of parameters a, b, both on the scale of risk ($p = P(D|X = x)$) and log odds ($\log(p/1 - p)$).*

value of b reflects increasing risk of D as exposure increases, and a negative value indicates decreasing risk as the level of exposure increases.

12.4.1 Interpretation of logistic regression parameters

We turn to interpretation of the two parameters, the intercept a and the slope b of the logistic regression model, Equation 12.3 or 12.4. We first consider the by-now familiar situation where the exposure variable X takes on only two values, say, $X = 1$ (exposed) and $X = 0$ (unexposed). We can easily understand the meaning of a and b in this context. First, when $X = 0$, we have $\log(p_0/1 - p_0) = a + (b \times 0) = a$. It follows that a is the log odds of D amongst the unexposed. In addition, comparing the exposed to the unexposed yields the Odds Ratio, OR, via

$$
\begin{aligned}
\log(OR) &= \log \left[\frac{\text{odds of } D | X = 1}{\text{odds of } D | X = 0} \right] \\
&= \log \left[\frac{p_1/(1 - p_1)}{p_0/(1 - p_0)} \right] \\
&= \log[p_1/(1 - p_1)] - \log[p_0/(1 - p_0)] \\
&= (a + b \cdot 1) - (a + b \cdot 0) \\
&= b.
\end{aligned}
$$

Thus, the slope parameter b is just the log Odds Ratio.

If X has several discrete (numerical) levels or is measured on a continuous scale, there is no change in the interpretation of a (the log odds of D when $X = 0$). To understand the slope parameter b, consider two exposure levels separated by one unit on the scale of X, say, $X = x + 1$ and $X = x$. Then the log Odds Ratio comparing these two exposure groups is

$$
\begin{aligned}
\log(OR) &= \log \left[\frac{(\text{odds of } D | X = x + 1)}{(\text{odds of } D | X = x)} \right] \\
&= \log \left[\frac{p_{x+1}/(1 - p_{x+1})}{p_x/(1 - p_x)} \right] \\
&= \log[p_{x+1}/(1 - p_{x+1})] - \log[p_x/(1 - p_x)] \\
&= [a + b \cdot (x + 1)] - [a + b \cdot x] \\
&= b.
\end{aligned}
$$

Thus, b is the log Odds Ratio associated with comparing two exposure groups whose exposure differs by *one unit on the scale of X*, that is, the log Odds Ratio associated with a unit increase in X. Again, the defining assumption of the logistic regression model is that this Odds Ratio, associated with a unit increase in X, does not depend on the choice of the baseline value X from which this unit increase is measured. For example, if X measures coffee consumption in cups/day, the model (Equation 12.4) indicates that the log Odds Ratio comparing exposures of 2 and 1 cups/day is b, as is also the log Odds Ratio comparing exposures of 5 and 4 cups/day; both these comparisons correspond to an increase in exposure of 1 unit on the selected scale. The value of b is therefore intimately connected to the particular exposure scale used. Different (albeit closely related) slope parameters would be needed if you measure the risk factor age (X) in years as against months; in the first case, a unit increase in X corresponds to a 1 year age difference, whereas with the second choice it corresponds to only a 1 month age difference.

Since the term $e^{-(a+bx)}$ is always positive, it is easy to see from Equation 12.3 that p_x must lie between 0 and 1 for any choice of the parameters a and b and at any level of the exposure X. Thus the logistic regression model does not suffer from the awkwardness of suggesting either a negative risk or a risk greater than one at some exposures. Further, it is relatively straightforward to estimate the logistic regression *slope* parameter from data generated from any design, including a case-control study, as discussed in Chapter 13.3.

12.5 Simple examples of the models with a binary exposure

Before we go further it is helpful to apply the various regression models to a population with a simple binary exposure. We use the example introduced in Table 3.1 relating a mother's marital status with subsequent infant mortality (D), with the relevant information repeated in Table 12.1 for convenience. Since there are only two levels of this exposure, we can code them as $X = 1$ (unmarried mother) and $X = 0$ (married mother). Since it is always possible to draw a straight line through 2 points, we can link the risks at $X = 0$ and $X = 1$ using any of the regression models introduced earlier in the chapter. Another way of saying this is that there is no substance to the regression assumption here, as there are only two possible levels of exposure.

Specifically, since $p_1 = 16,712/1,213,854 = 0.0138$ and $p_0 = 18,784/2,897,205 = 0.0065$, it follows that the linear regression model is given by

$$p_x = 0.0065 + 0.0073x.$$

Note that the slope 0.0073 is just the Excess Risk for infant mortality for an unmarried mother. Similarly, for the log linear model we have $a = \log p_0 = \log 0.0065 = -5.0385$ and $b = \log(\frac{p_1}{p_0}) = 0.7531$, so that this model is given by

$$\log(p_x) = -5.0385 + 0.7531x.$$

Table 12.1 *1991 U.S. infant mortality by mother's marital status*

Infant Mortality	Mother's Marital Status		Total
	Unmarried	Married	
Death	16,712	18,784	35,496
Live at 1 year	1,197,142	2,878,421	4,075,563
Total	1,213,854	2,897,205	4,111,059

Source: National Center for Health Statistics.

Again, this yields the Relative Risk associated with an unmarried status of $e^{0.7531} = 2.12$. For the probit regression model we have $p_0 = 0.0065 = \Phi(a)$, so that $a = -2.4847$. Similarly, $\Phi(a + b) = 0.0138$, so that $a + b = -2.2038$ yielding $b = 0.2808$. Therefore, the probit regression model is given by

$$p_x = \Phi(-2.4847 + 0.2808x).$$

Finally, for the logistic regression model we have $a = \log(p_0/(1 - p_0)) = -5.0294$ and $b = \log(p_1/(1 - p_1)) - \log(p_0/(1 - p_0)) = 0.7602$. This gives the logistic regression model:

$$\log\left(\frac{p_x}{1 - p_x}\right) = -5.0320 + 0.7604x,$$

yielding an Odds Ratio of $e^{0.7604} = 2.14$.

Note that in all four of these models, the positive values of the slope coefficient b reflect the increasing risk for infant mortality as you move from the group of married mothers ($X = 0$) to unmarried mothers ($X = 1$). Figure 12.5 shows how each of these four models exactly "fits" the population information, in that the regression curves pass through the known risks at $X = 0$ and $X = 1$. Of course, in this case there is no meaning for risks at any other values of X since none logically exist. However, in Section 12.6.1 we consider a more complex example with several levels of exposure.

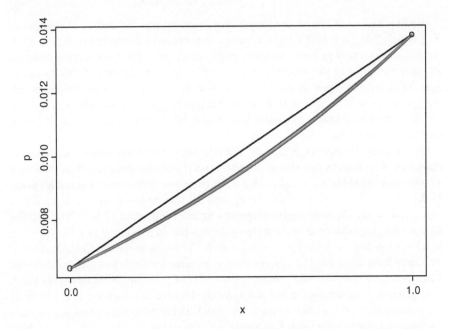

Figure 12.5 *Fitted versions of the linear, log linear, probit, and logistic regression models for infant mortality, based on a binary exposure variable, mother's marital status.*

It is, of course, only the simplicity of a binary exposure variable here that allows all four regression models to apply to the same population simultaneously. For more complex risk factor situations, the models will all be different (although, in rare disease situations like this example, the log linear and logistic regression models will be similar).

12.6 Multiple logistic regression model

Suppose we now have several risk factors that we wish to relate to the risk for D. For convenience we label these risk factors by $X_1, \ldots, X_k$; each of these factors may be discrete or continuous. At given "exposure" levels, say, $X_1 = x_1, \ldots, X_k = x_k$, we use $p_{x_1, \ldots, x_k}$ to denote $P(D|X_1 = x_1, \ldots, X_k = x_k)$.

The most obvious way to extend the simple logistic regression model to accommodate k risk variables is merely to add new linear terms on the right-hand side of the model given by (12.4). That is, a version of the multiple logistic regression model is given by:

$$\log \left(\frac{p_{x_1, \ldots, x_k}}{1 - p_{x_1, \ldots, x_k}} \right) = \log(\text{odds of } D|X_1 = x_1, \ldots, X_k = x_k)$$

$$= a + b_1 x_1 + b_2 x_2 + \cdots b_k x_k. \qquad (12.5)$$

Expressing this in terms of the risk yields

$$p_{x_1, \ldots, x_k} = \frac{1}{1 + e^{-(a + b_1 x_1 + b_2 x_2 + \cdots + b_k x_k)}}. \qquad (12.6)$$

Holding $X_2, \ldots, X_k$ fixed, the pattern that describes how the risk of D changes as X_1 (alone) changes is still a logistic curve, as previously illustrated in Figure 12.4. Further, this is true if each risk factor is examined in turn, each time keeping constant all other variables in the model. Let us consider the implications of this model in terms of how we interpret the parameters, now $a, b_1, \ldots, b_k$. As for the simple model, if $X_1 = 0, X_2 = 0, \ldots, X_k = 0$, we have that $\log(p_{0, \ldots, 0}/(1 - p_{0, \ldots, 0})) = a$. So, a is just the log odds of D at the baseline level where *all* the risk variables are at zero on their respective scales.

For the slope parameters, $b_1, \ldots, b_k$, consider the comparison of two groups whose risk factor X_1 differs by one unit on the scale of X_1, and who share identical values for all other risk variables $X_2, \ldots, X_k$. That is, suppose one group has risk variables given by $X_1 = x_1 + 1, X_2 = x_2, \ldots, X_k = x_k$, and the second group has $X_1 = x_1, X_2 = x_2, \ldots, X_k = x_k$. Then, the logistic regression model (Equation 12.5) tells us that the difference in log odds of D in these two groups is just $[a + b_1(x_1 + 1) + b_2 x_2 + \cdots + b_k x_k] - [a + b_1 x_1 + b_2 x_2 + \cdots + b_k x_k] = b_1$. Thus, b_1 is the log Odds Ratio that compares the risks of these two groups; that is, b_1 is the log Odds Ratio associated with a unit increase in the scale of X_1, *holding all other risk variables in the model constant*.

In general, b_j is the log Odds Ratio associated with a unit increase in the scale of X_j, holding all other variables in the model fixed. The impact of the linear assumption here is again that this log Odds Ratio does not depend on the value of X_j from which the one unit increase is made. But there is now an additional assumption regarding the Odds Ratio associated with changes in X_j, namely, that the log Odds Ratio (and therefore also the Odds Ratio) associated with changes in X_j is not affected by the values (held fixed) for the other variables in the model. That is, the multiple logistic regression model in Equation 12.5 or 12.6 assumes that there is no (multiplicative) interaction between X_j and the other variables. In turn, this is also assumed for each other risk factor so that this model assumes no interactive effects whatsoever amongst the exposure variables. In Chapter 14.2, we extend this simple version of the multiple logistic regression model to allow for interactive effects of various kinds.

Knowledge of the slope parameters, $b_1, \ldots, b_k$, allows us to compute the Odds Ratio comparing any two groups with specified risk factors. Symbolically, if our reference group has $X_1 = x_1, X_2 = x_2, \ldots, X_k = x_k$, and, for the second group, $X_1 = x_1^*, X_2 = x_2^*, \ldots, X_k = x_k^*$, the log Odds Ratio comparing the risk in these two groups is $b_1(x_1^* - x_1) + b_2(x_2^* - x_2) + \cdots + b_k(x_k^* - x_k)$, so that the Odds Ratio is then

$$OR = e^{b_1(x_1^* - x_1) + b_2(x_2^* - x_2) + \cdots + b_k(x_k^* - x_k)}. \tag{12.7}$$

12.6.1 The use of indicator variables for discrete exposures

In discussing logistic regression models, we noted how a two-state exposure variable can be accommodated through the use of a binary exposure variable X. For discrete variables that can assume more than two values, there are two available alternatives. First, we can impose a numerical scale on the differing discrete exposure states, as discussed in Chapter 11.3.1. This, of course, introduces an assumed monotonic dose-response effect. So, for example, with the data on body weight and incidence of CHD given in Table 9.2, we can code the body weight variable as $X = 0$ for <150 lb, $X = 1$ for 150^+ to 160 lb, $X = 2$ for 160^+ to 170, $X = 3$ for 170^+ to 180, and, finally, $X = 4$ for >180 lb. Then, the logistic model

$$\log\left(\frac{p_x}{1 - p_x}\right) = a + bx \tag{12.8}$$

induces the assumption that not only does the risk (of CHD) increase (or decrease) as body weight increases, but the relative change in risk as you go from the group with $X = 0$ to those with $X = 1$ as measured by the Odds Ratio (in fact, e^b) is *exactly the same* as going from $X = 3$ to $X = 4$, for example. As noted, this reflects the regression assumption. Different numerical codings of the body weight levels for X would introduce similar assumptions about comparisons of the original weight groups.

The second approach to discrete exposures avoids the imposition of a monotonic dose-response in the regression model through use of *indicator* (or "*dummy*") variables. For an exposure with K distinct levels, one level is first chosen as the baseline or reference group. Refer to that level as level 0, with the other $K - 1$ levels referred to as level 1, level 2, and so on up to level $K - 1$. Then define $K - 1$ binary exposure variables as follows:

- $X_1 = 1$ if an individual's exposure is at level 1, and $X_1 = 0$ otherwise.
- $X_2 = 1$ if an individual's exposure is at level 2, and $X_2 = 0$ otherwise.
- ...
- $X_{K-1} = 1$ if an individual's exposure is at level $K - 1$, and $X_{K-1} = 0$ otherwise.

Knowledge of these $K-1$ indicator variables for an individual uniquely identifies their original exposure level, and vice versa. For any individual, only one of the indicator variables can be nonzero. Only for individuals whose exposure is at the baseline, level 0, are all $K-1$ indicators equal to 0.

With these variables now defined, we can use the multiple logistic regression model

$$\log \left(\frac{p_{x_1,\ldots,x_{K-1}}}{1 - p_{x_1,\ldots,x_{K-1}}} \right) = a + b_1 x_1 + b_2 x_2 + \cdots + b_{K-1} x_{K-1}.$$

Note the interpretation of the separate regression parameters with this particular choice of variables $X_1, \ldots, X_{K-1}$. First, a is the risk when $X_1 = X_2 = \cdots = X_{K-1} = 0$, that is, the risk in the baseline exposure group. Formally, the first slope coefficient b_1 is the log Odds Ratio associated with a unit increase in X_1, holding $X_2, \ldots, X_{K-1}$ fixed. But the only way to increase X_1 by 1 unit and keep all other variables constant is to move from the baseline exposure level ($X_1 = 0$, all other X_ks are 0) to level 1 ($X_1 = 1$, all other X_ks are 0). Thus, b_1 is the log Odds Ratio comparing exposure level 1 to the baseline level 0. Analogously, b_j is the log Odds Ratio comparing level j to the baseline level 0 for any j between 1 and $K-1$. Since the b_js are unconstrained in the model, this regression structure does not therefore impose *any* restrictions, such as a monotonic dose-response, on the risks in the various exposure groups.

In the body weight example, we need four indicator variables:

1. $X_1 = 1$ if body weight is 150^+ to 160 lb, and $X_1 = 0$ otherwise
2. $X_2 = 1$ if body weight is 160^+ to 170 lb, and $X_2 = 0$ otherwise
3. $X_3 = 1$ if body weight is 170^+ to 180 lb, and $X_3 = 0$ otherwise
4. $X_4 = 1$ if body weight is >180 lb, and $X_4 = 0$ otherwise

to use with the logistic regression model

$$\log \left(\frac{p_{x_1,x_2,x_3}}{1 - p_{x_1,x_2,x_3}} \right) = a + b_1 x_1 + b_2 x_2 + b_3 x_3 + b_4 x_4. \tag{12.9}$$

The intercept coefficient still gives the log odds of D in the baseline group (≤ 150 lb); b_1 is the log Odds Ratio comparing the group who weigh between 150 and 160 lb to those who weigh less than or equal to 150 lb, b_2 is the log Odds Ratio comparing the group who weigh between 160 and 170 lb to those less than or equal to 150 lb, b_3 is the log Odds Ratio comparing the group who weigh between 170 and 180 lb to those less than or equal to 150 lb, and finally b_4 is the log Odds Ratio comparing those who weigh more than 180 lb to those less than or equal to 150 lb. The use of indicator variables in this manner does not impose any restrictions on these Odds Ratios or on the pattern of underlying risks in the four weight groups. Thus, the logistic model (Equation 12.9) is able to exactly match any pattern of observed risks in the five body weight groups.

Knowledge of the slope coefficients associated with the indicator variables again permit us to compute Odds Ratios that compare groups other than the baseline group. For example, using the model (Equation 12.9), the Odds Ratio comparing those who

Table 12.2 *Body weight and coronary heart disease*

		CHD Event		
		D	not D	
Body weight (lb)	≤150	32	558	590
	150⁺–160	31	505	536
	160⁺–170	50	594	644
	170⁺–180	66	501	567
	>180	78	739	817
		257	2897	3154

Table 12.3 *Two logistic regression models, (12.8) and (12.9), for the Western Collaborative Group Study data on body weight and incidence of CHD (the variable X codes body weight by $0, 1, \ldots, 4$ for the five categories; $X_1, \ldots, X_4$ are indicator variables for the same categories, using the group with body weight ≤150 lb as the baseline*

Model	Parameter	Estimate	OR
(12.8) $\log\left(\frac{p}{1-p}\right) = a + bx$	a	−2.839	—
	b	0.180	1.198
(12.9) $\log\left(\frac{p}{1-p}\right) = a + b_1 x_1 + \cdots + b_4 x_4$	a	−2.859	—
	b_1	0.068	1.070
	b_2	0.384	1.468
	b_3	0.832	2.297
	b_4	0.610	1.840

weigh more than 180 lb to those who weigh between 160 and 170 lb is simply $e^{b_4 - b_2}$, using Equation 12.7. The choice of the reference group in defining models like Equation 12.9 is completely arbitrary; for reporting purposes, it is helpful if it represents some normative or baseline level of exposure. When we turn to estimation of logistic regression model parameters in the next chapter, it is often useful to select the reference group to contain a substantial fraction of the sample so that comparisons can be estimated with reasonable precision. In particular, if there is hardly any sample in the reference group, then all slope coefficient estimates will have large standard deviations because of the lack of information at the baseline.

We illustrate the fit of models (Equations 12.8 and 12.9) to the Western Collaborative Group Study data on body weight given in Table 11.3, reproduced for convenience in Table 12.2. Estimation of the coefficients of the models based on these data is considered in detail in the next chapter. Table 12.3 provides the results of such estimation; note, however, that since the logistic model (Equation 12.9) fits the observed risks exactly, as discussed above, we can obtain the coefficient estimates for this model directly from Table 12.2. For example, the intercept a in Equation 12.9 matches the log odds of the observed risk in the baseline group, here, from Table 12.2, given by $\log((32/590)/(558/590)) = \log(0.0542/0.9458 = \log 0.0573 = -2.859$. Similarly,

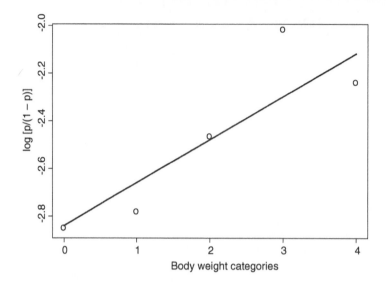

Figure 12.6 *Plot of a fitted logistic model, (12.7), to data relating body weight to incidence of CHD.*

the log odds of CHD in the group with body weight between 160 and 170 lb, i.e. $X_1 = 1$, is $\log((31/536)/(505/536)) = -2.791$. Thus, the log Odds Ratio comparing this weight level to the baseline group is just the difference in these log odds, and so is given by $-2.791 - (-2.859) = 0.068$. The corresponding Odds Ratio is then $e^{0.068} = 1.070$. The remaining estimates in Table 12.3 for the model (Equation 12.9) can be calculated in exactly this manner.

Note the different estimates of Odds Ratios comparing different levels of body weight that arise from fitting Equations 12.8 and 12.9. As noted above, the Odds Ratio comparing those with body weight between 160 and 170 lb to those with weight ≤ 150 lb is 1.070, as calculated above, or from e^{b_1}. On the other hand, this change in body weight corresponds to a 1 unit change in X in Equation 12.8 (going from $X = 0$ to $X = 1$), so that the estimated Odds Ratio from this model is $e^b = e^{0.180} = 1.198$. Similar comparisons can be made for other weight groups, and the differences between the two models is considered in greater detail in Chapter 13.2; see, in particular, Table 13.4.

Comparing the two models graphically, Figure 12.6 combines the third plot of Figure 11.2 (giving the estimated odds based on Equation 12.9) with a fitted version of the model of Equation 12.8. In plotting the model (Equation 12.9), we merely need to reproduce the log odds for each weight category as calculated above; equivalently we can compute the estimates of $a, a + b_1, \ldots, a + b_4$ from Table 12.3. In fitting the model (Equation 12.8), each observed odds influences the estimates of a and b, with greater weight being given to those with higher precision. Confidence interval bars centered on the estimated odds would emphasize this issue, although we have chosen not to use them here as the precision is roughly the same across the five weight categories.

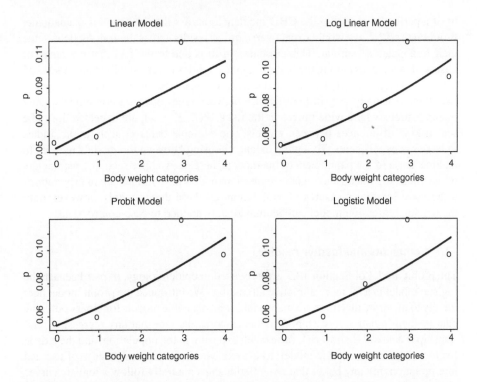

Figure 12.7 *Plot of fitted linear, log linear, probit, and logistic models, to data relating body weight to incidence of CHD, with risk (p) as the scale for the Y-axis.*

The observed incidences (or odds, or log odds) of CHD in the five body weight categories are, of course, exactly fit by model Equation 12.9, which involves four indicator variables. This model contains five parameters, the four slope parameters, plus the intercept, which allows an exact match to the five observed odds. This exact fit is analogous to a simple logistic model that always exactly fits incidences for an exposure with two levels, as noted in Section 12.5 (a straight line can always be chosen to pass through any two given points). On the other hand, the logistic regression model Equation 12.8 does not fit the observed log odds exactly, although the fit appears reasonable from Figure 12.6. A formal statistical comparison of the two models is described in Chapter 13.2.

As a final illustration, Figure 12.7 describes four fitted models, the linear, log linear, probit, and logistic model, where in each case the Y-axis gives the estimated risk $\hat{P}(D|X)$, where X denotes the simple ordered scale of body weight from 0 to 4 used in Figure 12.6. In both Figures 12.6 and 12.7, the observed data were used to choose the "best" fitting version of the relevant models. How the "best" version of a particular model is selected is the topic of the next chapter. At this point, note, however, that there is very little difference *between* the best fitting versions of the four models considered in terms of how well they match the estimated risks at the five body weight categories. In the next chapter, we discuss methods to assess whether the fit of a particular model to the CHD incidences across these categories is adequate. From Figure 12.7, we would expect very similar results across the four models, since their fit appears so similar. This closeness in fit is due to the fact that the range of observed incidences among the body weight categories is very small, from about 0.05 to 0.12, as is typical to many chronic disease investigations. Over such small ranges in risk, there is usually very little difference between types of regression models. Only in applications where wide ranges in the risks, $P(D|X = x)$, are expected does one see striking differences between models, one example being concentration studies in bioassay experiments. To a great extent, choosing between the models reduces to making sense of the parameters of the models; here, as we have seen, the parameters of the linear, log linear, and logistic regression models have immediate interpretations in terms of familiar measures of association. Of these three models, however, only the logistic regression model can be immediately applied to case-control data.

12.7 Comments and further reading

The probit model of Section 12.3 is rarely used in epidemiology, in part because the logistic model is a far more attractive alternative. We introduce the probit model here merely to illustrate that there are many viable and plausible models for binary outcome data beyond logistic regression. This underscores the fact that any regression relationship is a *model* for how risk varies with exposure in the population, and the reason for focusing on the logistic model, to the exclusion of others, is its ease of use and interpretation, not any belief that risk relationships naturally follow a logistic curve.

Each of the models in Sections 12.1 to 12.4 assumes linearity in the exposure scale but invokes a different pattern for the risk scale in which this linearity operates. Each of these models is a special case of a *generalized linear model*; an introduction to such models is given in Dobson (2001). The various transforms of the risks used, such as the log risk or log odds, are known as the *links* of the model. While the linear, log, and log odds links are the most commonly used, other versions appear in specialized examples. For example, Jewell and Shiboski (1990) use the complementary log–log link, $\log(-\log(1 - p(D|X)))$, to study the risk of HIV transmission among sexual partners, where X is the log of the number of infectious contacts; this provides a natural way to extend an assumption of constant risk per contact.

Choice of the link function is quite a different issue from selecting a scale for the exposure variable, X. The latter is also a crucial component of any regression structure, since, for example, the model $\log(p_x/1 - p_x) = a + bx$ may differ substantially from $\log(p_x/1 - p_x) = a + b \log x$, although both are logistic regression models. We discuss statistical approaches to the choice of exposure scale in Chapter 15.1.

12.8 Problems

Question 12.1

Suppose you have a single categorical risk factor measured at three levels ($L =$ low, $M =$ medium, $H =$ high). A risk model can be constructed by the following technique.

Pick one of the three categories as a reference group. Let $X_1 = 1$ for the first comparison group and $X_1 = 0$ otherwise. Let $X_2 = 1$ for the remaining comparison category and $X_2 = 0$ otherwise. A logistic regression model, $\log(p_{x_1,x_2}/(1 - p_{x_1,x_2})) = a + bx_1 + cx_2$, can then be used to link the incidence proportion at each level of the risk factor to the values of X_1 and X_2.

1. Carry out the above plan, indicating the X_1 and X_2 coding for each category, L, M, and H. Interpret the parameters in terms of either the incidence proportions for the L, M, and H categories or relevant Odds Ratios.

2. Are there any structural relationships imposed on the incidence proportions in the three categories by your logistic model?

3. How would you handle a risk factor with four categories this way?

Question 12.2

In Question 12.1, the labeling of categories as low, medium, and high suggests that the risk factor possesses a natural order. Suppose you code the risk factor through a single variable X that assumes the values 0 (L), 1 (M), and 2 (H).

1. Describe an appropriate logistic model for this situation, providing the interpretation of the parameters.

2. Are there any structural relationships imposed on the incidence proportions in the three categories by your logistic model?

Question 12.3

The Western Collaborative Group Study collected information on diastolic and systolic blood pressure (at baseline) as predictors of subsequent coronary heart disease. A logistic regression analysis was performed. The results for the fitted model are summarized in Table 12.4. Recall that these findings give the results for incidence after about 8.5 years of follow-up.

1. Calculate the Odds Ratio per unit increase for each measure of blood pressure in turn, from the model only including that variable.

2. Calculate the Odds Ratio per unit increase for each blood pressure measure from the joint model. (When calculating the Odds Ratio for one variable, consider the other variable fixed.) Interpret the joint model.

3. Calculate the log odds of risk ($\log(p/1 - p)$) and risk (p) from the fitted joint model for the combinations of values of diastolic and systolic blood pressure as proscribed in Table 12.5.

4. Using the results from (3), plot risk on the vertical scale and diastolic blood pressure on the horizontal scale, with one risk "curve" for each of the four levels of systolic pressure.

5. Similarly, now plot risk on the vertical scale and systolic blood pressure on the horizontal scale, with one risk "curve" for each of the four levels of diastolic pressure.

Table 12.4 *The Western Collaborative Group Study: Relationships between systolic and dias-tolic blood pressure and incidence of coronary heart disease after 8+ years of follow-up*

Predictors in Logistic Model		Intercept	Risk Factor Diastolic (mmHg)	Systolic (mmHg)
Diastolic alone	Logistic coefficient	−5.2217	0.0336	
	SD of logistic coefficient	0.5116	0.0060	
	p-value of Wald test	<0.0001	<0.0001	
Systolic alone	Logistic coefficient	−5.9265		0.0267
	SD of logistic coefficient	0.4970		0.0037
	p-value of Wald test	<0.0001		<0.0001
Diastolic and systolic	Logistic coefficient	−5.9143	−0.0006	0.0270
	SD of logistic coefficient	0.5307	0.0097	0.0060
	p-value of Wald test	<0.0001	0.95	<0.0001

Note: SD = standard deviation.

Table 12.5 *Various levels of dyastolic and systolic blood pressure at which to compute estimated risk of CHD*

Diastolic (mmHg)	Systolic (mmHg) 100	120	140	160
100				
90				
80				
70				

Question 12.4

Using the fitted joint model from Question 12.3 that relates the diastolic and systolic blood pressure at baseline to subsequent risk of CHD, and your calculations of risk at various blood pressure levels, estimate the Odds Ratio for CHD that compares the following groups of individuals: (1) individuals with diastolic = 100 mmHg and systolic = 100 mmHg, against individuals with diastolic = 70 mmHg and systolic = 160 mmHg; and (2) individuals with diastolic = 90 mmHg and systolic = 100 mmHg, against individuals with diastolic = 80 mmHg and systolic = 140 mmHg.

CHAPTER 13

Estimation of Logistic Regression Model Parameters

Now that we have spent some effort developing an understanding of various simple versions of the logistic regression model, we are eager to apply the model to examples. We want to know, for example, answers to the following: Does logistic regression really describe how body weight influences the risk of CHD? What happens when we add behavior type into the model? How about the level of coffee drinking and incidence of pancreatic cancer? Before going into further issues, such as confounding and interaction, in the context of logistic regression, we first consider estimation of the parameters of a specific population model using randomly sampled data. Initially we direct our attention to population-based and cohort designs. In Section 13.3 we extend estimation techniques to allow for case-control data.

13.1 The likelihood function

Before launching into estimation of a complex regression model, we introduce some ideas for an extremely simple case with which we are familiar, namely, estimation of a single probability or proportion. We will look at this problem with some specific data in mind. In Chapter 3.3, we considered estimation of the probability of being an unmarried mother to a newborn infant in the U.S. in 1991; specifically, we estimated the proportion of newborns in 1991 whose mothers were unmarried at the time of birth, based on a simple random sample of size 100 that yielded 35 infants with unmarried mothers. Given this data, let us ask questions about the unknown population proportion that we again label p for convenience. That is, p is the proportion of newborns in 1991 whose mothers were unmarried at the time of birth.

How possible or likely do we think it is that p could be zero? The answer is immediate: not likely at all, in fact, impossible, since we observed 35 unmarried mothers. How about $p = 1$? Again, this is impossible because we observed 65 married mothers. More realistically, what do we think about $p = 0.5$? This possibility seems at least plausible given the data. And $p = 0.5$ seems more reasonable than $p = 0.6$, although we cannot entirely rule out the latter value. Probably most of us would also say that $p = 0.5$ is more likely to be true than $p = 0.1$. Going through a series of these potential values for the unknown parameter p, we could plot a graph of our rough quantitative sense of plausibility or "likeliness" of a value of p against p. Such a graph might look something like Figure 13.1. As an estimate of the parameter p it seems reasonable to choose that value where the "likeliness" is maximized, that is, the most "likely" value that p might be, given the data.

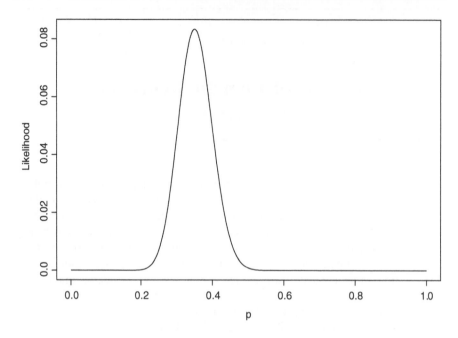

Figure 13.1 *Plot of likelihood function for an unknown population proportion, p, of a newborn having an unmarried mother, based on data with 35 observed births with unmarried mothers from a sample of 100.*

So far, this idea of "likeliness" is subjective. We can formally quantify such a concept through use of the *likelihood function* of p, defined by

$$L = P(\text{data}|p).$$

Here, $P(\text{data}|p)$ is based on an appropriate probability model assumed to have generated the data; in the case of our simple random sample of 100 live births, the number of infants with unmarried mothers in the sample follows a binomial sampling distribution with Binomial parameter p (assuming that the population size is very large, as we did in Chapter 3.3). We observed 35 unmarried mothers in the sample, so that $L = \binom{100}{35}p^{35}(1-p)^{65}$. It is often easier to deal with the log of the likelihood function, $\log L$, here given by $\log L = \log\binom{100}{35}+35\log p+65\log(1-p)$. Figure 13.1 is a plot of the likelihood function against p; Figure 13.2 provides the analogous plot of the log likelihood function.

The maximum of the likelihood function occurs at the same value of p as the maximum of the log likelihood function. In our example, the maximum occurs when $p = 0.35$, which is a reasonable and familiar estimate for a population proportion based on a simple random sample.

The log likelihood function is enormously useful. The estimator of p defined by the value where the (log) likelihood function takes its maximum is known as the *maximum likelihood* estimator of p. The log likelihood function not only defines the maximum

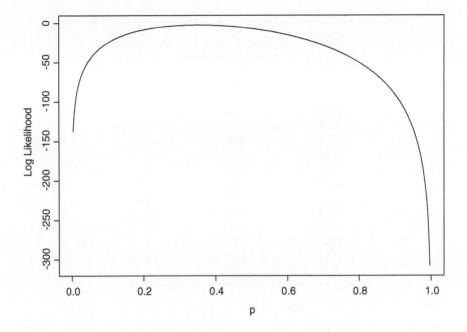

Figure 13.2 *Plot of log likelihood function for an unknown population proportion, p, of a newborn having an unmarried mother, based on data with 35 observed births with unmarried mothers from a sample of 100.*

likelihood estimator $\hat{p}$, it also gives information about the precision of the estimator. Qualitatively, this can be seen by considering the shape of the log likelihood function close to where the maximum occurs. If the likelihood climbs (and falls) gently both toward and away from its peak, it means that there are other values of p relatively far from $\hat{p}$ that give almost the same value of the likelihood function. This suggests that the sampling variability of $\hat{p}$ is high, reflecting that we must consider a sizeable range of values as plausible estimates of p, that is, that have a similarly high level of likelihood as $\hat{p}$. On the other hand, if the log likelihood function has a very sharp peak, meaning that the likelihood drops quickly as p moves away from $\hat{p}$, then we obtain a much lower value for the sampling variability of $\hat{p}$. This indicates that only values of p in a narrow range around the maximum likelihood estimate give a value of the likelihood close to the maximum, that is, seem reasonable given the data. In sum, how quickly the slope of the log likelihood function changes near the peak provides direct information on the sampling variability, needed for calculation of a confidence interval associated with the maximum likelihood estimate $\hat{p}$.

13.1.1 The likelihood function based on a logistic regression model

In this section, we discuss construction of the likelihood function for data that have been sampled from a population where it is assumed that a logistic regression model holds. For simplicity, assume that we have a single exposure variable measured

Table 13.1 *Extract of data from the Western Collaborative Group Study*

ID Number	Body Weight (lb) (X)	CHD (D)
2001	150	0
2002	160	0
2003	160	0
2004	152	0
2005	150	1
2006	204	0
2007	164	0
2008	150	0
2009	190	0
2010	175	0
2011	167	0
2013	156	0
2014	173	1
2017	180	0
2018	150	0

by X and that the risk for the outcome D follows the logistic regression model $\log(p_x/(1 - p_x)) = a + bx$, where $p_x = P(D|X = x)$, as usual. The ideas easily extend to both more complex logistic regression models and to the other regression models introduced in Chapter 12. Initially we focus on data generated from a population-based or cohort design. In Section 13.3 we extend these ideas to case-control samples.

The likelihood function is already more complicated than described in Section 13.1, since it depends on two unknown parameters, a and b, rather than just one. Other than the fact that the plot of the likelihood function is now three-dimensional, this does not introduce any additional conceptual complexity, although locating the maximum is a more difficult proposition. But first we describe the likelihood function, most easily illustrated through an example. Table 13.1 shows a small part of the Western Collaborative Group Study data set, 15 individuals in the sample, with information on outcome (CHD) and body weight. In the table, the coding for CHD is simply $D = 0$ for any individual who did not develop CHD during follow-up, and $D = 1$ for any individual who did. Here X represents the risk factor, body weight (in lb), measured at the beginning of follow-up.

Note that the observation corresponding to ID number 2001 is an individual with body weight 150 lb who did not develop CHD during follow-up. Thus, assuming the simple logistic regression model (Equation 12.3), the likelihood of this observation is just $P(D = 0 \ \& \ X = 150) = P(D = 0|X = 150)P(X = 150) = e^{-(a+150b)}/(1 + e^{-(a+150b)}) \times P(X = 150)$. Similarly, the likelihood of the observation number 2002 is $P(D = 0 \ \& \ X = 160) = P(D = 0|X = 160)P(X = 160) = e^{-(a+160b)}/(1 + e^{-(a+160b)}) \times P(X = 160)$. On the other hand, for individual number 2005, the likelihood contribution is $P(D = 1 \ \& \ X = 150) = P(D = 1|X = 150)$

$\times P(X = 150) = 1/(1 + e^{-(a+150b)}) \times P(X = 150)$, since this individual was a D. The individual observations are independent of each other, and so it follows that the complete likelihood function is a product of all these terms, one for each data point in the data set. That is,

$$L = \prod_{i=1}^{n} P(D_i|X = x_i)P(X = x_i),$$

where the index i runs over all individuals in the sample, and D_i and x_i are the outcome and body weight, respectively, for the ith individual. The terms involving $P(X = x_i)$ do not depend on a and b and so can be ignored when maximizing L. We are then faced with finding the values of a and b that maximize the following function of a and b:

$$L^* = \prod_{i=1}^{n} P(D_i|X = x_i) = \frac{e^{-(a+150b)}}{1 + e^{-(a+150b)}} \times \frac{e^{-(a+160b)}}{1 + e^{-(a+160b)}} \times \cdots .$$

In what follows, it will be this function of the (unknown) regression parameters that we will refer to as the likelihood of the model. For more complex logistic regression models, such as those given in Equations 12.5 and 12.6, there is a similar expression for the likelihood where the $(a + bx)$ terms in L^* are replaced by linear terms that depend on all the relevant covariates in the model, the right-hand side of Equation 12.5.

Unfortunately, in general, there are no simple formulas for the values of a and b that maximize L^*. On the other hand, standard (iterative) numerical techniques can quickly locate this maximum, yielding the maximum likelihood estimates of a and b based on the entire data set.

To illustrate these calculations, we consider fitting the simple logistic regression model (Equation 12.4) to the full sample from the Western Collaborative Group Study, with the risk factor X representing body weight (in lb), measured on a continuous scale. There is no grouping now imposed on body weight; in fact, there are 124 distinct values of body weight observed amongst the 3154 sampled individuals, ranging from 78 to 320 lb. The maximum likelihood estimates are given by $\hat{a} = -4.215, \hat{b} = 0.010$. The maximized value of the log likelihood $L^* = -884.5$. Figure 13.3 shows the plot of the observed proportion of CHD cases against each of the 124 distinct body weight values, on the scale of risk (p_x), together with the fitted logistic model. One drawback of the plot of the observed risks is that it does not convey either the sample numbers contributing to these estimates, or the underlying levels of precision of the plotted points; some weight values comprise but one individual. In addition, without grouping, it is much more difficult to assess the adequacy of the fit of the logistic model due to the volatility of observed risks, which are often just zero or one, particularly if there are few individuals at a given body weight. Goodness of fit for a chosen model is discussed in more detail in Chapter 15.

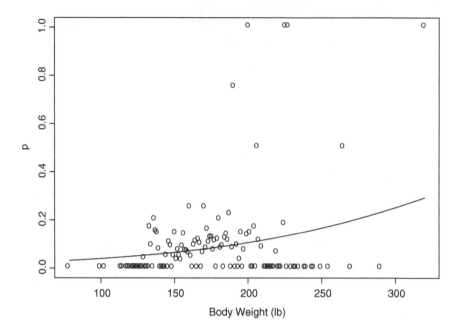

Figure 13.3 *Plot of estimated CHD incidence at all distinct body weight levels against body weight, with fitted simple logistic model.*

13.1.2 Properties of the log likelihood function and the maximum likelihood estimate

In addition to point estimates of logistic regression coefficients, the likelihood function can also be used to give related confidence intervals and hypothesis testing methods in a variety of situations. For the simple logistic regression model of Chapter 12.4, a confidence interval for either a or b can be derived from the fact that (almost) all maximum likelihood estimates have approximately Normal sampling distributions when the overall sample size is large (or both sample sizes are large for cohort or case-control designs). This remarkable property is actually a consequence of the central limit theorem which we most often encounter in studying the sampling distribution of averages. Often, this Normal approximation can be improved by estimating a transformed version of the parameter in question. (We discovered this when estimating confidence intervals for the Odds Ratio in Chapter 7.) In the case of the logistic regression model, the coefficients a and b are already on a log scale with reasonably symmetric sampling distributions, obviating the need for a transformation. To use the Normal approximation, it is necessary to derive an estimate of the variance of the sampling distribution of either $\hat{a}$ or $\hat{b}$. Such estimates are available based on the "steepness" of the likelihood function near the point estimates $\hat{a}$ and $\hat{b}$, as we described qualitatively in the last section. In sum, analysis of the likelihood function yields the point estimate $\hat{b}$ and an estimate of its sampling variance, $\hat{V}_b$.

Then, two-sided $100(1 - \alpha)\%$ confidence limits for b are given by

$$\hat{b} \pm z_\alpha \sqrt{\hat{V_b}},$$

where z_α is the $(1 - \frac{\alpha}{2})$th percentile of the standard Normal distribution. A similar approach works for a confidence interval for a, with $\hat{a}$ and $\hat{V_a}$ replacing $\hat{b}$ and $\hat{V_b}$, respectively. Since, for example, b represents the log Odds Ratio associated with a unit increase in X, we will usually prefer to report such confidence intervals in terms of e^b, the Odds Ratio for a unit increase in X. These, of course, are immediately obtained from the corresponding confidence interval for b by exponentiating, as described in Chapter 7 for a single Odds Ratio. This approach to calculating confidence intervals for the regression coefficients extends directly to the multiple logistic regression model of Chapter 12.6.

Many natural null hypotheses of interest are specified by setting one or more parameters in the regression model to zero. For example, in the context of the simple logistic model for one exposure variable X, given by $\log(p_x/(1 - p_x)) = a + bx$, the null hypothesis $H_0 : b = 0$ is equivalent to independence of D and X. The natural alternative hypothesis is then $H_A : b \neq 0$; if X is a simple binary exposure variable, this alternative corresponds to D and X not being independent (as in the χ^2 test for independence of Chapter 6). On the other hand, if X is a continuously scaled or ordered categorical exposure, this alternative corresponds to the existence of a trend in the risk as X increases (in fact, a linear trend on the log odds scale), as in the test for trend of Chapter 11.3.

Three likelihood based methods can be used to test this simple null hypothesis in the context of the logistic regression model:

- **The Wald Method.** Akin to the technique used to calculate a confidence interval for b, this method simply computes the test statistic $z_b = \hat{b}/\sqrt{\hat{V_b}}$ by dividing the maximum likelihood estimate of b by an estimate of its standard deviation $\sqrt{\hat{V_b}}$. Under the null hypothesis, $H_0 : b = 0$, the Wald statistic z_b will approximately follow a standard Normal distribution in large samples. Comparison with tables of the standard Normal distribution thus yields a p-value. Often the Wald statistic is squared and then compared to a χ^2 distribution with one degree of freedom.

- **The Score Method.** If the maximum likelihood estimator of b is close to the null hypothesis value $b = 0$, we would expect the slope of the log likelihood function to be small at $b = 0$. (The slope is exactly zero at $\hat{b}$; see Figure 13.2.) The test statistic for the score method is the value of the slope of the log likelihood function at $b = 0$, divided by an estimated standard deviation of the sampling distribution of this slope. This statistic can then be compared to tables of a standard Normal distribution in large samples. Again, the score statistic is often squared and compared to a $\chi^2_{(1)}$ distribution.

- **The Likelihood Ratio Method.** With this technique, we compare the value of the maximized log likelihood (at $\hat{b}$) with the smaller value of the log likelihood at $b = 0$. If the likelihood is much smaller at $b = 0$, this provides evidence that $\hat{b}$ is considerably more plausible as an estimate of b than the (null) hypothesized value $b = 0$, yielding a small p-value, questioning the validity of the null hypothesis.

On the other hand, if the values of the two likelihood calculations, at $\hat{b}$ and at $b = 0$, are similar, we deduce that $b = 0$ is almost as reasonable an estimate of b as the maximum likelihood estimator, suggesting that the data provide little evidence against $b = 0$, with a correspondingly large p-value. The likelihood ratio test statistic is the difference in the log likelihoods at $\hat{b}$ and $b = 0$ (and is thus the logarithm of the *ratio* of the likelihoods), *multiplied by 2*. In large samples, the sampling distribution of this statistic is closely approximated by a χ^2 distribution with one degree of freedom, assuming the null hypothesis is correct.

These techniques usually lead to very similar p-values. Differences between the methods are probably an indication of small samples, where exact procedures are required. We illustrate some of these methods in the examples later in the chapter. In using likelihood-based methods, we often encounter one additional piece of terminology; the value $-2\times$ (maximized log likelihood) is commonly referred to as the *deviance*. The numerical value of the deviance, like the likelihood, carries no absolute meaning, whereas differences in the deviance give the likelihood ratio. Since it is relative sizes of the likelihood that permit model comparisons, it does not matter whether you work with $\log L$ or $\log L^*$, since the difference between the terms disappears in such comparisons.

13.1.3 Null hypotheses that specify more than one regression coefficient

Consider again the analysis of the relationship between body weight and CHD based on the grouped data of Table 12.2. Suppose we use indicator variables, rather than an ordered scale, to describe the level of body weight. That is, we use the four indicator variables, X_1, X_2, X_3, X_4, defined in Chapter 12.6.1, and then fit the logistic regression model (Equation 12.9), given by $\log(p_{x_1,x_2,x_3,x_4}/(1 - p_{x_1,x_2,x_3,x_4})) = a + b_1x_1 + b_2x_2 + b_3x_3 + b_4x_4$. One null hypothesis of interest here is that body weight and CHD incidence are independent. In terms of this logistic regression model, this null hypothesis is expressed by $H_0 : b_1 = b_2 = b_3 = b_4 = 0$. The corresponding alternative hypothesis is that at least one of the slope coefficients is nonzero, reflecting that body weight is associated with CHD. This is, in fact, exactly the null and alternative hypotheses for the overall test of association described in Chapter 11.1.

Our null hypothesis here specifies that four regression coefficients are zero, a more complex situation than we considered in Section 13.1.2. Each of the three testing methods, the Wald, score, and likelihood ratio, can be adapted to accommodate this kind of null hypothesis. The simplest and most useful is the likelihood ratio method, which we now describe in more detail.

Consider two regression models for CHD incidence, labeled by Model I and Model II for convenience. Suppose also that Model I is *nested* within Model II; that is, Model I is a special case of Model II, described by placing simple constraints on the parameters of Model II. For example, in modeling body weight, Model II might be given by Equation 12.9, and one possible Model I might be

$$\log \left(\frac{p_{x_1,x_2,x_3,x_4}}{1 - p_{x_1,x_2,x_3,x_4}} \right) = a. \tag{13.1}$$

This model, of course, claims that CHD incidence is the same for all levels of body weight, that is, that body weight and CHD are independent. Thus, Model I corresponds to our null hypothesis and Model II to the alternative. Model I is nested within Model II; we can see that Model I is a special case of Model II since it corresponds to setting $b_1 = b_2 = b_3 = b_4 = 0$ in Equation 12.9.

Consider the calculation of the maximized log likelihood under Model I (in our example, involving computation of $\hat{a}$ and evaluation of the log likelihood at $\hat{a}$), and under Model II (involving computation of $\hat{a}$, $\hat{b}_1$, $\hat{b}_2$, $\hat{b}_3$, and $\hat{b}_4$, and subsequent evaluation of the log likelihood at these values). (Note that the intercept estimates $\hat{a}$ will be different under the two models and have different interpretations.) The maximized log likelihood under Model II will necessarily be larger than under Model I since it is a more general model.

Under the null hypothesis that the two models are equivalent (i.e., $b_1 = b_2 = b_3 = b_4 = 0$), the test statistic given by

$$2 \times (\text{the max. log likelihood in Model II} - \text{the max. log likelihood in Model I})$$
$$(13.2)$$

follows a sampling distribution approximated by a χ^2 distribution in large samples. The appropriate number of degrees of freedom for the χ^2 distribution is the difference in the number of degrees of freedom for the two models. In our example, Model I has one degree of freedom (a is arbitrary) and Model II has five (each of a, b_1, b_2, b_3, b_4 is arbitrary), so that the null hypothesis sampling distribution for the likelihood ratio test statistic is $\chi^2_{(4)}$, a χ^2 distribution with four degrees of freedom. The number of degrees of freedom is often just the difference in the number of free parameters in the two nested models, or the number of parameters that must be set to zero to obtain Model I as a special case of Model II. This procedure generalizes the likelihood ratio method of Section 13.1.2.

The likelihood ratio technique for this specific example is illustrated in the next section. Additional applications of the likelihood ratio procedure will appear in subsequent examples. We stress that comparative use of maximized log likelihoods does not work for nonnested models. One sure sign that your models are not nested is if they contain the same number of free parameters. Sometimes the nesting and appropriate parameterization may be difficult to see at first glance. This is discussed in Section 13.4 for the example on coffee drinking and incidence of pancreatic cancer.

13.2 Example—the Western Collaborative Group Study: part 7

We now illustrate some of the ideas regarding logistic regression modeling that we have introduced so far, using data from the Western Collaborative Group Study, which we previously analyzed with a variety of stratification methods. For convenience, Table 13.2 provides the coding used for a variety of measures of body weight. Table 13.3 shows the results from fitting several logistic regression models to this data, focusing on the separate roles of behavior pattern and body weight.

We first look at behavior pattern defined by the binary exposure variable X, which takes the value 1 for Type A individuals and the value 0 for Type B individuals.

Table 13.2 *Coding for variables in Western Collaborative Group Study data*

$$X = \begin{cases} 1 & \text{Type A behavior pattern} \\ 0 & \text{Type B behavior pattern} \end{cases}$$

Wt = Body weight (lb), on continuous scale

$Nwt = (Wt - 150)/20$

$Mwt = (Wt - 170)/20$

$$Z_1 = \begin{cases} 1 & 150 < Wt \leq 160 \\ 0 & \text{otherwise} \end{cases}$$

$$Z_2 = \begin{cases} 1 & 160 < Wt \leq 170 \\ 0 & \text{otherwise} \end{cases}$$

$$Z_3 = \begin{cases} 1 & 170 < Wt \leq 180 \\ 0 & \text{otherwise} \end{cases}$$

$$Z_4 = \begin{cases} 1 & 180 < Wt \\ 0 & \text{otherwise} \end{cases}$$

$$Z = \begin{cases} 0 & wt \leq 150 \\ 1 & 150 < Wt \leq 160 \\ 2 & 160 < Wt \leq 170 \\ 3 & 170 < Wt \leq 180 \\ 4 & 180 < Wt \end{cases}$$

Table 13.3 *Some simple logistic regression models for the Western Collaborative Group Study*

(No.) Model	Parameter	Estimate	SD	OR	p-value	max. log likelihood
(1) $\log\left(\frac{p}{1-p}\right) = a$	a	-2.422	0.065	—	<0.001	-890.6
(2) $\log\left(\frac{p}{1-p}\right) = a + bx$	a	-2.934	0.115	—	<0.001	
	b	0.864	0.140	2.373	<0.001	-870.2
(3) $\log\left(\frac{p}{1-p}\right) = a + b_1 z_1 +$	a	-2.859	0.182	—	<0.001	
$\cdots + b_4 z_4$	b_1	0.068	0.259	1.070	0.793	
	b_2	0.384	0.234	1.468	0.101	
	b_3	0.832	0.224	2.297	<0.001	
	b_4	0.610	0.217	1.840	0.005	-879.9
(4) $\log\left(\frac{p}{1-p}\right) = a + bz$	a	-2.839	0.132	—	<0.001	
	b	0.180	0.046	1.198	<0.001	-882.8
(5) $\log\left(\frac{p}{1-p}\right) = a + b(wt)$	a	-4.215	0.512	—	<0.001	
	b	0.010	0.003	1.010	<0.001	-884.5
(6) $\log\left(\frac{p}{1-p}\right) = a + b(nwt)$	a	-2.651	0.096	—	<0.001	
	b	0.208	0.058	1.232	<0.001	-884.5

Note: SD = standard deviation; variables are defined in Table 13.2.

Model (1) of Table 13.3 simply fits a constant risk for everyone in the population. The maximum likelihood estimate of a is just $\log(\hat{p}/(1 - \hat{p}))$ where $\hat{p} = 257/3154 = 0.0815$, the sample proportion of CHD occurrences in the sample of 3154 individuals (see Table 7.4). Note that $\log(.0815/.9185) = -2.422$, as seen from the fitted logistic regression model.

Model (2) of Table 13.3 adds to Model (1) the variable X for behavior type. Since X is a binary exposure variable, the logistic regression model does not impose any structure on the risks of CHD for the two behavior types. The estimate of b is 0.864, so that the estimated Odds Ratio for a unit increase in X_1, that is, comparing Type A individuals to Type Bs, is just $e^b = 2.373$, as can directly be obtained from the 2×2 table, Table 7.4. Specifically, this table gives $\widehat{OR} = (178 \times 1486)/(1411 \times 79) = 2.373$. In addition $\widehat{Var}(\log \widehat{OR}) = 1/178 + 1/1411 + 1/79 + 1/1486 = 0.0197$; note that this yields a standard deviation of $\sqrt{0.0197} = 0.140$, agreeing exactly with $\widehat{SD}(\hat{b})$ from the maximum likelihood fit of the regression model. From Table 13.3, we also have a 95% confidence interval for b given by $0.864 \pm (1.96 \times 0.140) = (0.590, 1.138)$; the corresponding confidence interval for e^b, the Odds Ratio, is then $(1.80, 3.12)$, exactly what we obtain from the procedure described in Chapter 7.1.2. This illustrates that the simple procedures in Chapter 7 are, in fact, applications of maximum likelihood techniques.

With regard to testing the null hypothesis $b = 0$, in Model (2), against the alternative hypothesis $b \neq 0$, the Wald method gives the test statistic $z_b = 0.864/0.140 = 6.17$, which yields a p-value of 7×10^{-10} when compared to tables of a standard Normal distribution. Equivalently, the Wald statistic squared is 38.1, giving the identical p-value from tables of the χ^2 distribution with one degree of freedom. Alternatively, the likelihood ratio test statistic can be computed by comparing the first two models of Table 13.3 (since the first model is nested within the second), giving the value $2[-870.2 - (-890.6)] = 40.8$, which again produces an extremely small p-value when compared to tables of the χ^2 distribution with one degree of freedom (the difference in the number of degrees of freedom of Models (1) and (2)). These test statistics yield very similar results, as expected. Both the Wald and likelihood ratio test procedures provide alternatives to the simple χ^2 test procedure described in Chapter 6; for the data of Table 7.4, this gave a χ^2 test statistic equal to 39.9, as computed in Chapter 7.2.1. The χ^2 test is not identical to any of the three maximum likelihood approaches discussed in Section 13.1, but it yields a test statistic that is very close to any of these methods when the sample size is large.

We now turn to the other models of Table 13.3, which focus on the role of body weight in the incidence of CHD. The variable body weight (at initiation of follow-up) is a continuous (interval-scaled) variable, measured on the scale of pounds. This variable is denoted by Wt, as indicated in Table 13.2. Four indicator variables, $Z_1, \ldots, Z_4$, are used, as discussed in Section 12.6.1, to capture body weight categorized into five intervals (Table 13.2), with the lowest weight group, $Wt \leq 150$, acting as the baseline or reference category. The variable Z (Table 13.2) is used to code body weight into a simple ordered scale $0, 1, \ldots, 4$, as we used in Chapter 11.4 and Figure 12.6.

The estimated intercept in Model (3) of Table 13.3 is $\hat{a} = -2.859$; this is, of course, the estimated log odds of CHD for individuals whose body weight is ≤ 150 lb (for whom $Z_1 = Z_2 = Z_3 = Z_4 = 0$). This estimate is identical to $\log \hat{p}/(1 - \hat{p})$ where $\hat{p} = 32/590$, the sample proportion of CHD cases in the first row of Table 12.2. Also, $\hat{b}_1 = 0.068$ gives the estimated log Odds Ratio comparing individuals whose weight lies between 150 and 16 lbs with the reference group; the corresponding Odds Ratio is $e^{\hat{b}_1} = 1.070$. Again this estimated Odds Ratio can be computed directly, from the first two rows of Table 12.2, as $\widehat{OR} = (31 \times 558)/(32 \times 505) = 1.070$. Similar calculations can be made for each of the other body weight categories in turn. The fact that the estimated regression coefficients can again be calculated directly from the grouped data is a consequence of the fact that Model (3) of Table 13.3 makes no regression assumption about the log odds of CHD in the various body weight groups. Note that confidence intervals can be computed directly from the estimated standard deviations of the corresponding slope estimates. For example, the estimated log Odds Ratio comparing the heaviest group (>180 lb) to the reference group is 0.610 with an associated 95% confidence interval given by $0.610 \pm (1.96 \times 0.217) = (0.185, 1.035)$; in terms of the Odds Ratio, the confidence interval is $(e^{0.185}, e^{1.035}) = (1.203, 2.816)$. Again, this could have been calculated directly from Table 12.2 using the techniques of Chapter 7.1.2.

Risk comparisons between other body weight categories are more complex when using the logistic regression structure. If one wishes to estimate the Odds Ratio comparing the category with body weight from 160^+ to 170 lb to those with weight between 150 and 160 lb, this can be done directly from the second and third rows of Table 12.2. From the fit of Model (3), the estimated log Odds Ratio is straightforward, since it is given by $\hat{b}_2 - \hat{b}_1 = 0.384 - 0.068 = 0.316$, with associated Odds Ratio $= e^{.316} = 1.371$. The confidence interval for this log Odds Ratio depends on the sampling variance of $\hat{b}_2 - \hat{b}_1$; this is just $Var(\hat{b}_2) + Var(\hat{b}_1) - 2Cov(\hat{b}_1, \hat{b}_2)$, the third term appearing because the estimates of $\hat{b}_1$ and $\hat{b}_2$ are correlated, being based on the same data (here, they use the same reference group). The results of fitting Model (3) immediately yield $Var(\hat{b}_2) = 0.234^2 = 0.055$, and $Var(\hat{b}_1) = 0.259^2 = 0.067$. However, an estimate of the covariance term has to be separately computed from the log likelihood function; here the estimate is 0.033 (not reported in Table 13.3). Thus, an estimate of the variance of $\hat{b}_2 - \hat{b}_1$ is then $0.055 + 0.067 - (2 \times 0.033) = 0.056$, with resulting standard error $= \sqrt{0.056} = 0.236$. This provides a 95% confidence interval for $b_2 - b_1$, the log Odds Ratio desired, of $0.316 \pm (1.96 \times 0.236) = (-0.148, 0.779)$. The corresponding confidence interval for the Odds Ratio is then $(e^{-0.148}, e^{0.779}) = (0.863, 2.180)$. We can easily check that these are exactly equivalent to the results obtained directly from Table 12.2.

For Model (3) of Table 13.3, the null hypothesis that $b_1 = b_2 = b_3 = b_4 = 0$ is equivalent to independence of CHD and body weight (as measured by these indicator variables), with the alternative being that at least one of the slope coefficients is nonzero. This is exactly the null and alternative hypotheses of the test of overall association of Chapter 11.1. We can most easily use the likelihood ratio method as a basis for this test in the regression approach. Model (1) is nested within Model (3) (set $b_1 = b_2 = b_3 = b_4 = 0$); the likelihood ratio test statistic is therefore $2[-879.9 - (-890.6)] = 21.4$, giving a p-value of 0.0003 when compared to tables of the χ^2 distribution with 4 degrees of freedom. This agrees exactly with

Table 13.4 *Comparison of estimated odds ratios for various body weight levels against the reference group, based on two logistic regression models for the Western Collaborative Group Study*

Model	Odds Ratios for Various Levels of Z Compared to $Z = 0$				
	$Z = 0$	$Z = 1$	$Z = 2$	$Z = 3$	$Z = 4$
$\log\left(\frac{p}{1-p}\right) = a + b_1 z_1 + \cdots + b_4 z_4$	1.000	1.070	1.468	2.297	1.840
$\log\left(\frac{p}{1-p}\right) = a + bz$	1.000	1.197	1.433	1.716	2.054

the results of the overall χ^2 test of association of Chapter 11.1, as described in Chapter 11.4.

To carry out an analogous test for trend (see Chapter 11.3), we can use the variable Z of Table 13.2. Model (4) describes the incidence of CHD in terms of Z, assuming that there is a trend in the risk as Z increases (specifically, a linear trend on the log odds scale). Note that the interpretation of a as the log odds of CHD amongst individuals whose body weight is less than 150 lb is the same as for Model (3); however, the estimate $\hat{a}$ is slightly different because, instead of just the first (as in Model (3)), all body weight categories now contribute to the estimate through the regression assumption. The slope estimate is $\hat{b} = 0.180$ with $e^{\hat{b}} = 1.198$. This is the estimated Odds Ratio associated with a unit increase in Z, giving the Odds Ratio for comparing individuals whose weight lies between 150 and 160 lb ($Z = 1$) to the reference group with weight ≤ 150 lb ($Z = 0$). It is also the estimated Odds Ratio comparing individuals with weight greater than 180 lb to those whose initial weight was between 170 and 180 lb, and so on. Both Models (3) and (4) yield estimates of the Odds Ratio associated with any weight group as compared to the reference group; these estimates based on the different models are given in Table 13.4 and provide the input for Figure 12.6, although the estimated log odds for each body weight category, using Models (3) and (4), are plotted there. These Odds Ratios are not constrained in Model (3) of Table 13.3, but are in the fourth model through the linearity assumption relating the log odds of CHD incidence to the ordered variable Z. The estimated Odds Ratios of the constrained Model (4) reasonably match the unconstrained Odds Ratio estimates of Model (3), except in the highest two weight categories, where Model (4) requires the Odds Ratios to continue increasing though the data reflect a drop in risk, perhaps artifactually; see Figure 12.6 for a visual illustration of this point.

Note that a test of the null hypothesis $H_0 : b = 0$ in Model (4) (against the alternative that $b \neq 0$) is a test for trend in the risk of CHD over the levels of body weight that is analogous to the test of Chapter 11.3. In fact, this test is based on assumed linearity on the log odds scale rather than the original risk scale—the top left and bottom right plots of Figure 12.7 show that we might expect these two approaches to give similar results. For Model (4), the Wald test statistic is $z_b^2 = (0.180/0.046)^2 = 15.2$ with an associated p-value $= 0.0001$. A similar result follows from the likelihood ratio test statistic comparing the nested Models (1) and (4), given by $2 \times [-882.8 - (-890.6)] = 15.6$, yielding a similarly small p-value. There is thus considerable evidence of an increasing trend in the incidence of CHD as body weight increases.

Does the simpler two-parameter Model (4) fit the data from the five weight strata adequately? Since Model (4) is a special case of Model (3) [putting $b_2 = 2b_1$, $b_3 = 3b_1$, and $b_4 = 4b_1$ in Model (3) gives Model (4)], we can use the likelihood ratio test statistic to address this question. The likelihood ratio test statistic is $2 \times [-879.9 - (-882.8)] = 5.8$. Comparison with a χ^2 distribution with 3 degrees of freedom [the difference in the degrees of freedom of Models (3) and (4)] yields a p-value of .12. This is, of course, analogous to the goodness of fit test (see Chapter 11.3.2), which gave the test statistic 6.0 when applied to the same data (see Chapter 11.4). There is therefore insufficient evidence to indicate that the simpler trend Model (4) inadequately describes the CHD incidence levels over the different body weight groups.

Finally, we look at Models (5) and (6) of Table 13.3, which relate true interval-scaled exposure variables to the log odds of CHD incidence. Model (5), which fits the raw body weight variable directly, has already been discussed briefly in Chapter 13.1.1 and illustrated in Figure 13.3. Note the marked increase in the standard deviation of the intercept estimate as compared with Model (4), for instance. This is explained by the interpretation of a in Model (5)—that it is the log odds of CHD incidence when $Wt = 0$, that is, for individuals whose initial body weight is 0 lb! Since there are no data on any individual with a body weight anywhere near to zero, this estimate is therefore based on considerable extrapolation from the region where actual body weights are observed. As such, the estimate correctly carries with it a large amount of uncertainty that is reflected in the high standard deviation. On the other hand, the slope coefficient, b, has a much smaller estimated value in the fifth model than we saw earlier. Again, this is largely due to the scale of Wt, since $\hat{b}$ is the estimated log Odds Ratio associated with an increase of one unit in Wt, that is, 1 lb! While we could consequently estimate a more meaningful log Odds Ratio by calculating $20\hat{b}$, say, associated with an increase in body weight of 20 lb, we can directly achieve more interpretable parameters by measuring body weight on a "regularized" scale. This is achieved in Model (6) by fitting the variable $Nwt = (Wt - 150)/20$. Now the 0 value of Nwt corresponds to a body weight of 150 lb, and a unit increase in Nwt corresponds to an increase of 20 lb in body weight.

13.3 Logistic regression with case-control data

Suppose we use a case-control design to study a population for which we assume a logistic regression model describes how the risk of disease (D) depends on (the numerical level of) an exposure variable, X. For simplicity, we suppose that there is just one exposure variable as this illustrates both the issues and solution to the analysis of case-control data. As an example, consider the study of coffee drinking (X) and pancreatic cancer (D) (which we will analyze numerically in Section 13.4). In the population, the logistic regression assumption gives $\log(p_x/(1 - p_x)) = a + bx$, where $p_x = P(D|X = x)$ as usual. We now consider how the likelihood techniques for estimating a and b, described in Section 13.1, apply to data arising from a case-control sample from this population. At first blush, the sampling method appears to cause a problem in that the construction of the likelihood function now depends on computation of terms such as $P(X = 3|D)$ for a sampled individual with $D = 1$ and $X = 3$. Thus, the likelihood depends on a and b in a more complex way than with population-based or cohort sampling. Recall that conditional probabilities such as $P(D = 1|X = 3)$ cannot be calculated from case-control data because of the design's manipulation of the frequency of cases $(D = 1)$ and controls $(D = 0)$.

For a binary exposure, the impact of case-control sampling turned out not to matter because of the properties of the Odds Ratio (Chapters 5.3 and 7.1), so that we were able to treat case-control data comparably to the other designs. Dare we close our eyes, cross our fingers, and do the same now with an interval-scaled exposure and logistic regression model parameters to estimate? Case-control sampling leads to a distortion of the relative frequency of cases and controls in the sample at each level of exposure X. We might assume that this will foul up the relationship between $P(D|X)$ and X in the sample, so that a population logistic regression model will no longer be appropriate. Before we abandon hope, however, we will look more closely at the distortion introduced by case-control sampling.

Suppose π_{case} is the probability of an individual being sampled given that they are a case; that is, $\pi_{case} = P(\text{sampled}|D)$. Similarly, define $\pi_{control} = P(\text{sampled}|\bar{D})$. In case-control sampling these selection probabilities, or *sampling fractions*, are not related to exposure level; that is, they do not depend on X. We now divide the subpopulation who share exposure level $X = x$ into four distinct groups based on (1) their disease status and (2) whether they are included in the sample or not. We can also measure the relative frequency of these groups in this subpopulation. For example, the probability of being a case and being sampled, amongst individuals with exposure $X = x$, is just $P(D \& \text{sampled} |X = x) = P(D|X = x)P(\text{sampled}|D, X = x) = \pi_{case} p_x$. The four groups and their respective proportions within the subpopulation with exposure $X = x$ are then

- Individual is a case and is sampled: proportion $= \pi_{case} p_x$.
- Individual is a case and is not sampled: proportion $= (1 - \pi_{case}) p_x$.
- Individual is a control and is sampled: proportion $= \pi_{control}(1 - p_x)$.
- Individual is a control and is not sampled: proportion $= (1 - \pi_{control})(1 - p_x)$.

Of course, we only see sampled individuals. The relative probability of being a case or control—a D or a $\bar{D}$— at exposure level $X = x$ and *conditional on being sampled* is just

$$P(D|X = x, \text{ sampled }) = \frac{\pi_{case} p_x}{\pi_{case} p_x + \pi_{control}(1 - p_x)}, \qquad (13.3)$$

based on the first and third proportions above.

This indicates directly how case-control sampling modifies the "apparent" risk at exposure level $X = x$ in that $P(D|X = x, \text{ sampled}) \neq p_x$, the population risk when $X = x$, unless $\pi_{case} = \pi_{control}$, that is, unless cases and controls are sampled at the same frequency. This situation is, of course, unlikely to be true, since the whole point of a case-control design is to oversample cases relative to controls. But look at how this distortion of p_x plays out when you compare different levels of X. Recall that, in the population, we assume that $\log (p_x/(1 - p_x)) = a + bx$. We have $1 - P(D|X = x, sampled) = [\pi_{control}(1 - p_x)]/[\pi_{case} p_x + \pi_{control}(1 - p_x)]$ from (Equation 13.3), so that, for sampled individuals,

$$\log \left(\frac{P(D|X = x, sampled)}{1 - P(D|X = x, sampled)} \right) = \log \left(\frac{\pi_{case} p_x}{\pi_{control}(1 - p_x)} \right)$$

$$= \log \left(\frac{\pi_{case}}{\pi_{control}} \right) + \log \left(\frac{p_x}{1 - p_x} \right)$$

$$= \log \left(\frac{\pi_{case}}{\pi_{control}} \right) + a + bx$$

$$= a^* + bx,$$

where $a^* = \log(\pi_{case}/\pi_{control}) + a$.

As expected, the outcome-dependent sampling has caused the log odds of the risk in the sample to differ from what it is in the population. But the difference is very specific, namely, the intercept term is now a^* rather than a, but the slope term b is exactly the same. We expect a change in the intercept because it measures the log odds of disease when $X = 0$; if, as is usual, π_{case} is much bigger than $\pi_{control}$, the intercept in the sample will be much larger than in the population [since then $\log(\pi_{case}/\pi_{control})$ will be a large positive number]. The fact that the slope coefficient b is not affected by case-control sampling is an extension of what we already observed about the Odds Ratio, namely, that this measure is not distorted by case-control sampling.

The implication of this analysis is that if we treat case-control data as if it were generated by a population-based design by fitting a logistic regression (as in Section 13.1.1), then the estimate of the slope coefficient b will be a reasonable estimate of the underlying parameter in our Target Population. On the other hand, the intercept estimate will be substantially distorted and cannot be treated as an estimate of the intercept in the population. Hypotheses and parameters can be investigated as before, so long as they do not directly involve the intercept term a.

This justification for the application of logistic regression techniques to case-control data does not quite reflect the exact form of case-control sampling defined in Chapter 5. There, as is customary, the sample sizes of cases and controls are fixed by design, where the sampling fraction description used in this section allows for a random number of cases and controls, albeit with respective sample size expectations given by $N\pi_{case}$ and $N\pi_{control}$, where N is the population size. Nevertheless, Prentice and Pyke (1979) showed that, in the situation with fixed sample sizes, we can still apply estimation techniques for population-based or cohort studies directly to case-control data as long as we acknowledge that any calculations involving the intercept term a directly will be distorted. This excludes estimation of the risk of D at any particular exposure level, since this involves a (see Equations 12.3 and 12.6). However, since we are often most interested in relative comparisons, such as Odds Ratios, which depend solely on the slope coefficients of the logistic model, this restriction is not a fatal flaw.

The results of Prentice and Pyke (1979) apply directly to the (log) likelihood function so that estimates of the standard deviations of slope coefficients and hypothesis testing techniques like the likelihood ratio method (as described in Section 13.1 and illustrated in Section 13.2) can also be used with case-control data. To see these in action in this context, we return to our example on pancreatic cancer.

13.4 Example—coffee drinking and pancreatic cancer: part 5

We use the findings of the last section to estimate various logistic regression models based on data associating coffee drinking to incidence of pancreatic cancer (e.g., Table 11.2). For convenience, Table 13.5 gives details on several coding schemes that capture coffee consumption. Table 13.6 describes coefficient estimates for several logistic regression models, using various choices for quantifying coffee drinking. We do not report the maximum likelihood estimates of the intercept terms a in any of these models since they do not provide estimates of the population log odds of disease for the relevant baseline group, as discussed in Section 13.3.

Point estimation, confidence intervals, and hypothesis testing for the Odds Ratio associated with a binary measure of coffee consumption (described in Chapter 7.1.3 using basic methods) can all be alternatively achieved using Models (1) and (2) of Table 13.6. In particular, the estimate of the Odds Ratio associated with coffee drinking is given by e^b in Model (2) which yields $e^{1.012} = 2.751$. A 95% confidence interval for this log Odds Ratio is simply $1.012 \pm (1.96 \times 0.257) = (0.508, 1.516)$; this

Table 13.5 *Various coding schemes for data relating coffee consumption to pancreatic cancer incidence as given in Tables 7.2 and 11.2*

$$X = \begin{cases} 1 & \text{Coffee drinker } (\geq 1 \text{ cups per day}) \\ 0 & \text{Coffee abstainer } (0 \text{ cups per day}) \end{cases}$$

$$Z_1 = \begin{cases} 1 & \text{1–2 cups per day} \\ 0 & \text{otherwise} \end{cases}$$

$$Z_2 = \begin{cases} 1 & \text{3–4 cups per day} \\ 0 & \text{otherwise} \end{cases}$$

$$Z_3 = \begin{cases} 1 & \geq 5 \text{ cups per day} \\ 0 & \text{otherwise} \end{cases}$$

$$Z = \begin{cases} 0 & \text{0 cups per day} \\ 1 & \text{1–2 cups per day} \\ 2 & \text{2–3 cups per day} \\ 3 & \geq 5 \text{ cups per day} \end{cases}$$

$$Y = \begin{cases} 1 & \text{Female} \\ 0 & \text{Male} \end{cases}$$

Table 13.6 *Logistic regression models relating coffee to incidence of pancreatic cancer*

Model (No.)	Parameter	Estimate	SD	OR	p-Value	Max. Log Likelihood
(1) $\log\left(\frac{p}{1-p}\right) = a$	a	—	—	—	—	−661.9
(2) $\log\left(\frac{p}{1-p}\right) = a + bx$	a	—	—	—	—	
	b	1.012	0.257	2.751	<0.001	−652.8
(3) $\log\left(\frac{p}{1-p}\right) = a + b_1z_1 +$	a	—	—	—	—	
$b_2z_2 + b_3z_3$	b_1	0.910	0.268	2.484	0.001	
	b_2	1.108	0.278	3.029	<0.001	
	b_3	1.091	0.284	2.978	<0.001	−651.8
(4) $\log\left(\frac{p}{1-p}\right) = a + bz$	a	—	—	—	—	
	b	0.234	0.070	1.263	0.001	−656.3

Note: SD = standard deviation; variables are defined in Table 13.5.

translates into a confidence interval of (1.662, 4.552) for the Odds Ratio. The Wald test statistic for the null hypothesis $b = 0$ in Model (2), that is, independence of coffee drinking and pancreatic cancer, is $z_b = 1.012/0.257 = 3.94$. This statistic squared is 15.5, yielding a p-value of 8×10^{-5}. The analogous likelihood ratio test statistic is $2 \times [-652.8 - (-661.9)] = 18.2$, giving a smaller p-value. These can be directly compared to the simple χ^2 test statistic for independence of 16.6, given in Chapter 7.1.3.

Similarly, an overall test of association between coffee drinking and pancreatic cancer, using all four measured levels of consumption, can be carried out by comparing Models (1) and (3). The likelihood ratio test statistic is simply $2 \times [-651.8 - (-661.9)] = 20.2$, which, when compared to a χ^2 distribution with 3 degrees of freedom, yields a p-value of 1.6×10^{-4}. Again, this can be compared with the overall χ^2 test for association statistic of 18.6, calculated in Chapter 11.2.

A test for trend in incidence over the four ordered coffee consumption categories can be investigated using the variable Z of Table 13.5 and Model (4) of Table 13.6. The Wald test of $b = 0$ in Model (4) gives $z_b^2 = 11.2$, and the likelihood ratio statistic comparing Models (4) and (1) is $2 \times [-656.3 - (-661.9)] = 11.3$. Both these statistics give essentially the same p-value, approximately 8×10^{-4}. These almost exactly replicate the (linear) test for trend χ^2 statistic of 11.3 given in Chapter 11.5.

A goodness of fit statistic for the adequacy of Model (4) in describing the variation in risk over the four consumption categories can be computed by comparing Models (3) and (4), using the likelihood ratio test statistic of $2 \times [-651.8 - (-656.3)] = 8.9$. Comparing this to a χ^2 distribution with 2 degrees of freedom gives a p-value of .012, again similar to the goodness of fit statistic of 7.3 from Chapter 11.5, reflecting that a linear trend in log odds does not describe the pattern of risk effectively. In Chapter 11.5, we discussed the possibility of a threshold relationship between consumption and pancreatic cancer incidence. This might be fit using the model

$$\log \left(\frac{p_{z_1,z_2,z_3}}{1 - p_{z_1,z_2,z_3}} \right) = a + bz_1 + bz_2 + bz_3,$$

for the three indicator variables. This model allows the incidence of pancreatic cancer to differ for coffee drinkers as compared to nondrinkers, but assumes that the risk does not depend on the level of consumption. Of course, this is simply Model (2) in disguise, and as it is nested within Model (3) we can compare Models (2) and (3) using the likelihood ratio technique. In other words, this is a test of the null hypothesis $H_0 : b_1 = b_2 = b_3$ in Model (3). The likelihood ratio test statistic is $2 \times [-651.8 - (-652.8)] = 1.9$, giving a p-value of 0.38 in comparison to a χ^2 distribution with 2 degrees of freedom (the difference in the degrees of freedom between the two models is 2). Thus, the threshold model of a common risk for all the coffee consumption groups (above zero cups per day), albeit higher than the abstainers, fits the observed pattern of risks in the four consumption groups closely. Although we cannot directly compare Models (4) and (2)—they are not nested, having the same number of free parameters or degrees of freedom—their separate comparison to the more general Model (3) strongly suggests that Model (2) fits the data substantially better than Model (4). Figure 13.4 reproduces Figure 11.3 and adds the fitted versions of Models (2) and (4), visually demonstrating the superior fit of the threshold model.

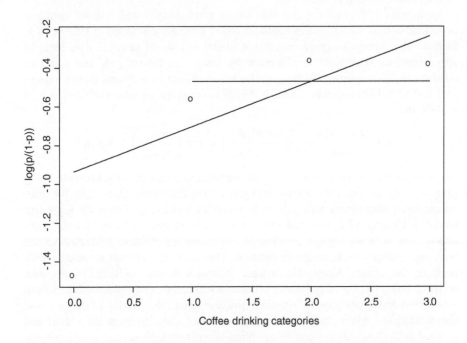

Figure 13.4 *Plot of observed log odds* $(\log(p/(1 - p)))$ *for incidence of pancreatic cancer, with fitted log odds for threshold model and trend model (Models (2) and (4) of Table 13.6, respectively).*

Note that Model (2) fits the observed log odds for the coffee abstainers exactly, so that its fitted log odds of disease in this group is the plotted point in the "zero" coffee drinking category.

13.5 Comments and further reading

Clayton and Hills (1993) provide further introduction to the use of the likelihood function. Maximum likelihood techniques can also be used to estimate the parameters in the other regression models of Chapter 12. However, only the logistic regression model has the property that the slope coefficients can be estimated directly from case-control data without additional information; however, knowledge of the sampling fractions, or equivalently of the population frequency of disease ($P(D)$), is sufficient to construct parameter estimates for other models. Scott and Wild (1997) describe an iterative technique for estimating regression parameters from case-control data for an arbitrary generalized linear model using maximization of a population-based likelihood as the primary component.

Although in both Tables 13.3 and 13.6 we used simple category scores to examine the roles of body weight and coffee drinking, it is usually preferable to deal directly with the ungrouped interval-scaled version of the exposure if possible, as in Models (5) and (6) of Table 13.3. The direct approach produces more precise estimates of exposure effects (Greenland, 1995).

Application of logistic regression to case-control designs with risk-set sampling or to case-cohort studies raises identical issues to those discussed in Chapter 7.5. In particular, fitting a logistic regression model to risk-set sampled data requires appropriate accounting for stratification, by design, on time at risk, and therefore involves methods specifically designed for matched data to be discussed in Chapters 16.5 and 17.3. For case-cohort data, it is easy to adapt the argument of Section 13.3 to show that

$$\log\left(\frac{P(case|X = x, sampled)}{P(cohort|X = x, sampled)}\right) = \log\left(\frac{\pi_{case}}{\pi_{cohort}}\right) + \log p_x$$

where in the data $P(case)$ refers to being sampled as a case and $P(cohort)$ to being sampled in the cohort. This extends the idea of using the sample Odds Ratio for case-cohort data with a binary exposure. If the conditional risks, p_x, follow the log-linear model of Chapter 12.2, this then induces a logistic regression model for the case-cohort data, with the logistic coefficients estimating log Relative Risks, associated with unit changes in X, in the population. This approach extends to models with multiple risk factors. Again, the variance estimates for the coefficients associated with maximum likelihood estimation require modification as the naïve variances from straightforward application of logistic regression ignore the overlap of the case and cohort samples. Alternatively, we can ignore cases sampled from the cohort and proceed as for classical case-control sampling, where now logistic regression estimates correspond to population log Odds Ratios. If the outcome is rare, these two approaches essentially coincide. One advantage of the case-cohort design, as compared to classical case-control sampling, is that the cohort part of the data provides direct estimates of the intercept parameter or, equivalently, the risk of D at any selected value of the risk factors, X.

As for stratification techniques, interpretation of a logistic regression effect as causal depends on an assumed causal graph linking exposure to outcome with the assumption that there are no excluded confounding variables. In this chapter, we have focused on a single explanatory variable, but in the next chapter we turn to the modeling of several exposure variables simultaneously, using the multiple logistic regression model (Chapter 12.6).

13.6 Problems

Question 13.1

Consider a cohort study of a population designed to investigate the incidence of lung cancer as it relates to age (X), sex (Y), and smoking status (Z). Suppose each of these variables was coded as follows: $X = 0$ (age $\leq$40 years), $X = 1$ (age >40 years); $Y = 0$ (male), $Y = 1$ (female); $Z = 0$ (nonsmoker), $Z = 1$ (ever smoked).

The following logistic regression model is used to describe the relationship between incidence of lung cancer and these explanatory variables:

$$\log \left(\frac{p_{x,y,z}}{1 - p_{x,y,z}} \right) = a + bx + cy + dz,$$

where $p_{x,y,z}$ represents the incidence proportion of the disease for the group of individuals with $X = x$, $Y = y$, and $Z = z$, with each of x, y, z either 0 or 1.

1. How many parameters are in the model?
2. Given the model, what is the incidence proportion (in terms of the parameters) for females, age $\leq$40 years, who don't smoke?
3. Given the model, what is the incidence proportion (in terms of the parameters) for females, age >40 years, who smoke?
4. What is the Odds Ratio that compares the incidence in the group in (3) with the incidence in the group in (2)?
5. In terms of the parameters of the model, write down the null hypothesis that states that there is no relationship between age and risk of lung cancer, having adjusted for sex and smoking status.
6. In terms of the parameters of the model, write down the null hypothesis that states that males and females share the same risk for lung cancer, controlling for age and smoking status.

Question 13.2

"Husbands and wives, little children lost their lives"

Refer again to the data set *titanic*, found by going to http://www.crcpress.com/ e_products/downloads/. Using a logistic regression model, examine and interpret the impact separately of (1) the sex of a passenger, (2) his or her age, (3) his or her place of embarkment, and (4) his or her ticket class on risk of death in the disaster. For age, use the continuous scale and assume linearity; note that there is missing age data on 263 of the 1309 passengers. For ticket class, use both indicator variables and an ordered scale and assess whether the latter provides an adequate fit.

Question 13.3

The data set *wcgs*, at http://www.crcpress.com/e_products/downloads/, contains data from the Western Collaborative Group Study that has been extensively analyzed in many chapters. Using this data set, examine the variable giving the number of cigarettes smoked per day. You will observe a substantial amount of "digit preference" in individual responses. Bearing this in mind, choose eight to ten ordered categories for this variable. Then, fit logistic regression models that relate baseline cigarette smoking to the risk of CHD during follow-up, using (1) indicator variables and (2) a suitably defined ordered scale. Investigate whether a linear term in the ordered scale, in a logistic model, provides an adequate fit to the CHD incidence data using suitable plots and a likelihood ratio test statistic.

Question 13.4

Using the data set *wcgs*, found at http://www.crcpress.com/e_products/downloads/, fit a logistic regression model that relates diastolic and systolic blood pressure, at baseline, to subsequent risk of CHD. Compare your results to those reported in Question 12.2.

CHAPTER 14

Confounding and Interaction within Logistic Regression Models

The previous two chapters introduced the logistic regression model and provided the necessary tools to fit such models to data, including that arising from case-control designs. Chapters 13.2 and 13.4 contrasted results from this approach with those previously obtained for categorical exposures. Although we briefly tackled the modeling of an interval-scaled exposure (body weight) in Table 13.3, we so far seem to have introduced the heavy machinery (of regression) merely to do a job effectively performed by hammers and screwdrivers (simple categorical methods of Chapters 7 to 11). What's the point? Are we just trying to complicate matters for effect? Well, of course not. While the previous chapters introduced logistic regression, linking these simple cases with our previous work, we now want to take advantage of the generality of regression methods so that we can achieve the goals we promised, in particular, simultaneous adjustment of several risk factors and confounders using a modest number of degrees of freedom.

The multiple logistic regression model of Chapter 12.6 allows for the evaluation of several risk factors at the same time, albeit assuming that there is no multiplicative interaction. We now use the machinery at close to its full capacity by (1) addressing the assessment of confounding within logistic regression models and (2) extending the multiple logistic regression model to allow for interaction.

14.1 Assessment of confounding using logistic regression models

For simplicity, first focus on two risk factors X_1 and X_2 where it is plausible to assume that there is no (multiplicative) interaction between X_1 and X_2. All of the ideas of this section extend directly to the situation where there are many risk factors under examination. Consider the following two logistic regression models:

$$\log\left(\frac{p_{x_1}}{1 - p_{x_1}}\right) = a + bx_1 \tag{14.1}$$

$$\log\left(\frac{p_{x_1,x_2}}{1 - p_{x_1,x_2}}\right) = a^* + b^*x_1 + cx_2, \tag{14.2}$$

where, as before, $p_{x_1} = P(D|X_1 = x_1)$ and $p_{x_1,x_2} = P(D|X_1 = x_1, X_2 = x_2)$.

As the notation suggests, there is a distinction between the two slope coefficients, b and b^*, associated with the variable X_1 in these models. Since X_2 is not included in the model (Equation 14.1), the coefficient b yields the log Odds Ratio associated with a unit increase in X_1, ignoring any potential confounding role of X_2

(or any other variable, for that matter). On the other hand, b^* in Equation 14.2 gives the log Odds Ratio associated with a unit increase in X_1, *holding the variable X_2 fixed*. As noted in Chapter 12.6, the model (Equation 14.2) specifically excludes the possibility of (multiplicative) interaction between X_1 and X_2.

The log Odds Ratio, given by b^* in Equation 14.2, measures the effect of a unit increase in X_1, in any population group that shares a common value of X_2. Thus, this measure of association of X_1 and D directly accounts for the possible confounding effects of X_2. This observation has several implications: first, for simple categorical exposures, the maximum likelihood estimate of b^* is an alternative estimator to both the Woolf and Mantel–Haenszel procedures of Chapter 9.2 for estimating a common (log) Odds Ratio, accounting for the presence of a possible confounding variable. Maximum likelihood is a slightly different technique and so will usually yield similar, but not identical, results to these earlier approaches, particularly if the sample size is large. Second, with categorical risk factors, a test of the null hypothesis $H_0 : b^* = 0$ (against the alternative $H_A : b^* \neq 0$) in Equation 14.2 is analogous to the Cochran–Mantel–Haenszel test of association from Chapter 9.1.1, in that it examines the association between X_1 and D, controlling for the possible confounding effects of X_2.

Finally, for arbitrary exposure variables, comparison of estimates of the two parameters, b and b^*, allows us to assess the extent of confounding of the X_1–D relationship induced by X_2, assuming that the trend models (Equations 14.1 and 14.2) adequately describe exposure effects. Within the context of the two models, the two parameters b and b^* being equal is equivalent to collapsibility of the effect of X_1 across levels of X_2, as discussed for categorical variables in Chapter 8.4. Subject to having an appropriate causal graph underlying the models (Equations 14.1 and 14.2), we can then use estimates of b and b^* as an empirical description of confounding, as we did in Chapter 9.5.2. This, of course, assumes that collapsibility of the Odds Ratio is roughly equivalent to the absence of confounding, which is reasonable if the disease is rare. The relevant causal graph not only accounts for the causal direction of associations, but also protects us from the inadvertent and incorrect view of confounding if X_2 is a collider.

Subject to these constraints, this empirical judgment of confounding corresponds to the approach of Chapter 9.5.2 and can be summarized as follows: if the maximum likelihood estimates $\hat{b}$ and $\hat{b}^*$ are very similar, then there is little confounding of the X_1–D relationship by X_2. If the estimates are markedly different, then the data indicate that X_2 has an important confounding effect, and we normally then prefer to account for X_2 in our analysis, reporting the results of fitting Equation 14.2 rather than Equation 14.1. In choosing between the unadjusted and adjusted estimates, the same pragmatic approach of Chapter 9.5.2 can be used effectively.

Note that the estimated standard errors of the maximum likelihood estimates, $\hat{b}$ and $\hat{b}^*$, will also be different, and the analysis of Chapter 9.5.1 indicates that variability will be higher for $\hat{b}^*$ than for $\hat{b}$. This is the "price" we pay to account for confounding bias. Sometimes the increase in standard error can be substantial, an issue we discuss further in Section 14.5 on *collinearity*. Nevertheless, the loss in precision is likely to be less than when using an adjusted estimate based on stratification by X_2, and often substantially less in cases where many confounding variables must be included. Usually we can effectively control for the effects of a confounder X_2 using very few

Table 14.1 *Additional logistic regression models for the Western Collaborative Group Study*

Model (No.)	Parameter	Estimate	SD	OR	p-Value	Max. Log Likelihood
(7) $\log\left(\frac{p}{1-p}\right) = a + bx$	a	−3.330	0.204	—	<0.001	
$+ c_1 z_1 + \cdots + c_4 z_4$	b	0.843	0.141	2.324	<0.001	
	c_1	0.059	0.261	1.061	0.820	
	c_2	0.355	0.235	1.426	0.131	
	c_3	0.798	0.225	2.220	<0.001	
	c_4	0.561	0.218	1.752	0.010	−860.6
(8) $\log\left(\frac{p}{1-p}\right) = a + bx$	a	−3.311	0.161	—	<0.001	
$+ cz$	b	0.843	0.141	2.323	<.001	
	c	0.168	0.047	1.183	< 0.001	−863.5
(9) $\log\left(\frac{p}{1-p}\right) = a + bx$	a	−4.607	0.524	—	<0.001	
$+ c(wt)$	b	0.849	0.140	2.337	<0.001	
	c	0.010	0.003	1.010	0.001	−864.8
(10) $\log\left(\frac{p}{1-p}\right) = a + bx$	a	−3.140	0.134	—	<0.001	
$+ c(nwt)$	b	0.849	0.140	2.337	<0.001	
	c	0.196	0.059	1.216	0.001	−864.8

Note: Variables are defined in Table 13.2.

degrees of freedom (only one in Equation 14.2), as opposed to stratification, where the degrees of freedom "used up" are one less than the number of strata of X_2. The difference in the degrees of freedom between the two approaches quickly increases as we add confounders to the model.

14.1.1 Example—the Western Collaborative Group Study: part 8

Table 14.1 gives the results of fitting several logistic regression models to examinine the roles of behavior type and initial body weight simultaneously. The coding for the referenced variables is given in Table 13.2.

Model (7) of Table 14.1 includes body weight in terms of the four indicator variables that we considered in Model (3) of Table 13.3. Note that Model (7) provides an estimated Odds Ratio of $e^b = e^{0.843} = 2.32$ associated with behavior type, controlling for the effects of body weight. Since behavior type is binary, we can compare this estimate with the Woolf estimate of 2.26 and the Mantel–Haenszel estimate of 2.32 (both given in Chapter 9.2.3) for the same Odds Ratio. We can test the null hypothesis $H_0 : b = 0$ in the context of Model (7) via the Wald method, which gives the test statistic $z_b = 0.843/0.141 = 6.0$ (with $z_b^2 = 35.9$). Alternatively, we can compute the likelihood ratio test statistic by comparing the maximized likelihood for Model (7), −860.6, with that obtained from the nested Model (3) of Table 13.3 (that is, −879.9), which excludes behavior type. This gives a likelihood ratio test statistic of $2 \times [-860.6 - (-879.9)] = 38.6$, yielding a p-value of 5×10^{-10} in comparison with tables of the χ^2 distribution with 1 degree of freedom. A similarly small p-value is obtained from the Wald test statistic. Again, this yields very similar results to the Cochran–Mantel–Haenszel test statistic for the same null hypothesis, computed as 37.6 in Chapter 9.2.3. All results point to the sizeable impact of behavior type on CHD incidence, controlling for the potential confounding effects of body weight.

To assess the extent of confounding here, we compare the unadjusted estimate of the Odds Ratio for behavior type, calculated for Model (2) of Table 13.3 as $OR = 2.373$, with the adjusted version of the same Odds Ratio, estimated in Model (7) of Table 14.1 as $OR = 2.324$. This comparison reflects little confounding due to body weight, despite the strong association of body weight with CHD. Based on the discussion of Chapter 8 in general, and Chapter 9.2.3 specifically, this implies little association between body weight and behavior type observed in the data. Of course, this observation can be confirmed directly.

We can also perform similar analyses that use fewer degrees of freedom to quantify the role of body weight. For example, to assess the adjusted effect of behavior type on CHD, we can compare Model (8) of Table 14.1 with Model (4) of Table 13.3, or Models (9) and (10) with Models (5) and (6), respectively. Very similar estimates of the Odds Ratio (relating behavior type to CHD) are found by any of these approaches, in large part because there is little confounding due to body weight, however it is coded. This has the consequence that, with interest focusing on behavior type, it does not really matter how we model body weight nor whether we model it appropriately.

The estimated standard error associated with the estimate $\hat{b}$ in Model (7) of Table 14.1 is slightly larger than the corresponding standard error in the unadjusted estimate in Model (2) of Table 13.3, as expected due to having to control for the effects of body weight in Model (7). In Model (7), the adjustment is made through use of an additional 4 degrees of freedom (the four indicator variables) and is equivalent to simple stratification on body weight into five strata. Thus, in terms of precision, this approach gains nothing over the stratified analysis of Chapter 9. The regression approach encourages us to model the role of body weight more succinctly, say, with just one additional degree of freedom, as in Models (8), (9), or (10). Table 14.2 gives the estimated standard errors for the log Odds Ratio associated with behavior type for each of these models [Model (10) is identical to Model (9)].

As we can see, the simpler models, (8) and (9), regain some of the precision lost to stratification. The effects here are extraordinarily subtle since both (1) the level of stratification is very modest and (2) body weight is unassociated with behavior type. However, this table represents the fundamental advantage of regression modeling over stratification, namely, that regression models are more parsimonious, thereby allowing more accurate measures of the effects of interest. We see much greater gains

Table 14.2 *Comparison of estimated standard errors of estimate $\hat{b}$ of the log odds ratio for behavior type, based on logistic regression Models (2), (7), (8), and (9) of Table 13.3 and Table 14.1*

Model No.	(2)	(7)	(8)	(9)
Estimated standard error of b	0.14021	0.14067	0.14054	0.14048

from regression models when they contain a large number of extraneous variables in the model and, thus, use far fewer degrees of freedom than stratification. We return to this issue in Chapter 15.

14.2 Introducing interaction into the multiple logistic regression model

All logistic regression models with more than one exposure variable considered to date have been based on the multiple logistic regression model (Equation 12.5 or Equation 12.6) and assume no (multiplicative) interaction amongst the various risk factors. We now show how to extend this model to allow for the possibility of interaction effects.

For simplicity, we begin with the simplest situation, where interest focuses on the impact of two risk factors, X and Z, on an outcome D. As noted, the model $\log(p_{x,z}/(1 - p_{x,z})) = \log(\text{odds of } D|X = x, Z = z) = a + bx + cz$ assumes no interaction between X and Z. To incorporate interaction, we simply need to add to this model an additional derived covariate, W, defined by $W = X \times Z$. We then fit the following model:

$$\log \left(\frac{p_{x,z}}{1 - p_{x,z}} \right) = a + bx + cz + dw \equiv a + bx + cz + d(x \times z). \quad (14.3)$$

The interpretation of the intercept coefficient remains as before, namely, the log odds of D when both X and Z are zero. However, the meaning of the slope coefficients is somewhat different, as we now explore.

Consider two groups of individuals whose risk factor X differs by one unit on the scale of X and who share identical values for the other risk variable Z. That is, suppose one group has risk variables given by $X = x + 1, Z = z$, and the second group has levels given by $X = x, Z = z$. Then, the logistic regression model (Equation 14.3) indicates that the difference in log odds of D in these two groups is just

$$[a + b(x + 1) + cz + d(x + 1) \times z] - [a + bx + cz + d(x \times z)] = b + dz.$$

This, as before, is the log Odds Ratio associated with a unit increase in X, but now this log Odds Ratio depends on the fixed level of Z; in other words, it is modified by Z. This is exactly what we want, since this explicitly allows for (multiplicative) interaction.

Suppose both X and Z are binary and coded with values 0 and 1 to describe their two levels. For a concrete example, let X denote coffee consumption and Z be the binary covariate sex in studying pancreatic cancer incidence. We can interpret that when $Z = 0$ (males, say), the log Odds Ratio comparing the two levels of X, coffee drinkers to abstainers, is just b. This is similar to our earlier interpretation of b, except we are now restricting this log Odds Ratio to only those in the population for whom $Z = 0$, i.e., males. On the other hand, when $Z = 1$ (females), the log Odds Ratio comparing the two levels of X is given by $b + d$. Thus, the parameter d measures the difference in the log Odds Ratios associated with X (coffee drinking) between males and females (the $Z = 0$ and $Z = 1$ strata). Further, testing the null hypothesis $H_0 : d = 0$ against the alternative $H_A : d \neq 0$ provides a test of the evidence for heterogeneous Odds Ratios, that is, for (multiplicative) interaction. Similarly, in Equation 14.3, the log Odds Ratio comparing the two sexes is c for coffee abstainers ($X = 0$) and $c + d$ for coffee drinkers ($X = 1$).

Now suppose the second risk factor can assume several (say, K) discrete levels; these can be incorporated into the model through a set of indicator variables, $Z_1, \ldots, Z_{K-1}$, as discussed in Chapter 12.6.1. For an example that matches this situation, let X denote behavior type, with $Z_1, \ldots, Z_{K-1}$ capturing the five categories of body weight ($K = 5$) given in the WCGS study. To allow for the possibility that the log Odds Ratio associated with behavior type is different in each of the K strata defined by the levels of body weight, we must add $K - 1$ product terms to obtain the analog of Equation 14.3, each extra derived covariate comprising the product of X and one of the $K - 1$ indicator variables, $Z_1, \ldots, Z_{K-1}$. That is, we fit the following model:

$$\log \left(\frac{p_{x,z_1,\ldots,z_{K-1}}}{1 - p_{x,z_1,\ldots,z_{K-1}}} \right) = a + bx + c_1 z_1 + \cdots + c_{K-1} z_{K-1}$$
$$+ d_1(x \times z_1) + \cdots + d_{K-1}(x \times z_{K-1}).$$

With this model, similar calculations show that the log Odds Ratio comparing the two levels of X (type A and type B) is

- b for the reference group of Z (i.e., weight below 150 lb, $Z_1 = \cdots = Z_{K-1} = 0$)
- $b + d_1$ for the next level of Z (i.e., weight between 150 and 160 lb, $Z_1 = 1$)
- $b + d_2$ for the next level of Z (i.e., weight between 160 and 170 lb, $Z_2 = 1$)
- $b + d_3$ for the next level of Z (i.e., weight between 170 and 180 lb, $Z_3 = 1$)
- $b + d_4$ for the next level of Z (i.e., weight greater than 180 lb, $Z_4 = 1$)

This achieves the goal of permitting a different Odds Ratio for X at each level of Z. Testing the null hypothesis $H_0 : d_1 = d_2 = \cdots = d_{K-1} = 0$ assesses the homogeneity, or lack thereof, of these K Odds Ratios for X, thus providing a test of (multiplicative) interaction between X and Z.

Alternatively, we can use an ordered scale for the K levels of Z, coded in an appropriate fashion, say, $Z = 1, 2, \ldots, K - 1$. If we then fit the model

$$\log \left(\frac{p_{x,z}}{1 - p_{x,z}} \right) = a + bx + cz + d(x \times z),$$

the log Odds Ratio associated with X, behavior type, is still b when $Z = 0$ (i.e., weight below 150 lb), but is $b + d$ when $Z = 1$ (i.e., weight between 150 and 160 lb), $b + 2d$ when $Z = 2$ (i.e., weight between 160 and 170 lb), etc., up to $b + (K - 1)d$ when $Z = K - 1$. This model therefore allows the log Odds Ratios for X to vary across the levels of Z, but these (log) Odds Ratios must increase or decrease linearly in terms of the ordered scale for Z. Now, a test of the null hypothesis $H_0 : d = 0$ against $H_A : d \neq 0$ is a test of interaction that focuses solely on evidence that the log Odds Ratio for X increases or decreases over levels of Z (according to a linear trend), thereby providing a targeted test, precisely of the kind desired in Chapter 10.3.4.

Before turning to some illustrative examples, we consider one further situation—when both risk factors X and Z carry continuous scales. One possible logistic regression model for X and Z that permits interaction is given by:

$$\log\left(\frac{p_{x,z}}{1 - p_{x,z}}\right) = a + bx + cz + d(x \times z).$$

Now the log Odds Ratio associated with a unit increase in X is given by $b + dz$ at a fixed level of the second risk factor $Z = z$. Thus, this model allows the Odds Ratio associated with X to vary across the levels of Z, but again only according to a linear trend on the scale of Z. As a variant of this model, we may wish to fit Z as a "main effect" invoking its continuous scale, but use indicator variables for a grouped version of Z in the interaction terms to avoid the trend assumption in the interactive effects. By this point, it should be apparent that the logistic regression model is extraordinarily flexible with regard to modeling the way in which risk varies according to one or several explanatory variables.

As a final comment to this section, it is, in principle, possible to examine *higher order* interaction terms involving three risk factors, say, X_1, X_2, and X_3. A second-order interaction term examines the extent to which the nature of the interaction, or effect modification, between X_1 and X_2 is itself modified by the levels of X_3! Such higher order interactive effects are rarely studied with epidemiological data, in part because it is difficult to interpret them, and also due to the fact that there is even less power, or precision, available to assess them than regular (first order) interaction effects.

14.3 Example—coffee drinking and pancreatic cancer: part 6

Table 14.3 provides results from fitting additional logistic regression models to the coffee drinking and pancreatic cancer data, some of which include interactive effects.

Models (5) and (6) use a simple dichotomous scale for coffee consumption. Note that Model (6) includes an interaction term between this binary exposure and sex. This model now indicates that an estimate of the Odds Ratio for coffee drinkers, as compared to abstainers, is $e^b = e^{0.984} = 2.676$ for males and $e^{b+d} = e^{0.984-0.050} = 2.545$ for females. Since both risk factors are binary here, the linear assumption of the regression model places no constraints on the Odds Ratios; so these results exactly match the stratified estimates of Table 9.3. Note that e^d is not truly an Odds Ratio as reported in Table 14.3, but is instead the *ratio* of the female and male Odds Ratios, so that a value close to 1, here 0.951, reflects that the two Odds Ratios are similar.

The consistency of these male and female Odds Ratios can be examined formally by testing the null hypothesis $H_0 : d = 0$ in Model (6). The Wald test statistic for this hypothesis is given by $z_d = -0.050/0.520 = -0.096$. The square of this is 0.01, yielding a p-value of 0.92. Alternatively, this null hypothesis can be assessed by comparing Models (5) and (6) using the likelihood ratio test statistic, which is just $2 \times (-648.116) - (-648.121) = 0.01$, extremely close to the Wald statistic. Both indicate that the Odds Ratios associated with coffee drinking are essentially equivalent for males and females, allowing for sampling variation.

Table 14.3 *Additional logistic regression models relating coffee to incidence of pancreatic cancer*

Model (No.)	Parameter	Estimate	SD	OR	p-Value	Max. Log Likelihood
(5) $\log\left(\frac{p}{1-p}\right) = a + bx + cy$	a	—	—	—	—	
	b	0.957	0.258	2.603	< 0.001	
	c	−0.406	0.133	0.667	0.002	−648.1
(6) $\log\left(\frac{p}{1-p}\right) = a + bx + cy$	a	—	—	—	—	
$+ d(x \times y)$	b	0.984	0.388	2.676	0.011	
	c	−0.359	0.501	0.698	0.474	
	d	−0.050	0.520	0.951	0.923	−648.1
(7) $\log\left(\frac{p}{1-p}\right) = a + b_1z_1 + b_2z_2$	a	—	—	—	—	
$+ b_3z_3 + cy$	b_1	0.867	0.269	2.379	0.001	
	b_2	1.073	0.279	2.923	< 0.001	
	b_3	0.990	0.286	2.691	0.001	
	c	−0.404	0.135	0.668	0.003	−647.3
(8) $\log\left(\frac{p}{1-p}\right) = a + b_1z_1 + b_2z_2$	a	—	—	—	—	
$+ b_3z_3 + cy$	b_1	1.033	0.402	2.809	0.010	
$+ d_1(z_1 \times y) + \cdots + d_3(z_3 \times y)$	b_2	0.935	0.418	2.547	0.025	
	b_3	0.956	0.414	2.602	0.021	
	c	−0.359	0.501	0.698	0.474	
	d_1	−0.352	0.542	0.704	0.517	
	d_2	0.281	0.561	1.324	0.617	
	d_3	0.132	0.580	1.141	0.820	−645.1
(9) $\log\left(\frac{p}{1-p}\right) = a + bz + cy$	a	—	—	—	—	
	b	0.206	0.071	1.229	0.004	
	c	−0.398	0.134	0.672	0.003	−651.8
(10) $\log\left(\frac{p}{1-p}\right) = a + bz + cy$	a	—	—	—	—	
$+ d(z \times y)$	b	0.097	0.093	1.102	0.297	
	c	−0.809	0.269	0.445	0.003	
	d	0.254	0.143	1.289	0.076	−650.2

Note: Variables are defined in Table 13.5.

A similar analysis is available from Models (7) and (8) but with coffee consumption now coded with three indicator variables to capture four distinct levels of exposure. To capture the possibility of different Odds Ratios for males and females at each nonzero level of consumption, we need three interaction variables as shown for Model (8). Here, a test of interaction considers the null hypothesis $H_0 : d_1 = d_2 = d_3 = 0$ and is most easily examined through the 3 degree of freedom likelihood ratio test that compares Models (7) and (8). The likelihood ratio test statistic here is $2 \times (-645.1) - (-647.3) = 4.3$, which gives a p-value of 0.23. So there is somewhat more (although hardly convincing) evidence that the *pattern of risks* over the four exposure groups is different for males and females. Similarly, we can consider Models

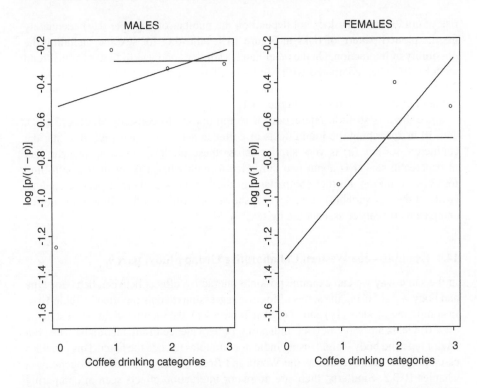

Figure 14.1 *Plot of observed log odds (log(p/(1 − p))) for incidence of pancreatic cancer, with fitted log odds for logistic models (of Table 14.3) based on coffee consumption, by sex: Model (8), plotted points; model(6), horizontal lines with plotted points for coffee drinking category 0; and model (10), sloped lines.*

(9) and (10), where the coffee consumption categories are given the ordered codes 0,1,2,3.

The various comparisons of coffee consumption effects across the two sexes are illustrated in Figure 14.1. Comparing the patterns of plotted points ("o") is the interaction effect assessed by comparing Models (7) and (8) (p-value = 0.23); comparing the slopes of nonhorizontal lines is the interaction effect achieved by comparing models (9) and (10) (p-value = 0.08); and comparing the horizontal lines (and the point at $z = 0$), given by the threshold model, is the interaction effect achieved by comparing Models (5) and (6) (p-value = 0.92).

We treat with caution the suggestion of interaction when an ordered code is used for consumption [Models (9) and (10)], since we already know that the threshold model fits the overall data better than the logistic model with the ordered code (although there is a hint that the ordered model fits the data for females better than for males). Formally, we can consider the goodness of fit of Model (6), nested within the more general Model (8), that gives a likelihood ratio test statistic of $2 \times (-645.1) - (-648.1) = 6.0$ with a p-value of 0.2; this indicates that the threshold model (which states that the risk of coffee drinking does not depend on the number of cups per day) adequately fits the plotted pattern of risks in Figure 14.1, adjusting for sex and including the possibility of interaction. On the other hand, a similar goodness of fit test for the trend model (10), when compared with Model (8), has a likelihood ratio test statistic of $2 \times (-645.1) - (-650.2) = 10.2$ with a p-value of 0.04, reflecting some inadequacy in the fit of the sloped lines in Figure 14.1.

Since there is so little interaction, it is appropriate to consider Models (5), (7), and (9) in describing the joint effects of coffee consumption and sex. Note that the coefficient for sex (c) is very similar across these models, reflecting that the risk of pancreatic cancer is about two thirds for women what it is for men, controlling for coffee drinking. Further comparison of these models to their respective analogs (without the sex variable) in Table 13.6 shows only little confounding of the coffee and pancreatic cancer association by sex.

14.4 Example—the Western Collaborative Group Study: part 9

In the same way we can examine possible interactive effects between behavior type and body weight using the series of logistic regression models reported in Table 14.4. In comparing Models (11) and (7) (from Table 14.1), the likelihood ratio test statistic ($= 4.0$) yields a p-value of 0.41, indicating little evidence of interaction between behavior type and body weight, using indicator variables to code the latter. This provides essentially the same results as the Woolf and Breslow–Day tests of homogeneity in Chapter 10.3.3. Similarly, there are no major interaction effects seen in comparing Models (8) and (13) where body weight is given an ordered categorical code, or Models (9) and (14) where body weight carries its original continuous scale.

In Model (12), the main effects of body weight are incorporated using four indicator variables, but a targeted interaction term is now added using the ordered categorical version of body weight. Thus, the test of the null hypothesis, $H_0 : d = 0$, looks for evidence that the log Odds Ratio for behavior type changes linearly as body weight increases. From Models (7) and (12), the 1 degree of freedom likelihood ratio test statistic is 0.36; so a linear pattern is clearly not apparent in the data. However, if the hypothetical variable from Table 10.8 is substituted for body weight, we obtain exactly the same likelihood ratio test statistic (4.0) for the overall examination of heterogeneity (with p-value 0.41), but a test statistic of 3.1 for the linear trend in log Odds Ratios over increasing levels of the hypothetical variable. This linear trend test statistic gives a p-value of 0.08 indicating that the observed trend in Odds Ratios is more suggestive of an interaction effect. With this hypothetical variable, the targeted test of interaction is much more powerful in detecting a pattern, as discussed in Chapter 10.3.4.

14.5 Collinearity and centering variables

In comparing Models (9) and (14) of Tables 14.1 and 14.4, respectively, we noted very little interactive effect either through the very small estimated interaction coefficient d in Model (14), or by comparison of the almost identical maximized

Table 14.4 *Logistic regression models that investigate interactive effects in the Western Collaborative Group Study*

Model (No.)	Parameter	Estimate	SD	OR	p-Value	Max. Log Likelihood
(11) $\log\left(\frac{p}{1-p}\right) = a + bx$	a	−3.418	0.321	—	<0.001	
$+ c_1 z_1 + \cdots + c_4 z_4$	b	0.975	0.391	2.652	0.013	
$+ d_1(xz_1) + \cdots$	c_1	0.122	0.455	1.130	0.789	
$+ d_4(xz_4)$	c_2	0.769	0.393	2.157	0.050	
	c_3	0.829	0.400	2.291	0.038	
	c_4	0.473	0.398	1.605	0.235	
	d_1	−0.095	0.555	0.910	0.865	
	d_2	−0.653	0.491	0.521	0.184	
	d_3	−0.050	0.484	0.952	0.918	
	d_4	0.112	0.477	1.118	0.815	−858.6
(12) $\log\left(\frac{p}{1-p}\right) = a + bx$	a	−3.237	0.252	—	<0.001	
$+ c_1 z_1 + \cdots + c_4 z_4$	b	0.697	0.282	2.007	0.013	
$+ d(xz)$	c_1	0.022	0.267	1.022	0.935	
	c_2	0.279	0.266	1.321	0.295	
	c_3	0.680	0.297	1.974	0.022	
	c_4	0.399	0.346	1.491	0.248	
	d	0.061	0.102	1.063	0.550	−860.4
(13) $\log\left(\frac{p}{1-p}\right) = a + bx$	a	−3.226	0.220	—	<0.001	
$+ cz + d(xz)$	b	0.714	0.275	2.042	0.010	
	c	0.133	0.081	1.142	0.100	
	d	0.054	0.099	1.055	0.588	−863.4
(14) $\log\left(\frac{p}{1-p}\right) = a + bx$	a	−4.999	0.884	—	<0.001	
$+ c(wt) + d(x \times wt)$	b	1.440	1.088	4.220	0.186	
	c	0.012	0.005	1.012	0.017	
	d	−0.003	0.006	0.997	0.583	−864.7
(15) $\log\left(\frac{p}{1-p}\right) = a + bx$	a	−3.193	0.168	—	<0.001	
$+ c(nwt) + d(x \times nwt)$	b	0.930	0.205	2.534	<0.001	
	c	0.241	0.101	1.272	0.017	
	d	−0.068	0.124	0.934	0.583	−864.7

Note: Variables are defined in Table 13.2.

log likelihoods for the two models. Close similarity between the maximized log likelihoods reflects that the two models are essentially indistinguishable, leading us to conclude that there is no evidence of (multiplicative) interaction between behavior type and body weight. Despite the equivalence of the two models, the estimated slope coefficient, $\hat{b}$, for X (behavior type) is somewhat different, and, even more strikingly, the associated estimated standard deviation of $\hat{b}$ increases more than seven-fold, from 0.140 to 1.088! The other coefficients are reasonably similar between the two models as are their respective standard deviations; but how can the addition of the trivial interaction term with such a small estimated slope $\hat{d} = -0.003$ have such an impact on $\hat{b}$ and its standard deviation? Note that the naïve p-value associated with the Wald test of $H_0 : b = 0$ is also enormously affected, changing from approximately 10^{-9} in Model (9) to 0.2 in Model (14), so that careless examination of Model (14) might suggest that there is no apparent association between behavior type and CHD incidence, a conclusion clearly at odds with what we infer from Model (9).

Here, thoughtful consideration of the context of the model, yielding the correct interpretation of the coefficient b in each of the models, provides the answer to this seeming paradox. In Model (9), the coefficient b is just the log Odds Ratio comparing Type A and Type B individuals, assumed constant over all body weights; this is estimated with considerable accuracy, as shown by the estimated standard deviation. On the other hand, in Model (14), due to the presence of the added interaction term, the interpretation of b is now the log Odds Ratio comparing Type A and Type B individuals, *restricted to those individuals whose body weight is 0 lb* ($Wt = 0$). This is clearly estimated by extreme extrapolation from the observed data, where almost all weights lie between 100 and 250 lb (see Figure 13.3). Although this extrapolation is explicitly based on Model (14), it naturally carries considerable uncertainty since the value $Wt = 0$ is so far from the bulk of the data (and impossible!). Thus we see a very high standard deviation associated with b in Model (14). For the same reason, the Wald test statistic associated with b in Model (14) also has a high p-value since it is testing the null hypothesis of independence of behavior type and CHD for individuals with zero body weight.

In statistical terms, this phenomenon is described by the term *collinearity*. Collinearity refers to the situation where two (or more) explanatory variables are highly correlated; in such situations, maximum likelihood, or any estimation technique for that matter, is unable to precisely distinguish between very different values of the coefficients, thereby leading to high standard deviations. This is most easily understood in the extreme case where there are two *identical*—perfectly correlated—independent variables, X_1 and X_2 such that $X_1 = X_2$. Suppose the true population regression model can be described by $\log(p/(1 - p)) = a + b_1 X_1 + b_2 X_2 = 1 + 2X_1$, that is, $b_1 = 2, b_2 = 0$. But since $X_2 = X_1$, the same model can be written identically as $\log(p/(1 - p)) = 1 + X_1 + X_2$ (i.e., $b_1 = 1, b_2 = 1$), or $\log(p/(1 - p)) = 1 + 2X_2$ (i.e., $b_1 = 0, b_2 = 2$), or even $\log(p/(1 - p)) = 1 + 200X_1 - 198X_2$ (i.e., $b_1 = 200, b_2 = -198$). Thus, no data from such a population allow precise determination of a particular set of b_1 and b_2 values that accurately fit the observations, since an infinite array of different combinations fits identically well. Our example is clearly extreme, but it indicates the fundamental difficulty in accurate coefficient estimation when there are collinear explanatory variables.

In the example of Model (14) with the Western Collaborative Group Study, the two variables X (the binary indicator of behavior type) and the constructed interaction term $X \times Wt$ are highly correlated. Their estimated correlation is, in fact, 0.98! This collinearity explains the high standard deviation associated with the slope estimate $\hat{b}$ in Model (14) of Table 14.4.

For general risk factors, there is no obvious fix to this level of collinearity. With observational data and absent external insight, we cannot tell which of the collinear variables is the "right" one that "causes" the outcome D. We must pragmatically choose a single member of the collinear variables to include in a logistic regression model, and then exclude other variables that are highly correlated with the one we have selected. However, in the case of constructed variables, such as the interaction term in the above example, there is a simple direct fix that avoids the confusing elevation of standard errors found in Model (14).

14.5.1 Centering independent variables

We already indicated that "regularizing" some independent variables leads to more interpretable coefficients in logistic regression models. By regularization, we mean a simple linear rescaling of the variable so that its zero value corresponds to values commonly seen in the data, and so that a unit increase in the transformed variable reflects a nontrivial change in risk. With body weight, we achieve this through the definition of the variable Nwt given in Table 13.2. The choice here of 150 lb as the "center" of the data is subjective and chosen for convenience. The median of the observed values of body weight, $med(Wt) = 170$ lb, is an alternative choice; for example, we could use the variable given by $Wt^* = [Wt - med(Wt)]/20$. If we use the rescaled version over the original, particularly for the constructed interaction product term, a substantial amount, if not all, of the collinearity is removed. It is important to stress that this leads to an identical but *reparameterized* version of the same model, with parameters that now can be estimated from the data with reasonable accuracy.

The value of centering is illustrated by Model (15) of Table 14.4. Replacing Wt with the rescaled variable Nwt makes absolutely no difference in the model; that is, Model (15) is identical to Model (14); it merely uses a different set of parameters. We obtain the exact same assessment regarding interaction—that there is very little—but now we see only a slight increase in the standard deviation of b in Model (15) (from 0.140 to 0.205) as compared with the original Model (9). The p-value associated with the Wald test of $H_0 : b = 0$ is now only slightly changed from that of Model (9), and we are not subject to the confusion of Model (14). The reason for the reduction in collinearity is that, with centering, the correlation between X and Nwt is 0.57, substantially lower than for X and Wt. There is no need to center the covariate X behavior type since its zero value (Type B) is observed for a substantial fraction of the sample.

14.5.2 Fitting quadratic models

In Chapters 12 and 13, we investigated the relationship between body weight and CHD incidence in the Western Collaborative Group Study, giving particular attention to a logistic regression model that is linear in body weight; see Figure 12.6 and Table 13.4. We noted, both graphically and through a formal goodness of fit test, that the linear model provides an adequate description of the relationship, at least for the five grouped body weight categories. By extension, it is thus plausible that a linear model in the continuous variable representing body weight (either Wt or Nwt) is also appropriate; in fact, these are Models (5) and (6) of Table 13.3. To further investigate whether there is some curvature in the relationship, it is helpful to fit a *quadratic* relationship between body weight and CHD incidence, that is, the model

$$\log\left(\frac{p}{1-p}\right) = a + b(wt) + c(wt)^2. \tag{14.4}$$

Note that this quadratic model can be rewritten as $\log[p/1-p] = a+(b+c(wt))(wt)$, showing that it allows the log Odds Ratio associated with a unit increase in body weight to change with body weight itself. That is, the quadratic model allows body weight to modify the effect of body weight. If the coefficient c is positive, then the rate at which the log odds of D changes (with body weight) increases as body weight increases; alternatively, for a negative c, the rate at which the log odds of D changes (with body weight) decreases as body weight increases. Using either the Wald or likelihood ratio test, the null hypothesis $H_0 : c = 0$ can be examined for evidence regarding whether the quadratic model fits the data better than the simpler linear model.

Table 14.5 provides the results of fitting quadratic model (14.4) in Wt, i.e., Model (16). The Wald test statistic for $H_0 : c = 0$ is given by $-0.0000637/0.0000755 = -0.84$, with a p-value of 0.4. A similar result is achieved via the likelihood ratio test statistic, obtained from comparing Model (5) of Table 13.3 with Model (16), that is, $2 \times (-884.1) - (-884.5) = 0.8$. Both tests indicate little evidence of a quadratic effect, confirming our earlier and cruder assessment of the adequacy of a linear model.

In particular, the tests show that Models (5) and (16) are almost identical. Yet, once more we see an unexpected change in the size of the linear coefficient $\hat{b}$ and, of more importance, an almost tenfold increase in the standard deviation, from 0.003 to 0.028. The reason again is collinearity, here between Wt and $(Wt)^2$; the sample correlation of these two explanatory variables is 0.99. Since the variable $(Wt)^2$ is a constructed covariate, we can again use centering to reduce or eliminate collinearity. Model (17)

Table 14.5 *Logistic regression models that investigate a quadratic relationship between body weight and CHD incidence in the Western Collaborative Group Study*

Model (No.)	Parameter	Estimate	SD	OR	p-Value	Max. Log Likelihood
(16) $\log\left(\frac{p}{1-p}\right)$	a	-6.302	2.507	—	0.012	
$= a + b(wt) + c(wt)^2$	b	0.034	0.028	1.034	0.222	
	c	-0.00006	0.00008	1.000	0.398	-884.1
(17) $\log\left(\frac{p}{1-p}\right)$	a	-2.683	0.105	—	<0.001	
$= a + b(nwt) + c(nwt)^2$	b	0.291	0.113	1.338	0.010	
	c	-0.025	0.030	0.975	0.398	-884.1
(18) $\log\left(\frac{p}{1-p}\right) = a + b(mwt)$	a	-2.442	0.066	—	<0.001	
	b	0.208	0.058	1.232	<0.001	-884.5
(19) $\log\left(\frac{p}{1-p}\right)$	a	-2.417	0.072	—	<0.001	
$= a + b(mwt) + c(mwt)^2$	b	0.240	0.070	1.272	0.001	
	c	-0.025	0.030	0.975	0.398	-884.1

Note: Variables are defined in Table 13.2.

of Table 14.5 uses the normalized body weight variable Nwt, where the 0 value is 150 lb. The correlation of Nwt and $(Nwt)^2$ is 0.80; so some lingering collinearity effects remain. The standard error of $\hat{b}$ goes from 0.058, in Model (6) of Table 13.3, to 0.113 in Model (17), still substantially better than when we used the original body weight. The choice of 150 lb as the 0 value of Nwt was subjective. We can use the sample median of observed body weights, 170 lb, to define an alternative centered version of body weight, given by $Mwt = (Wt - 170)/20$. Models (18) and (19) in Table 14.5 give the linear and quadratic models relating Mwt to CHD incidence. We stress that Models (16), (17), and (19) are identical and yield exactly the same analysis of the impact of a quadratic model. However, the parameters used in each model are different, and estimates of the slope coefficients b used in Models (18) and (19) suffer least from the addition of an unnecessary quadratic term. Now, as you move from Model (18) to (19), the standard deviation of $\hat{b}$ increases only from 0.058 to 0.070. Here, the sample correlation between Mwt and $(Mwt)^2$ is just 0.30, so that almost all of the effects of collinearity are removed.

This discussion regarding the possible detection and use of a quadratic rather than linear model in describing the effects of an explanatory variable is part of a broader issue regarding the choice of appropriate exposure scales for a logistic regression model. For example, why not use log(body weight) instead of the raw weight, and so on. We return to this issue in Chapter 15 in consideration of this and other goodness of fit issues.

Now we return briefly to the general issue of collinearity for distinct explanatory variables (rather than constructed variables like those used to model interaction and quadratic effects). Although, as noted, centering does not address collinearity for distinct explanatory variables, there are statistical techniques available that allow construction of a set of newly defined and uncorrelated covariates from a set of original collinear variables. One such technique is *principal components*. However, the "new" explanatory variables for such methods are linear combinations of all the original covariates and thus can be difficult to interpret. This approach is often useful, however, in situations where several similar measures of exposure are available and exhibit a substantial amount of collinearity. For example, in assessing stress as an exposure, several different but related measurements may be available with no single one identified as the "correct" quantification of stress. Methods such as principal components then define uncorrelated "risk" scales that depend on combinations of the original measurements.

14.6 Restrictions on effective use of maximum likelihood techniques

In Chapters 13 and 14, we illustrated repeatedly how the logistic regression model is sufficiently flexible to implement all the stratification analyses of Chapters 9 to 11. We noted at the beginning of Chapter 12 that a stratification approach breaks down when the number of strata becomes large. How is this reflected in the use of logistic regression analyses?

Accommodation of a large number of strata, without making any regression assumptions regarding how the pattern of risk changes from stratum to stratum, requires use of a similarly large number of indicator variables (see Chapter 12.6.1) in an appropriate logistic regression model. Because there is one slope coefficient for every indicator variable, we are faced with estimation of an identically large number of parameters. At some point there are insufficient data to accurately estimate a large number of parameters using any estimation method, maximum likelihood in particular. Exactly how many parameters of a logistic regression model can be reasonably estimated with maximum likelihood is impossible to pin down. It depends not only on the overall sample size but also on other factors, as we have seen, such as marginal balance on the number of cases and controls, and on the distribution of exposure variables. As a rough rule of thumb, it is risky to fit more parameters than 10% of the sample size. We should even be cautious when the total number of parameters exceeds 10% of the number of cases (assuming the number of cases to be smaller than the number of controls).

The bottom line for maximum likelihood is thus similar to stratification methods in that the method fails when there are a very large number of unknown parameters to be estimated in a regression model. But as we pointed out in the beginning of Chapter 12, the whole point of regression models is to discover smooth models, that is, models that use assumptions of linearity and the like to reduce the number of parameters or degrees of freedom. Thus, in most epidemiological studies, the complexity of the regression model, and therefore the number of unknown parameters, will usually be relatively small compared to the available sample size. Of course, in choosing an appropriate regression model we look for one that fits the data reasonably well and does not miss important features of the relationship between exposure variables, confounders, and the outcome of interest. This is the topic of Chapter 15. However, sometimes we have to use models with a large number of parameters as for the analysis of highly stratified designs or matched data, introduced in Chapter 16. In these cases, we must abandon maximum likelihood as we have discussed it so far; fortunately, however, there is a simple modification to the procedure, known as *conditional maximum likelihood*, that allows us to estimate certain key parameters at the expense of ignoring those not of central interest. This procedure is described in Chapter 16.5. In addition, many software packages include exact procedures that are relevant for inference procedures based on small sample estimates of logistic regression coefficients (Hirji et al., 1987). Collett (2002, Chapter 9) provides a brief introduction to exact methods for logistic regression.

14.7 Comments and further reading

Throughout our discussion on estimation of the coefficients of a logistic regression model, we have assumed that exposure and disease measurements are correct and that all sampled observations contain complete information on each variable of interest. In practice, most epidemiological studies are subject to both measurement error and missing data. We highlighted earlier that the obvious strategy to deal with measurement error is to avoid it in the first place. The same applies to missing data: studies should be planned to minimize the possibility of missing measurements on any individual. That said, we now briefly discuss statistical approaches for dealing with the presence of both measurement error and missing data as they apply in estimating logistic regression models.

14.7.1 Measurement error

The SIMEX method of Chapter 7.5.1 is easily extended to studies where there is external information on the size of random measurement *nondifferential* error in one or more risk factors or confounders. SIMEX also applies when information on the variance of random measurement errors is derived from *replicates* of an exposure variable on sampled participants. Carroll (1998) gives a simple teaching example, based on data from the Framingham Heart Study, where he considers adjustments for error in measures of systolic blood pressure. MacMahon et al. (1990) discuss the effects of measurement error of systolic blood pressure in medical and epidemiological studies.

An alternative approach to SIMEX is available when the study contains exact measurements (the so-called "gold standard" measures) for the risk factor (otherwise measured with error) on a subsample of individuals. This often occurs when only a small number of "gold standard" measurements of a nutritional, environmental, or occupational exposure, X, can be afforded, but where an inexpensive proxy measure, X^*, such as a biomarker, is available for the entire sample. In such a study, we can use a regression model, usually linear regression, that predicts the "gold standard" variable X from the proxy X^* and other explanatory variables. Estimates of the parameters of this model can be calculated using the subsample for which both X and X^* are available. This regression function is then used to predict X on the rest of the sample for whom only data on X^* was collected. Subsequently, the logistic regression model for the disease outcome is estimated using the complete sample, as discussed in Chapter 13, with the predicted X rather than the proxy X^* as the exposure variable. This technique, known as *regression calibration*, was popularized for logistic regression by Rosner et al. (1989, 1990), who applied the method to biomarker information in the Nurses' Health Study. Variances of the slope coefficients estimated in this fashion can be estimated using large sample approximations or the bootstrap (Carroll et al., 1995).

The situation with mismeasured exposure, supplemented by some internal validation data, can also be viewed as a missing data problem since the "gold standard" measurement is missing for a substantial fraction of the sample. We turn to a broader view of missing data next, and also observe that differential measurement error is often best approached as a missing data problem. Neuhaus (1999) suggests methods for correcting the estimates of logistic regression model parameters in the presence of disease misclassification.

14.7.2 Missing data

One form of missing data, often referred to as *nonresponse*, occurs when information on all variables is missing for a subset of the sample. This most often arises when data are collected via some form of interview. Nonresponse is best handled under the rubric of *selection bias* since it effectively modifies the Study Population, as discussed in

Chapter 5, to include only respondents. A more pervasive kind of missing data is when only *some* variables have missing responses for a given individual, a situation commonly known as *item nonresponse*. For example, in the Western Collaborative Group Study (WCGS), a few participants did not have their serum cholesterol measured at baseline. In the case-control study of pancreatic cancer, it is plausible that laboratory measurement may be missing for some individuals, perhaps more often for controls if these variables were routinely included in medical records that are available for all cases. Item nonresponse arises for many reasons: (1) individuals may not respond to interview questions on specific variables, particularly if these relate to sensitive issues (household income, drug abuse, etc.), (2) medical or occupational records may be incomplete, (3) information on a variable may be unknown particularly if a proxy respondent provides data for the sampled individual, and (4) certain variables may be very expensive to measure for all participants. We do not deal here with missing outcome data, which has also been studied extensively (see, for example, Dodge (1985)).

Analyzing only those observations with complete data on the variables included in a logistic regression model is a common strategy to deal with item nonresponse. Whether and by how much item nonresponse distorts coefficient estimates in terms of their Target Population values depends on the probability that an individual's response is missing for the relevant variables. That is, how does the probability of a participant's serum cholesterol being measured in the WCGS depend on whether they develop disease, their behavior pattern, and perhaps the level of their serum cholesterol itself? What are the chances that observation of a blood sample measurement is missing for a case and control in the study of pancreatic cancer? A simplistic assumption is that variables have missing values *completely at random*, meaning that the probability of a variable's response being missing does not depend on any factors under study, including exposures, confounders, and outcome of interest. In this scenario, focusing solely on complete data does not introduce bias, although the analysis may be quite imprecise if there is enough missing data on multiple variables so that there are few observations with entirely complete information. Further, it is implausible that mechanisms that govern missing data are not themselves influenced by the levels of the factors being studied.

A weaker, and usually essential, assumption is that the data are *missing at random*, meaning that the probability that a specific variable X has a missing value for a study participant does not depend on the (unknown) value of X but only on variables, say, W and the outcome D, that are fully observed for that individual. This assumption is the analog of the randomization assumption underlying a study's ability to draw causal inference from observations of single counterfactuals (see Chapter 8.1.1). Distinction is often further made between differential "missingness" probabilities that depend on the disease outcome. Such differential probabilities of observing a specific variable often arise in case-control studies where (1) information on cases and controls are obtained from different sources and (2) controls differ from cases in their ability or interest in responding to specific questions.

Using only complete data produces satisfactory logistic regression estimates if the data are missing *nondifferentially*, even if the missingness probabilities are influenced by the values of all factors (including those with missing values), and thereby violate the "missing at random" assumption. This follows because in such cases, missingness alters the pattern of risk factors observed in the complete data but will not affect the pattern of disease incidence at different levels of these factors, and it is this pattern that is described by a logistic regression model. On the other hand, as just noted, differential missing values—that is where the probability that a risk factor is missing depends on an individual's disease status—are more common in practice. In such cases, there can be substantial bias in only using complete observations to estimate a logistic regression model (Vach and Blettner, 1991).

Several techniques have been suggested to allow for missing data on explanatory variables when fitting a logistic regression model (Vach, 1994, 1998) for which the data are missing at random. We mention several general strategies here, providing references for further reading. The first method is *single imputation*, where a "guessed" value is substituted for the missing covariate, and then standard methods are applied to the entire data set. For example, in the WCGS, we can substitute the sample mean serum cholesterol for any missing values. If the probabilities of a missing value do not depend on disease status, the imputed value can be based on a regression with the variable with missing values as the dependent variable, and with other fully observed covariates as predictors. For example, in the WCGS, we might use a different sample mean serum cholesterol for every age/weight category; this can be extended to a regression model where interval-scaled measurements of age, weight, smoking, and systolic blood pressure are used as predictors of serum cholesterol (fitting such a model on participants for whom all of these values are measured). Although variance estimates of the estimated coefficients are underestimated by this approach (as they do not account for variability in the imputed values), the underestimation is usually small (Vach, 1994; Vach and Schumacher, 1993). The bootstrap can be used as an alternative variance estimation method (Efron and Tibshirani, 1993). Single imputation can also be modified for missingness probabilities that vary by disease status (Vach and Schumacher, 1993).

Multiple imputation uses a similar tactic but repeats the imputation multiple times using *random guesses* for the missing value. These random guesses are generated by some form of sampling of known measurements for the variable subject to missingness (see Rubin and Schenker, 1991). However, both kinds of imputation strategies can be imprecise and continue to suffer from bias if the imputation strategy is misspecified.

A very different approach is based on fitting the relevant logistic regression model to only complete observations, but inversely weighting each individual based on estimates of the probability of observing all risk factors. That is, individuals with known serum cholesterol are given greater weight if their other factors (age, weight, etc.) are commonly associated with missing cholesterol values, and vice versa. The probability of having a complete serum cholesterol measurement can be estimated using the full data set with a separate logistic regression model where the outcome is binary—is the variable (serum cholesterol, here) missing for this individual or not—and fully observed covariates (age, weight, etc.) are used as predictors. If missingness is common in the sample, these inversely weighted estimates can again be quite imprecise.

A more complex strategy is to use maximum likelihood based on a likelihood function that allows for the presence of missing observations, assuming some model for the probability of values being missing. Unfortunately, this likelihood now depends on the distribution of the risk factors in the population, an issue that was easily avoided when no data were missing (see the comments regarding the use of L^*, as against L, in Chapter 13.1.1). Thus, estimates based on this likelihood function often require specification of properties of the risk factor distribution, using assumptions that may lead to bias if incorrect. Recent approaches use ideas from *semiparametric* theory to avoid making such assumptions. At the core of these methods is a broadly appropriate estimator, such as weighting the complete observations, which is then adjusted to both improve its precision and make the estimator robust against misspecification of either the risk model (logistic regression, here) or the model for missingness. This approach is covered in considerable detail in Robins and Rotnitzky (1995) and Rotnitzky and Robins (1997); the most general theory of these estimators, covering both missing data and causal inference, is in van der Laan and Robins (2002).

We end this brief discussion of missing data by highlighting a common technique that does *not* guarantee undistorted estimates. Investigators often incorporate individuals with missing values of a variable X by assigning a separate category when X is missing. For example, if X represents serum cholesterol with five categories, modeled using four indicator variables, then a sixth category (and additional indicator) is created for the missing X values. A similar missing indicator variable can be used when X is interval-scaled. Unfortunately, this does not remove bias in estimating the regression coefficient associated with other risk factors in the model, even when the X variable is missing completely at random. This inherent bias can easily be seen with a single additional exposure variable such as behavior type; with data on serum cholesterol missing completely at random, the complete observations yield an undistorted coefficient estimator for behavior type, adjusted for serum cholesterol, as noted above. However, in the part of the sample where serum cholesterol is missing, the logistic regression coefficient estimator for behavior type does not control for serum cholesterol and so will be distorted if serum cholesterol is a confounder. The overall estimator from the whole sample is then an average of these two estimators and remains biased. This distortion can be substantially greater if the X values are only missing at random. Furthermore, variance estimation for the estimated coefficient for behavior type, based on a logistic regression fit with the extra missingness category for serum cholesterol, can be much too small (Greenland and Finkle, 1995).

14.8 Problems

Question 14.1

A case-control study investigated the role of several reproductive risk factors for breast cancer. Part of the data relating to number of births is reported in Table 14.6. Suppose parity is coded by the variable $X = 1$ if parity is 0–1, and $X = 0$ if parity is ≥ 2. Similarly age is given the binary code via the variable $Z = 1$ if age is ≥ 40 years, and $Z = 0$ if age is <40 years. For both (1) and (2) below, do not use a logistic regression program, as all answers can be computed by simple calculator operations.

Table 14.6 *Case-control data on parity and breast cancer incidence, stratified by age*

Age			Breast Cancer	
			Cases	Controls
<40 years	Parity	0–1 births	24	58
		≥2 births	96	160
≥40 years	Parity	0–1 births	127	172
		≥2 births	353	718

1. Suppose age is ignored and the logistic model $\log(p/1 - p) = a + bX$ is fit to the data. What is the estimate of b?

2. Suppose the logistic model $\log(p/1 - p) = a + bX + cZ + d(XZ)$ is fit to the data. What are the estimates of b, c, and d?

Question 14.2

Referring again to the data set *oesoph*, found by going to http://www.crcpress.com/e_products/downloads/, now use logistic regression models to attack the problems raised in Questions 7.3, 9.2, 10.5, and 11.3. For each case, carefully state the appropriate logistic regression model and relevant hypothesis, both in the context of the problem and in terms of model parameters. Use both the Wald and likelihood ratio methods to carry out any hypothesis tests, and provide relevant estimated Odds Ratios (with 95% confidence intervals) where appropriate. In particular,

1. Investigate the relationship between alcohol consumption and incidence of esophageal cancer. Treat alcohol consumption as a dichotomous variable (≥80 g/day vs. <80 g/day), ignoring age. Compare your answer to that obtained in Question 7.3.

2. Investigate the relationship between alcohol consumption and incidence of esophageal cancer, controlling for the potential confounding effects of age. Treat alcohol consumption as a dichotomous variable (≥80 g/day vs. <80 g/day), and age as a dichotomous variable (25 to 54 years old or 55 to 75+ years old). Compare your answer to that obtained to Question 9.2. Give your assessment of the extent of confounding by age using the models fit in (1) and (2).

3. Investigate the evidence of (multiplicative) interaction between age and alcohol consumption in relation to incidence of esophageal cancer. Treat alcohol consumption and age as dichotomous variables as in (2). Compare your answer to that obtained in Question 10.5.

4. Investigate the relationship between alcohol consumption and incidence of esophageal cancer. First, treat alcohol consumption as a categorical variable with four categories (0 to 39 g/day, 40 to 79 g/day, 80 to 119 g/day, and ≥120 g/day), by using indicator variables for the various categories (select 0 to 39 g/day as the reference group); second, treat alcohol consumption as an ordered variable by appropriately

CONFOUNDING AND INTERACTION

coding the four categories of consumption. Compare the two analyses and discuss whether an increasing trend in risk, as alcohol consumption increases, adequately fits the pattern of risks for the four categories. Compare your interpretations with those from Question 11.3.

Question 14.3

Referring again to the data set *titanic*, found by going to http://www.crcpress.com/e_products/downloads/, expand the analysis of Question 13.2 by fitting a logistic regression model that includes both ticket class (use indicator variables) and fare (interpret the roles of both risk factors, and discuss confounding issues by comparison to your single variable models of Question 13.2). Repeat this analysis, but now adding the passenger's sex to the model; again comment on the issue of confounding. Now add the variable for place of embarkment and revise your interpretations as necessary.

Question 14.4

Referring again to the data set, *titanic*, found by going to http://www.crcpress.com/e_products/downloads/, expand the analysis of Question 14.3 by fitting logistic regression models that include both ticket class (examine both indicator variables and an ordered scale) and sex, allowing for the possibility of multiplicative interaction between the two variables. What is your assessment and interpretation of interaction? In the model with interaction, does the ordered scale for ticket class allow for an adequate fit as compared with using indicator variables? Compare with Question 13.2 and discuss.

Question 14.5

The data set *breastcancer*, found at http://www.crcpress.com/e_products/downloads/, contains data from a population-based study of 3303 women in Nashville with prior benign breast biopsies (Dupont and Page, 1985). Information on these previous biopsies included whether the biopsied lesion was proliferative or not, as well as the family history of breast cancer. Women with prior proliferative breast lesions were further classified by whether the lesions also displayed atypical hyperplasia. The women were then followed for around 17 years for subsequent incidence of breast cancer. Using logistic regression, examine the roles of proliferative breast disease, with and without atypical hyperplasia, and family history on the incidence of breast cancer. Consider interactive effects if and when appropriate.

CHAPTER 15

Goodness of Fit Tests for Logistic Regression Models and Model Building

Ideally, every epidemiological study would be designed and subsequently analyzed with attention given to a small set of risk factors, and a further set of possible confounding or interacting variables, with the roles of each of these variables identified *a priori*. In this case, it would make sense to build logistic regression models from the "bottom up," beginning with the few exposures of interest, and then examining the issues of confounding and interaction associated with extraneous variables, much as we have done in the two examples considered at length in Chapters 12 to 14. Unfortunately, in most cases selection and elucidation of the exact nature of suspected exposures is difficult in the design phase of a study; thus, many possible candidate exposure variables (e.g., possible proxies for some underlying proposed risk factor such as social support, or stress) are measured on sampled individuals. In these studies, we face the construction of a regression model with only limited prior knowledge to guide us. In this chapter, we consider three statistical issues that direct a sensible approach to regression model building: (1) choosing the scale of a selected explanatory variable, (2) general model building strategies, and (3) methods to assess whether a "final" model fits the sample data adequately. All of these ideas arise from the same questions about traditional regression analyses of continuous outcome variables, though details differ because of a binary outcome, D, here. We only touch on these topics, which are discussed further in monographs on logistic regression analysis, particularly Hosmer and Lemeshow (2000).

15.1 Choosing the scale of an exposure variable

Before tackling the issues of model building and goodness of fit, we look at the simplest possible example of regression model construction, where there is only one exposure variable of interest, X, and it is assumed to be continuously scaled. The most obvious logistic regression approach is to fit the simple model $\log[p/(1-p)] = a + bx$ that assumes that the risk of D changes linearly with X on the log odds scale. But this may not describe the relationship between X and the risk of D adequately in the sample, and thereby presumably the population. Perhaps the log odds of D changes linearly in the logarithm of X, a reasonable alternative, particularly if X measures the concentration of an exposure in some sense. We therefore need to determine which possible scales of exposure are the most appropriate in the context of a linear association with the log odds of D. This is a statistical approach to the choice of scale, not to be confused with or substituted for appropriate and effective exposure *measurement* as discussed in Chapter 2. Here, we focus solely on arithmetic changes in the measured scale of X.

15.1.1 Using ordered categories to select exposure scale

We implicitly used ordered categories in Chapters 13 and 14 when studying the role of body weight in CHD incidence in the Western Collaborative Group Study, and in modeling the effect of coffee drinking on pancreatic cancer. The strategy is straightforward:

- Divide the scale of X into four or five ordered categories so that there is roughly the same sample size in each category; this can be achieved by using quartiles or quintiles of the sample observations on X, although it is helpful to make the category boundaries meaningful in terms of the original scale of X if possible.
- Construct indicator variables to describe these categories as in Chapter 12.6.1.
- Also construct for X a simple ordered proxy, Z, that is constant within each category but reflects the original ordering of X; for example, one might use simply the values $Z = 0, 1, \ldots$; alternatively, for each category of X, assign Z the median value of X for all sample observations in the relevant category.
- Fit the logistic regression model using only the indicator variables.
- Fit the logistic regression model with the single explanatory variable Z.
- Compare the fit of these two models using both plots and formal comparison through the likelihood ratio test.
- If the fit of the model using Z is poor in comparison with the more general indicator variable model, evaluate the plots to suggest possible changes in the scale of Z (and thus X) that might improve the fit of a linear model.

In the Western Collaborative Group Study, Table 13.2 defines indicator variables needed to describe five categories for the risk factor body weight, and Table 13.3 gives details on the fit of the two relevant models in body weight, namely, Models (3) and (4). The bottom right-hand plot of Figure 12.7 provides a visual comparison of these two models (albeit plotted on the scale of risk rather than log odds). Finally, our discussion of goodness of fit (Chapter 13.2) shows that the linear model provides a reasonable fit to the observed pattern of risks over these five categories. We can reasonably infer from these results that a linear model in body weight, using the original scale [that is, Model (5) or (6) of Table 13.3], is appropriate for this data set.

We reach a somewhat different conclusion for the coffee consumption and pancreatic cancer example. Here, the relevant definitions are given in Table 13.5, the models in Table 13.6 [Models (2) and (3)], and the visual examination in Figure 13.4. In this case, a linear model in a simple ordered scale for consumption does not fit the data particularly well, as noted in Chapter 13.4; as an alternative, the models and figure suggest use of a simple non-linear transformation of consumption into a simple binary scale of $0 =$ abstainers and $1 =$ any coffee drinking (that is, the variable X of Table 13.5) to better describe the observed variation in pancreatic cancer risk over consumption categories.

15.1.2 *Alternative strategies*

There are several computing-intensive techniques that can assist in choosing an appropriate scale for X. The first of these uses the original data on an exposure X, then estimates the log odds at, or near, each X (collapsing values of X that are close together to give enough observations to allow estimation), and finally uses the idea of *smoothing* these estimates. Smoothing here refers to averaging estimates at nearby values of X to ensure that the estimated log odds of D changes regularly over small changes in X. The result is an estimate of a smooth pattern for the estimated log odds as X varies, a plot that can then be examined to see if it resembles linearity or suggests an alternative. This strategy may allow more subtle risk patterns to emerge than the formal grouping approach in Section 15.1.1.

A quite different approach uses what are known as *fractional polynomials* (Royston and Altman, 1994); these are functions of X that include simple powers, like X^2, X^3, or X^{-1}, square roots such as $X^{\frac{1}{2}} = \sqrt{X}$ and $X^{-\frac{1}{2}}$, and the logarithm function, $\log X$. Algorithms are available that systematically search through these functions—taken one at a time, two at a time, and so on—to find which fits the data most effectively using the likelihood function as a measure of fit.

Figure 15.1 illustrates these two approaches for the data relating body weight to CHD incidence in the Western Collaborative Group Study. The scatterplot fit uses

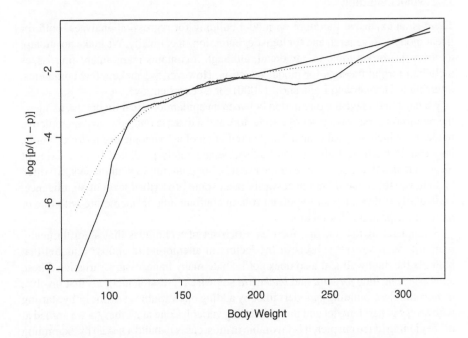

Figure 15.1 *Plot of estimated CHD incidence at all distinct body weight levels against body weight, with (1) fitted simple logistic model, (2) lowess smoothed scatterplot (jagged solid line), and simple fractional polynomial fit (dotted line).*

what is known as the *lowess* smoothing algorithm, which uses local quadratic functions to "average" log odds estimates in regions of similar values of X; the fractional polynomial was selected from eight possible transformations of the scale of body weight: $(Wt)^{-2}$, $(Wt)^{-1}$, $(Wt)^{-\frac{1}{2}}$, $\log(Wt)$, $(Wt)^{\frac{1}{2}}$, Wt, $(Wt)^2$, and $(Wt)^3$. The transformation $(Wt)^{-2}$ yielded the largest likelihood and was used in a linear model to give the dotted curve of Figure 15.1, of course with a negative estimated slope coefficient to reflect the increased risk of CHD as body weight increases.

The scatterplot smooth estimate and the fractional polynomial fit are extremely similar, both reflecting a slight leveling off in risk growth at the higher body weights, an observation made earlier based on the grouped measures of body weight. It is important to note that these plots tend to be highly variable at extreme body weights for which there are very few observations; for example, there are only 43 observations whose body weight is less than 130 lb, and only 4 less than 115 lb; similarly, only 6 weigh 250 lb or greater. Thus, discrepancies among the three curves for body weights less than 115 lb or greater than 250 lb can be safely ignored. For body weights represented by the vast majority of the sample, both curves are hard to distinguish from the linear model, a finding supported by more formal analysis of the likelihood function for the fractional polynomial fit. This analysis thus confirms the simpler approach of Section 15.1.1.

15.2 Model building

There is an extensive literature on model building for regression analyses, both for linear models, in general, and for logistic regression, specifically. We make no attempt to cover this broad topic in any detail, although it contains many interesting issues including formal theories for model selection. However, we make a few comments, referring to Hosmer and Lemeshow (2000) for an excellent overview.

We must first make the distinction between an epidemiological model, focusing on the relationship between a set of risk factors and a disease outcome, and a predictive model for which the goal is an accurate prediction of an outcome event (for example, how can 24-h survival after a heart attack be accurately predicted from a series of measurements made at the time of the event?). For epidemiological models, we often include variables that do not necessarily meet some proscribed level of significance, particularly if they play an important role in confounding or interacting with one or more of the primary risk factors.

Given a set of risk factors, there is a rich set of techniques that algorithmically search through various subsets of the factors in attempting to choose a model that both fits the data well and also does not include many unnecessary variables. These approaches include *forward* and *backward* stepwise regression methods that involve, at their simplest, building a model either by adding one variable at a time or by starting with a very general model and then excluding variables one at a time. As we argued at the beginning of the chapter, it is favorable in most cases to build a model by examining the risk factors in order of their primary interest, at each stage carefully considering relevant issues of scale choice, confounding, and interaction. Causal graphs often prove helpful in guiding this process. In this way, a coherent descriptive analysis of the role of various risk factors can be constructed to "annotate" the formal logistic regression model that is ultimately chosen.

In situations where there are a large number of risk factors without prior specification of their relevance, Hosmer and Lemeshow (2000) recommend the following strategy:

- Fit a simple logistic regression model for each risk factor separately using the original raw scale of the variable; this may be a categorical scale (for variables such as ethnicity, for example) or a continuous ordered scale, if this is natural. For continuous variables, the linearity assumption in the regression model is of little concern since the regression model will detect even nonlinear associations (see Chapter 11.3.1 and 11.3.2), unless the nonlinearity involves some form of "up and down" behavior in the risks; if the latter is suspected, then categorization or a different choice of scale can be used a priori.

- Keep those risk factors whose inclusion reaches a reasonably liberal significance level, such as 0.2.

- Fit a multiple logistic regression model using all retained risk factors from the univariate analyses, ignoring interaction for the time being.

- One by one, remove those risk factors that now appear to have lost their significance within the multivariate model, while checking via the likelihood ratio test that the reduced model does not fit the data significantly worse than the original multiple logistic model.

- Consider each risk factor, one at a time, that was originally discarded in the univariate analyses, to determine whether adding it now to the multivariate model is important.

- For the current set of included risk factors, consider the choice of scale using the ideas of Section 15.1, changing scale where appropriate.

- Consider interactions between pairs of included risk factors, preferably limiting this to a reasonable number of plausible interactive effects. Add interactions where they significantly add to the fit, or alter the interpretation of risk factors substantially.

- Assess the final model for goodness of fit to the data (Section 15.3).

We apply these ideas briefly to the Western Collaborative Group Study. Table 15.1 provides a list of risk factors for CHD together with their raw scales: these include age, height, blood pressure, serum cholesterol, and cigarette consumption, in addition to the two variables previously considered, behavior pattern and body weight. All variables represent measurements taken on participants at the beginning of follow-up. For simplicity we have not regularized these variables, although for many standardization provides for simpler interpretations of subsequent logistic regression coefficients.

Table 15.2 provides the results of univariate logistic regression analyses for each variable of Table 15.1 in turn. All of the variables show significant association with CHD incidence, except for height; similar results are achieved from either the Wald or likelihood ratio tests. The analysis of serum cholesterol is based on 3142 observations since 12 individuals have this measurement missing; this explains the lower value of

Table 15.1 *List of variables in Western Collaborative Group Study data*

$$X = \begin{cases} 1 \text{ Type A behavior pattern} \\ 0 \text{ Type B behavior pattern} \end{cases}$$

Ht = Height (in.)
Wt = Body weight (lb)
Sbp = Systolic blood pressure (mmHg)
Dbp = Diastolic blood pressure (mmHg)
$Chol$ = Fasting serum cholesterol (mg/100 ml)
$Ncigs$ = Number of cigarettes per day
Age = Age (years)

Table 15.2 *Results of univariate logistic regression models in the Western Collaborative Group Study*

Variable	Regression Estimate ($\hat{b}$)	Wald Statistic	p-Value	OR	Max. Log Likelihood
x	0.864	6.16	<0.001	2.373	−870.2
ht	0.027	1.06	0.29	1.028	−890.1
wt	0.010	3.57	<0.001	1.130	−884.5
sbp	0.027	7.27	<0.001	1.027	−866.2
dbp	0.034	5.61	<0.001	1.034	−875.8
chol	0.012	8.65	<0.001	1.013	−851.2
ncigs	0.023	5.74	<0.001	1.023	−875.0
age	0.074	6.58	<0.001	1.077	−869.2

Note: Model with only a constant has max. log likelihood = −890.6.

the maximized log likelihood when fitting this variable. The fraction of the sample with missing serum cholesterol data is sufficiently small to reasonably use the complete observations.

Table 15.3 now shows the fits of three multiple logistic regression models; all three omit the 12 individuals with the missing cholesterol information. Model (A) fits a multiple logistic regression model that includes all the variables from the univariate analyses of Table 15.2, except height. Each of the included variables remains strongly associated with CHD, except for diastolic blood pressure. Model (B) removes Dbp and basically shows no change in the maximized log likelihood. We thus eliminate diastolic blood pressure; in Model (C), we consider whether the reintroduction of height is of importance. There is essentially no improvement in the fit of model, and the height variable seems unimportant; further, there is no noticeable confounding of the other effects, except for a slight diminution of the weight effect [compare Models (B) and (C)]. At this point, it is plausible to continue with Model (B), removing both diastolic blood pressure and height from further consideration.

Table 15.3 *Some multiple logistic regression models for the Western Collaborative Group Study*

Model (Label)	Parameter	Estimate	Wald Statistic	p-Value	OR	Max. Log Likelihood
(A) $\log\left(\frac{p}{1-p}\right) = a + bx$	b	0.654	4.51	<0.001	1.924	
$+ c(wt) + d(sbp)$	c	0.009	2.74	0.006	1.009	
$+ e(dbp) + f(chol)$	d	0.018	2.78	0.006	1.018	
$+ g(ncigs) + h(age)$	e	−0.001	−0.06	0.95	0.999	
	f	0.011	7.25	<0.001	1.011	
	g	0.021	4.96	<0.001	1.021	
	h	0.064	5.34	<0.001	1.067	−790.5
(B) $\log\left(\frac{p}{1-p}\right) = a + bx$	b	0.654	4.51	<0.001	1.924	
$+ c(wt) + d(sbp)$	c	0.009	2.78	0.005	1.009	
$+ f(chol)$	d	0.017	4.26	<0.001	1.018	
$+ g(ncigs) + h(age)$	f	0.011	7.26	<0.001	1.011	
	g	0.021	5.01	<0.001	1.021	
	h	0.064	5.33	<0.001	1.067	−790.5
(C) $\log\left(\frac{p}{1-p}\right) = a + bx$	b	0.653	4.50	<0.001	1.922	
$+ c(wt) + d(sbp)$	c	0.008	2.06	0.039	1.008	
$+ f(chol)$	d	0.018	4.29	<0.001	1.018	
$+ g(ncigs) + h(age)$	f	0.011	7.27	<0.001	1.011	
$+ i(ht)$	g	0.021	4.93	<0.001	1.021	
	h	0.065	5.35	<0.001	1.067	
	i	0.016	0.49	0.63	1.017	−790.4

We now turn to consideration of the scales of each of the retained variables. Using the techniques of Section 15.1.1 reveals that the linear model in the original scale provides an adequate fit in each case (of course, behavior pattern need not be examined). In fact, dividing the observations into five groups, i.e., by quintiles, and comparing linear models to indicator variable models for the five categories gives large p-values for each retained variable, except for age where the p-value is 0.08. Examination of the coefficients of the indicator variables for the age categories, and the smoothed plot of the log odds against age (Section 15.1.2) both reveal a slight decline in risk as age increases from 39–41 to 41–44, before the risk rises sharply. No simple polynomials, fractional or otherwise, make a substantial improvement to a linear term in age. Since age is not a primary risk factor of interest, it is probably reasonable to proceed with the original variable; alternatively, we could proceed with a categorized version of age and use indicator variables to capture the complex pattern of risk observed.

Leaving age as it is, we now turn to examine possible interaction effects. Retaining six of the original risk factors, we use the same strategy as for the main effects and examine each of the 15 possible pairwise interactions in turn, using the likelihood ratio procedure to avoid collinearity problems. From this analysis, five interaction terms had p-values less than 0.2 and were retained. Adding all of these together to the model

Table 15.4 *Selected multiple logistic regression model for the Western Collaborative Group Study*

Model	Parameter	Estimate	Max. Log Likelihood
$\log\left(\frac{p}{1-p}\right) = a + bx$	b	0.671	
$+c(wt) + d(sbp)$	c	0.096	
$+f(chol)$	d	0.068	
$+g(ncigs) + h(age)$	f	0.065	
$+j(age \times chol)$	g	0.021	
$+k(wt \times sbp)$	h	0.167	
$+l(wt \times chol)$	j	-0.0004	
	k	-0.0003	
	l	-0.0002	-783.7

and then eliminating unnecessary interactions reduced the number of interactions to three (we now use a p-value of 0.1 as a criterion for continued inclusion). This final model is reported in Table 15.4.

A next step would be to center and regularize variables appropriately so that the coefficients and their estimated standard deviations are more readily interpretable. Interpretation of the final model, including interaction terms, is a crucial final step, although as we argued earlier, interpretation of effects is important throughout the model building process, particularly in suggesting relevant models.

15.3 Goodness of fit

Once we have a "final" model or any model of interest along the way, how can we assess whether it effectively describes the pattern of disease outcomes in the sample? For any given individual with a specified set of risk factors, the model provides an estimate of the probability of D, given the observed level of covariates. Specifically, suppose there are r risk factor terms in the logistic regression model under consideration (including all indicator variables and interaction terms), given by $X_1, \ldots, X_r$, where these variables incorporate any relevant scale changes; that is, the model is denoted by:

$$\log\left(\frac{p_{x_1,\ldots,x_r}}{1 - p_{x_1,\ldots,x_r}}\right) = \log(\text{ odds of } D|X_1 = x_1, \ldots, X_r = x_r)$$

$$= a + b_1 x_1 + b_2 x_2 + \cdots b_r x_r, \tag{15.1}$$

or, equivalently,

$$p_{x_1,\ldots,x_r} = \frac{1}{1 + e^{-(a+b_1 x_1 + b_2 x_2 + \cdots + b_r x_r)}}. \tag{15.2}$$

Then, an individual whose observed values of risk factors are $X_1 = x_1, \ldots, X_r = x_r$ has an estimated probability of disease, in the fitted version of the model,

Table 15.5 *Comparison of observed and expected frequencies to assess goodness of fit*

		Disease		
		D	not D	
Covariate pattern	1	$O_{11}(E_{11})$	$O_{01}(E_{01})$	m_1
	2	$O_{12}(E_{12})$	$O_{02}(E_{02})$	m_2
	$\cdots$	$\cdots$	$\cdots$	$\cdots$
	K	$O_{1K}(E_{1K})$	$O_{0K}(E_{0K})$	m_K
		n_D	$n_{\bar{D}}$	n

given by

$$\hat{p}_{x_1,\ldots,x_r} = \frac{1}{1 + e^{-(\hat{a}+\hat{b}_1 x_1+\hat{b}_2 x_2+\cdots+\hat{b}_r x_r)}}. \tag{15.3}$$

To assess the goodness of fit of our model, we now require methods to compare this model-based probability with the observed outcome for this individual, that is, $D = 1$ (incident case) or $D = 0$ (no disease). Performing this comparison for the entire sample is equivalent to looking at the *residuals* in a standard linear regression analysis. However, residuals are not as directly useful here since we only observe outcomes $D = 1$ or $D = 0$, so that residuals are always either $\hat{p}_{x_1,\ldots,x_r}$ or $1 - \hat{p}_{x_1,\ldots,x_r}$.

Nevertheless, m individuals with exactly the same pattern of covariates, $X_1 = x_1, \ldots, X_r = x_r$, all share the same estimated probability of disease, $\hat{p}_{x_1,\ldots,x_r}$, so that the *expected* number of cases anticipated amongst these m observations, based on the model (Equation 15.1), is just $m \times \hat{p}_{x_1,\ldots,x_r}$. This can then be compared to the observed number of cases in this group of m individuals. Performing this calculation for all distinct patterns of covariates leads to Table 15.5; here we assume that there are exactly K distinct risk factor patterns in the sample of size n.

If the risk factors are reasonably discrete, so that K is small compared to n, we can formally compare the observed and expected (based on the model) number of cases for each risk factor pattern, either by (1) fitting a logistic regression model with $K - 1$ indicator variables that capture the K levels of the risk factors, and then using the likelihood ratio test to compare this to the model under investigation, or by (2) using what is known as the *Pearson χ^2* test. The use of the likelihood ratio test in (1) is exactly the same goodness of fit test for a simple linear model that we used in Chapter 13.2 and 13.4 with only one categorical risk factor (see also Figure 13.4). Note that the degrees of freedom of the likelihood ratio test are $K - (r + 1)$, where r is the number of parameters in the model of interest.

The Pearson χ^2 test compares the observed and expected counts through

$$\chi^2_{Pearson} = \sum_{i=0}^{1} \sum_{j=1}^{K} \frac{(O_{ij} - E_{ij})^2}{E_{ij}},$$

using the notation of Table 15.5. Under the null hypothesis that Model 15.1 describes the population risk pattern, $\chi^2_{Pearson}$ will follow a sampling distribution that is approximated by a χ^2 distribution with $K - (r + 1)$ degrees of freedom, akin to the likelihood ratio test. In fact, these two tests will give similar results with large samples. The χ^2 test of Chapter 6 is a special case of the Pearson χ^2 test wherein the model assumption under consideration is independence between D and a single binary outcome E; see Chapter 6.4.1.

As for the likelihood ratio test (see Chapter 14.6), the validity of the Pearson χ^2 test depends on sufficiently large sample sizes in several of the risk factor categories. In most examples, however, the set of risk factors is sufficiently diverse, or some of the risk factors are continuous so that the total number of distinct covariate patterns may be very close to n, the sample size. For example, there are 3141 distinct levels of the set of risk factors, listed in Table 15.1, amongst the 3142 sampled individuals with complete data (recall that 12 individuals have missing data on the cholesterol variable and are thus excluded from this analysis). In such cases, these goodness of fit procedures cannot be used without further modification. One way to proceed is to group the set of possible risk levels into a much smaller set of categories to allow appropriate use of the Pearson χ^2 test. In principle, this can be achieved by a subjective choice of categories; in the following section, we introduce an objective form of categorization introduced by Hosmer and Lemeshow (2000).

15.3.1 The Hosmer–Lemeshow test

The categorization underlying the Hosmer–Lemeshow goodness of fit test depends on the predicted or estimated risk probabilities, Equation 15.3, for all individuals in the sample. Once each of these has been calculated, the categories are formed by ordering the predicted risks and dividing them into g groups based on this ordering. It is recommended to use at least $g = 5$ such ordered categories, and as many as $g = 10$ if the original sample size n is large enough. Thus, for $g = 10$, the sample is divided into deciles of risk based on the model under examination; Table 15.5 is constructed based on this categorization and the Pearson χ^2 test statistic computed. Assuming the null hypothesis that the model (Equation 15.1) applies in the population, this test statistic has been shown, using simulations, to have an approximate χ^2 sampling distribution with $g - 2$ degrees of freedom.

Table 15.6 gives the Western Collaborative Group Study version of Table 15.5, based on the logistic regression model of Table 15.4, which yields the estimated deciles of risk. The Hosmer-Lemeshow test statistic is then computed to be

$$\chi^2_{H-L} = \frac{(0 - 2.9)^2}{2.9} + \frac{(9 - 5.9)^2}{5.9} + \cdots + \frac{(76 - 82.5)^2}{82.5}$$
$$+ \frac{(315 - 312.1)^2}{312.1} + \frac{(305 - 308.1)^2}{308.1} + \cdots + \frac{(238 - 231.5)^2}{231.5}$$
$$= 8.58.$$

Comparing this with a χ^2 distribution with $10 - 2 = 8$ degrees of freedom yields a p-value of 0.38. Note that almost all of the test statistic arises from lack of fit at the two lowest and two highest deciles of risk; if these are separately combined into

Table 15.6 *Comparison of observed (expected) frequencies for model in Table 15.4 in deciles of risk*

		Disease		
		D	not D	
Level of risk	≤0.014	0 (2.9)	315 (312.1)	315
	0.014–0.024	9(5.9)	305 (308.1)	314
	0.024–0.033	10(8.9)	304 (305.1)	314
	0.033–0.043	9(12.0)	305 (302.0)	314
	0.043–0.057	16 (15.7)	298 (298.3)	314
	0.057–0.073	17 (20.2)	298 (294.8)	315
	0.073–0.096	27 (26.1)	287 (287.9)	314
	0.096–0.127	37 (34.8)	277 (279.2)	314
	0.127–0.188	56 (48.0)	258 (266.0)	314
	>0.188	76 (82.5)	238 (231.5)	314
		257	2885	3142

a single low and single high risk group, the fit improves even more. Thus, the main problem of the model is in distinguishing subtle differences between individuals at the very lowest and very highest levels of risk. In summary, there is no glaring lack of fit of the model of Table 15.4 as compared with the observed pattern of CHD events in the sample. With this level of goodness of fit, our interpretations of this model in the population are at least plausible.

For comparison, note that the Hosmer–Lemeshow test statistic for the model of Table 15.4, excluding the three interaction terms, is 11.7, with an associated p-value of 0.17. As an aside, we note that the Pearson χ^2 test statistic based on all 3141 distinct risk factor patterns is 2979.3, which, when nominally compared to a χ^2 distribution with 3131 degrees of freedom, yields a p-value of 0.97. Since all but one of the categories contain but a single observation, this is clearly a very misleading assessment of goodness of fit.

To complete this section, we return to our motivation for using regression models. Note that the model of Table 15.4 estimates the log Odds Ratio associated with behaviour type as 0.671 ($OR = 1.96$) with an estimated standard deviation of 0.146. Compare this to the simple estimate of 0.864 ($OR = 2.37$) with an estimated standard deviation of 0.140 (see Model (2) of Table 13.3): we have removed a sizeable amount of confounding at this juncture. However, the increase in the standard deviation reflects the "price" we pay for controlling for the effects of the other variables in the model in Table 15.4, including the interaction terms. However, this very modest loss of precision is considerably less than what we face if we try to achieve the same analysis through stratification methods. For instance, suppose we stratify each of the "extraneous" variables of Table 15.1 into five categories (using, say, the quintiles of the relevant variable) with the intention of estimating the log Odds Ratio for behavior pattern, controlling for the other variables though this stratification. Note that adjusting for one variable requires 5 strata, but two variables requires 25 strata, three need 125 strata, four 625 strata, and so on. But we have seven variables of interest to consider, that is, 78,125 strata! This analysis is clearly impossible with "only" 3154 data points. Further, stratifying on only three of these variables (age, weight, and systolic blood pressure, for example) leads to an estimated standard deviation of 0.148 for the log Odds Ratio for behavior pattern, already greater than what we obtained from the model of Table 15.4. The standard deviation quickly deteriorates when any additional stratification variables are considered. This quick comparison reflects the enormous advantage that regression models have over simple stratification approaches. The regression model, by using the power of the model assumptions, limits loss of precision from covariate adjustment; the key is, of course, to use the regression assumptions wisely by checking both the goodness of fit of the scale of individual variables, and the overall fit of the final model, using the techniques of this chapter.

15.4 Comments and further reading

We have barely scratched the surface on techniques that examine the adequacy of a model in describing patterns of risk. Overall goodness of fit approaches, including the Pearson and Hosmer and Lemeshow statistics, are unlikely to detect subtle but important discrepancies between the model and the data (Hosmer et al., 1997). Further, we should not assume that a "good" fitting model is necessarily "correct"; indeed, many quite distinct models that include different variables can lead to similar goodness of fit statistics. Any selected model must be subject to careful scrutiny to assess whether the associations and interactions between variables and the outcome bear reasonable interpretations. Causal graphs are important aids to ensure that we have not included variables on the pathway between exposure and disease, nor adjusted for colliders. In sum, goodness of fit procedures are unfortunately a very crude instrument in assessing the appropriateness and value of a specific model, and we must remain aware that models with similar fits may have strikingly different interpretations with regard to individuals in the population.

Further model checking includes examination of the impact of unusual values of one or more variables, sometimes referred to as "outliers." Univariate line or box plots of each variable in the model may reveal surprisingly large or small values of a variable. Joint scatter plots can also highlight outlying combinations of a pair of covariates. Extreme values deserve examination to assess their accuracy. More formal assessment of the extent to which a single individual influences the estimate of a coefficient of interest can be implemented by fitting the same model with the individual removed from the data to determine the resulting change in the estimate. For example, in the Western Collaborative Group Study, one individual has a reported baseline serum cholesterol level of 645 mg/100 ml, an extraordinarily extreme value (the next highest value is 414 mmHg)—this individual developed CHD during follow-up. However, omitting this individual from analyses made no appreciable difference to the results in either Table 15.2 or 15.3(a), with changes in coefficients, standard deviations, or Wald statistics usually occurring only in the third significant digit. Further details of this and other forms of sensitivity analysis are provided in Hosmer and Lemeshow (2000).

In addition, there is a wide variety of statistical *model selection* methods that are particularly designed to constrain the possibility of model *overfitting*, a situation where a model with multiple parameters apparently fits the data well (which it must to a large extent because the same data are used to estimate the "best" fitting version of the model) but will yield substantial error when applied to future observations. A useful statistical model selection technique is *cross-validation*, where the data are split into two parts, one used for estimation and the other for model validation. If such splitting and model checking is done many times, more accurate estimates of future error are possible. This form of model selection is particularly important if the logistic regression model will be used for prediction in other populations.

15.5 Problems

Question 15.1

Using the data set *titanic*, found by going to http://www.crcpress.com/e_products/ downloads/, use a logistic regression model to examine an appropriate scale for age in terms of assessing its role in determining the probability of dying. Recall that there is missing age data on 263 of the 1309 passengers. Use the approach of ordered categories and supplement your findings with a scatterplot plot smoother, such as lowess, and fractional polynomial fits. Repeat your analysis for each ticket class separately, and contrast your findings across these groups and against the results from the entire data set.

Question 15.2

Still using the data set *titanic*, use model building techniques to fit a suitably parsimonious logistic regression model for survival status using the explanatory variables sex, ticket class, and place of embarkment. As part of this exercise, fit the model with an indicator variable for all 18 distinct levels of the factors, and compare your selected model to this *saturated* model to assess goodness of fit. Now add the two continuous variables, age and ticket fare, to your analysis and again use model building techniques to select an appropriate parsimonious "final" logistic regression model. In this case, assess the goodness of fit of your model using the Hosmer–Lemeshow test statistic. For both cases, provide an interpretation of your chosen logistic regression model.

Question 15.3

Referring to the data set *oesoph*, found by going to http://www.crcpress. com/e_products/downloads/, use model building ideas to select an appropriate parsimonious logistic regression model relating the risk of esophageal cancer to the risk factors age, alcohol consumption, and tobacco consumption. In addition, fit the saturated model, based on these covariates, using indicator variables to capture their 96 distinct levels. Compare these two models using the likelihood ratio test statistic to assess goodness of fit. Interpret your findings.

CHAPTER 16

Matched Studies

At the beginning of Chapter 12, we noted that matching represents a design alternative to regression analysis that mitigates the loss of precision due to adjustment for several potential confounding variables. In this chapter, we describe matched designs and statistical techniques to analyze data arising from matched studies. We consider both frequency matching, where there are only a few distinct levels of the confounding variables in question, and pair matching, where there are very large numbers of possible confounding variable patterns. These designs represent extreme examples of the approach, and it should be recognized that there are intermediate variations.

16.1 Frequency matching

In the example relating coffee consumption to incidence of pancreatic cancer, the original design produced a roughly 1.75:1 ratio of controls to cases (Table 7.3), presumably reflecting the availability of cases and limitations on total sample size, although relatively marginal gains in precision could be expected from additional controls. If we expect to have to control for potential confounding effects of sex, we have no way of knowing how this carefully designed balance may be changed by stratification on sex. In fact, the balance is better in the male stratum (Table 9.3), but deteriorates to about 2.2:1 in the female stratum. Although the change in balance does not materially affect precision in estimates of the Odds Ratio, the investigator cannot be sure that a more serious loss of balance will not occur. Frequency matching provides control to the investigator over case-control marginal balance, in sex strata in this example.

In this study, there were 151 female and 216 male pancreatic cancer cases available for analysis. To ensure a balance of 1.75:1 in both sex strata, the investigator randomly samples 265 female and 378 male controls (since $265 \approx 1.75 \times 151$ etc.). We can view this design as simultaneous implementation of two separate case-control studies, one of males and one of females. Instead of the design only specifying the overall sample number of cases and controls, this frequency-matched design predetermines the case and control sample sizes (and thus the balance) in *each* stratum, the two sexes in this particular case. A frequency-matched cohort design is similar in that separate cohort studies are carried out in each stratum, determined by levels of the matching variables, thereby guaranteeing desired sample sizes and balance for the exposed and unexposed.

Thus, frequency matching requires (1) the specification of one or more potentially confounding variables, (2) the ability to stratify the sampling frame for the Study Population into separate categories according to levels of the prespecified confounding variables, and (3) implementation of a case-control (or cohort) design in each such stratum with investigator-determined samples sizes of cases and controls (or of each exposure category in a cohort design). It is important to control the balance in the choice of sample sizes in step (3) to achieve the objectives of frequency matching. Sample sizes may be zero at some levels of the matching factors when it is not possible to find cases or controls with those characteristics.

The impact of frequency matching on data analysis is immediate. For example, for a matched case-control study, it is no longer possible to estimate the conditional probabilities, $P(E|D)$ or $P(E|\bar{D})$, because manipulation of the sample sizes over levels of the matching factor, C, say, necessarily modifies the observed frequency of exposure in both cases and controls. This seems to present a serious obstacle, since it is exactly these conditional probabilities that form the basis for estimation of the Odds Ratio as described in Chapter 5.3. However, we can estimate conditional probabilities such as $P(E|D, C = c_i)$ and $P(E|\bar{D}, C = c_i)$, where c_i denotes a specific level of the matching variable C. These, in turn, allow estimation for the Odds Ratio associating E and D *after stratification on C*.

On the other hand, it is no longer possible with matched case-control data to estimate or evaluate the association of the matching factors, C, with the outcome, D; the frequency of cases and controls at each matching level is entirely determined by the design.

By definition, frequency matching uses only a few distinct levels of the matching factors so that stratification methods (see Chapters 9 and 10) can be used to examine the relationship between E and D. The logistic regression model can also be directly applied, as long as the matching variables defining strata membership are included in any model considered. In summary, the advantage of this design approach is that loss in precision due to adjustment for matching factors is potentially mitigated, with the price that all analyses include these design factors. We provide a more detailed study of the subtle differences between matched cohort and case-control studies in Section 16.7.

16.2 Pair matching

When the set of matching factors has a very high number of discrete levels, it follows that there will likely be few individuals sampled at any specific level. In the most extreme situation, there may be only two individuals sampled at any given fixed value of the matching factors. In cohort studies, we sample one exposed individual and one unexposed individual at each level of the matching factors. For a case-control study, one case and one control are sampled at each level. There have to be at least two individuals sampled to ensure balance on the appropriate marginal. This extreme form of design is known as *pair matching*. For the time being, we focus our discussion on matched case-control designs. Simple modifications can be made to cover matched cohort data.

As with frequency matched data, we can only conceive of estimating probabilities (with matched case-control data) that are conditional on both D (case or control status) *and* the matching factors, denoted by C. That is, we can try to estimate, for example,

Table 16.1 *Possible types of matched pair case-control data*

(1)

		Control	
		E	$\bar{E}$
Case	E	X	
	$\bar{E}$		

(both case and control are E)

(2)

		Control	
		E	$\bar{E}$
Case	E		X
	$\bar{E}$		

(case is E, control is $\bar{E}$)

(3)

		Control	
		E	$\bar{E}$
Case	E		
	$\bar{E}$	X	

(case is $\bar{E}$, control is E)

(4)

		Control	
		E	$\bar{E}$
Case	E		
	$\bar{E}$		X

(both case and control are $\bar{E}$)

$P(E|D, C = c)$. In principle, this is exactly what we want, since we are committed to estimating the D–E relationship, controlling for the effects of C, the matching variables. However, we are now in the uncomfortable situation of having data divided into a very high number of strata with only two observations in each stratum of C. This is exactly the scenario where some of our methods break down—in particular, the Woolf technique of Chapter 9 and the maximum likelihood approach of Chapter 13. As we indicate below, however, the Cochran–Mantel–Haenszel test and the Mantel–Haenszel estimates can be applied to such extremely stratified data, and there is a modification of the maximum likelihood methodology that also can be used with finely matched data. We now turn to a discussion of these ideas, beginning by noting simple ways of representing pair matched case-control data. For simplicity, for now we will consider the exposure of interest, E, as a simple binary variable.

Since there are only two observations in each C stratum (one D and one $\bar{D}$), there are only four possible patterns with regard to the measurement of the exposure status of each case-control pair. These four possibilities are listed in Table 16.1. For example, for a matched case-control pair of Type (1) in Table 16.1, both the case and control are exposed (E). In Section 16.3, we consider a matched case-control study of pregnancy histories and incidence of coronary heart disease in women, where the matching factors are age and location of residence; if E represents a history of at least one spontaneous abortion, then for a pair of Type (2), the CHD case had such a history whereas the control did not.

The data on all matched pairs can then be summarized by counting the number of matched pairs of each type, rather than listing each pair separately. We suppose that there are A pairs of Type (1) in Table 16.1, B pairs of Type (2), C pairs of Type (3), and D pairs of Type (4). The data can then be represented by a 2×2 classification of the exposure status of the case and control pair, as illustrated in Table 16.2. Here, N

Table 16.2 *Summarization of matched pair case-control data*

		Control	
		E	$\bar{E}$
Case	E	A	B
	$\bar{E}$	C	D
			N

Table 16.3 *Exposure patterns in the four types of matched pairs*

(1)	D	$\bar{D}$	
E	1	1	2
$\bar{E}$	0	0	0
	1	1	

(2)	D	$\bar{D}$	
E	1	0	1
$\bar{E}$	0	1	1
E	1	1	

(3)	D	$\bar{D}$	
E	0	1	1
$\bar{E}$	1	0	1
	1	1	

(4)	D	$\bar{D}$	
E	0	0	0
$\bar{E}$	1	1	2
E	1	1	

represents the total number of matched pairs in the data set, so that the total number of sampled individuals is $2N$.

Now, for a given level of the matching factors, say, $C = c_i$, the total number of exposed individuals in our matched pair (that is, 0, 1, or 2) will largely depend on the strength of the association between E and C. In our example, the number of women with a history of spontaneous abortion in a given pair may be dependent on their common age. This relationship is not of immediate interest, as we wish to understand the $D - E$ association (between spontaneous abortion history and CHD). Suppose we therefore look at the probability of the observed exposure pattern, *conditional on the total number of exposed individuals in the matched pair at $C = c_i$*. Note that it is only the exposure patterns that are random, since we have fixed the count of cases and controls (one each), at $C = c_i$, in the design. If we further condition on the number of exposed individuals at $C = c_i$, the only unknown is how those exposed individuals are related to disease status: do they arise from the case, control, both or neither? For example, a matched pair of Type (1) yields the first simple 2×2 table of Table 16.3, with the remaining 2×2 tables originating from the matched pairs of the other types.

Note that for the first and fourth types, where the case and control are both either exposed or unexposed, knowing the total number of exposed individuals allows you to fill in the entries of the corresponding 2×2 table in Table 16.3 without error. These matched pairs are known as *concordant* pairs; the case and control "agree" with regard to exposure history. On the other hand, there is still uncertainty as to the 2×2 table entries for matched pairs of Type (2) or (3), since knowing that there is one exposed and one unexposed member of each pair does not reveal which is case and

which is control. These *discordant* pairs are the sole source of information about the
D–E relationship once we condition on the total number of exposures in each pair.
With the notation of Table 16.2, there are therefore $B + C$ discordant pairs from our
original sample of N matched pairs.

For convenience, label the matched pairs by the index i, and for each pair write
$r_i = P(E|D, C = c_i)$, where c_i is the level of the matching factors for the ith pair.
Similarly, write $s_i = P(E|\bar{D}, C = c_i)$. The probability of observing a discordant pair
with the case being the exposed member [i.e., type (2)] is then $r_i(1 - s_i)$. Similarly, the
probability of observing a discordant pair with the control being the exposed member
[i.e., type (3)] is $(1 - r_i)s_i$. Thus, among discordant pairs at $C = c_i$, the probability that
the case is exposed for a randomly selected pair is $[r_i(1 - s_i)]/[r_i(1 - s_i) + (1 - r_i)s_i]$.
Dividing the top and bottom of this fraction by $(1 - r_i)s_i$ shows this probability to be
$\frac{r_i}{(1-r_i)} \frac{(1-s_i)}{s_i} / [\frac{r_i}{(1-r_i)} \frac{(1-s_i)}{s_i} + 1]$. But $\frac{r_i}{(1-r_i)} / \frac{(1-s_i)}{s_i} = OR_i$, the Odds Ratio relating D and
E when $C = c_i$ (see Chapter 4.4). Thus, the probability that the case in a randomly
selected discordant pair is exposed is just $OR_i/(1 + OR_i)$. This observation provides
the link between information on the discordant pairs to the Odds Ratio associating E
and D.

In general, it is possible that this Odds Ratio and thus the relative frequency of
discordant pairs corresponding to an exposed case will vary with c_i, the level of the
matching factors. This is, in fact, an issue of effect modification by the matching
factors. If we assume that there is no (multiplicative) interaction between the set
of matching factors and E, then OR_i does not vary with i, and so the proportion
of discordant pairs with an exposed case is the same regardless of the level of the
matching factor. Thus, if we use P to denote this constant proportion of discordant
pairs where it is the case that is exposed, we have shown that

$$P = \frac{OR}{1 + OR} \qquad (16.1)$$

where OR is the Odds Ratio for D associated with E, now assumed constant over
levels of the matching factors.

The relationship (16.1) allows us to address questions regarding the Odds Ratio
by restating them in terms of P, a simple population proportion. For example, since
there are $B + C$ discordant matched pairs, of which B correspond to the case being
exposed (see Table 16.2), P can be estimated directly by $\hat{P} = B/(B + C)$. Solving
Equation 16.1 for OR in terms of P allows us to translate this estimate "back" to an
estimate for OR. Specifically,

$$OR = \frac{P}{1 - P}, \qquad (16.2)$$

so that the corresponding estimate of the Odds Ratio is just

$$\widehat{OR} = \frac{\frac{B}{B+C}}{1 - \frac{B}{B+C}} = B/C. \qquad (16.3)$$

This is known as the *conditional maximum likelihood* estimate of the Odds Ratio,
as it results from applying maximum likelihood to the pairs data, *conditional* on the
number of exposed individuals in each pair.

A confidence interval for P can also be computed using any of the appropriate methods discussed in Chapter 3.3. If the limits of such an interval are (P_L, P_U), then this leads immediately to the confidence interval $[P_L/(1 - P_L), P_U/(1 - P_U)]$ for the Odds Ratio. It is worth remembering here that this Odds Ratio already adjusts for the potential confounding effect of any matching variable. In Section 16.4.1 we consider the possibility that matching variables might have a modifying effect on this Odds Ratio.

Finally, the null hypothesis that D and E are independent, having controlled for the effects of the matching variables, may be of interest, that is, $H_0 : OR = 1$. In terms of P from Equation 16.1, this is equivalent to $H_0 : P = 1/2$. Qualitatively, the null hypothesis therefore indicates that if D and E are independent, we should expect on the average the same number of exposed case discordant pairs as exposed control discordant pairs; that is, B should be close to C. Formally testing this null hypothesis is thus equivalent to testing whether a coin is fair ($P = 1/2$) on the basis of a series of independent tosses ($B + C$ "tosses," in this case).

Given the sample size $n = B + C$, the random variable B follows a binomial distribution with probability given by nP, treating the number of discordant pairs as fixed. Under H_0, $P = 1/2$, so the mean and variance of this binomial distribution are $(B + C)/2$ and $(B + C)/4$, respectively, the latter term following from the fact that the variance of the binomial distribution is $nP(1 - P)$. If $\hat{P} = B/B + C$ is far from $1/2$ [or, equivalently, B is far from its null mean, $(B + C)/2$] in terms of its known variance, there is concern about the plausibility of the null hypothesis that D and E are independent. We can then use exact calculations of the tail probabilities of this particular binomial distribution to yield an exact p-value. Alternatively, if $B + C$ is large enough, a Normal approximation to this binomial distribution with the same mean and variance can be used to compute a p-value associated with the null hypothesis of independence. For the approximation, we calculate

$$B - \left[\frac{(B + C)}{2}\right] \Big/ \sqrt{\frac{(B + C)}{4}} = (B - C)/\sqrt{B + C},$$

and compare this to tables of a standard Normal distribution. Equivalently, we can square this statistic to give

$$\chi^2_{McN} = \frac{(B - C)^2}{B + C}, \tag{16.4}$$

which approximately follows a χ^2 distribution with one degree of freedom if the null hypothesis is correct. This simple test of independence of D and E, based on matched pairs, is known as *McNemar's test* and is illustrated in Sections 16.3 and 16.6.

16.2.1 Mantel–Haenszel techniques applied to pair-matched data

An alternative approach to matched data is to apply stratified data techniques to the matched pairs, treating each pair as a separate stratum. If we assume no interaction between E and the matching factors, we might use either the Woolf or Mantel–Haenszel approaches discussed in Chapters 9.1 and 9.2. Recall, though, that the

Table 16.4 *Cochran–Mantel–Haenszel test statistic, and Mantel–Haenszel odds ratio estimator, calculations for matched pair data*

Pair Type	# Pairs of Type	a_i	A_i	V_i	$a_i d_i / n_i$	$b_i c_i / n_i$
(1)	A	1	1	0	0	0
(2)	B	1	1/2	1/4	1/2	0
(3)	C	0	1/2	1/4	0	1/2
(4)	D	0	0	0	0	0
Totals		$A+B$	$A + \frac{B+C}{2}$	$\frac{B+C}{4}$	$\frac{B}{2}$	$\frac{C}{2}$

Woolf technique fails when we have many strata each containing few observations. Matched pairs is thus the worst possible scenario in which to use the Woolf method, as there are only two observations in each stratum; so we reject that approach. On the other hand, the Mantel–Haenszel methods work effectively whatever the number of strata and whatever the pattern of sample sizes of each stratum, as long as we assume a reasonably large *total* sample size. We now look at the Cochran–Mantel–Haenszel test for independence of D and E, and the Mantel–Haenszel estimator of the Odds Ratio, as applied to matched pairs.

First, using the ideas of Chapter 9.1.1 and 9.2.2, Table 16.4 provides the necessary calculations for both the Cochran–Mantel–Haenszel test statistic and the Mantel–Haenszel estimator of the Odds Ratio. The results for a given stratum can only take on four different values, depending on the type of matched pair from Tables 16.1 or 16.2; thus, for example, the first row of Table 16.4 represents A 2 × 2 tables of Type (1) in Table 16.3. This is acknowledged in computing the totals row by multiplying the entries for each row by the number of pairs of the relevant type.

From Equation 9.1, the Cochran–Mantel–Haenszel test statistic is

$$\frac{\left((A+B) - \left(A + \frac{B+C}{2}\right)\right)^2}{\frac{B+C}{4}} = \frac{(B-C)^2}{B+C},$$

which is the just the McNemar test statistic. Thus, for matched pairs, the McNemar test is equivalent to the Cochran–Mantel–Haenszel test. Note the importance here of using the term $n_i^2(n_i - 1)$ instead of n_i^3 in the definition of V_i (see Chapter 9.1.2).

Similarly, the Mantel–Haenszel estimator (Equation 9.4) is here given by $(B/2)/(C/2) = B/C$, exactly the estimator given in (Equation 16.3). Thus, the Mantel–Haenszel estimator and the conditional maximum likelihood estimator agree exactly for matched pair data.

With more general finely matched data, for example (1:M matched case-control data where each case is matched to M controls) the conditional maximum likelihood and Mantel–Haenszel approaches do not coincide, although they usually give very similar results.

16.2.2 Small sample adjustment for odds ratio estimator

As for unmatched data, the Odds Ratio estimator, B/C, is slightly biased in small samples, again reflecting a slight overstatement on average of the true population Odds Ratio. A less biased estimator, provided by Jewell (1984), is defined by

$$\widehat{OR}_{SS} = \frac{B}{C+1}.$$

There is no need for small sample adjustments to the confidence interval procedures, since on the transformed scale of P—see Equation 16.1—the estimate $\hat{P}$ and its estimated variance are already unbiased. The discussion in Chapter 7.1.4 regarding caution in the use of small sample estimators applies equivalently here.

16.3 Example—pregnancy and spontaneous abortion in relation to coronary heart disease in women

Differences in heart disease mortality between men and women decline with increased age and suggest the possibility of endocrine factors in the etiology of CHD for women. Winkelstein et al. (1958) used a study of menstrual and pregnancy histories and their relationship to CHD incidence as a first approximation to possible endocrine effects. They carried out a matched pair case-control study where each CHD case was matched to a disease-free control by age and location of residence. Table 16.5 classifies the selected 50 matched pairs with regard to the history of spontaneous abortions for both the case and control in each matched pair. For example, there were 7 matched pairs in which the case had a history of three or more spontaneous abortions and the control had no history of any abortions. Table 16.6 summarizes this data, dichotomizing the risk factor into any or no history of spontaneous abortions (SA).

The techniques of Section 16.2 provide immediate insight into the relationship of this aspect of pregnancy history and CHD incidence. In particular, $\hat{P} = 18/23 = 0.783$; equivalently, $\widehat{OR} = 18/5 = 3.6$, reflecting a more than threefold increase in CHD risk associated with any history of spontaneous abortions, controlling for the effects of age and place of residence (assuming no interaction with these factors). The small sample estimator of the Odds Ratio is simply $\widehat{OR}_{SS} = 18/6 = 3.0$.

Table 16.5 *Matched pair case-control data on spontaneous abortions and coronary heart disease*

| | | Number of Spontaneous Abortions for Controls | | | |
		0	1	2	3+
	0	20	3	2	0
Number of spontaneous	1	7	0	2	1
abortions for cases	2	4	1	0	0
	3+	7	0	0	3

Source: Winkelstein et al., 1958.

Table 16.6 *Matched pair case-control data based on presence/absence of history of spontaneous abortion*

		Control		
		≥1 SA	No SA	
Case	≥1 SA	7	18	
	No SA	5	20	
				50

The more complex technique of Chapter 3.3 yields a 95% confidence interval for P of $(0.581, 0.903)$, whereas the exact interval is $(0.563, 0.925)$. Using Equation 16.2 then gives the corresponding confidence interval for the Odds Ratio as $(1.39, 9.35)$; the exact method gives $(1.29, 12.40)$. Finally, the McNemar test statistic (Equation 16.4) equals $(18 - 5)^2/(18 + 5) = 7.35$, giving a p-value of 0.007 when compared to a χ^2 distribution with 1 degree of freedom. There is thus substantial evidence of an important effect of a history of spontaneous abortions on CHD incidence after controlling for the effects of age and place of residence.

16.4 Confounding and interaction effects

So far, we have assumed that there is no interaction between the exposure and any of the matching factors. Although matched case-control data does not allow us to examine the association of any matching factor on the outcome, it is possible to investigate whether a matching variable modifies the effect of E on D. For example, we may wish to look at whether the effect of a history of spontaneous abortions on CHD incidence only occurs in relatively younger women. In this section, we first examine the possibility of such (multiplicative) interaction, and then continue by discussing the potential confounding and interactive roles of extraneous variables *not included as matching factors*. For this situation, we consider cigarette smoking as either a confounder or effect modifier of pregnancy history information.

16.4.1 Assessing interaction effects of matching variables

Taking the discordant pairs that are used to estimate the Odds Ratio, we divide these pairs into groups within which the matching factor of interest has some specified commonality (not necessarily at as fine a level as used in the matching). For example, in studying the possible relation of spontaneous abortions to CHD incidence, suppose we were interested in whether the relationship we observed in Section 16.3 is modified by age (at interview) or not. Since age is a matching factor, Table 16.7 separates the matched pair data from Table 16.5 into two groups, depending on whether the common age of the respondents in a matched pair is less than or equal to 65, or greater than 65. Note that 29 of the original pairs are associated with ages less than or equal to 65, and 21 arise from those whose age is greater than 65.

Table 16.7 *Matched pair case-control data on history of spontaneous abortion and CHD, stratified on age*

Age ≤65		Control			Age >65			Control	
		≥1 SA	No SA					≥1 SA	No SA
Case	≥1 SA	5	10		Case	≥1 SA		2	8
	No SA	2	12			No SA		3	8
				29					21

Table 16.8 *Examination of interactive effect of age on the association between occurrence of spontaneous abortions and CHD incidence*

		Age ≤65	Age >65
Discordant pairs	Case exposed	10	8
	Control exposed	2	3

Now we simply estimate the Odds Ratio associated with the occurrence of one or more spontaneous abortions for each of the two age groups, as we did for the entire data set. Thus, for the group whose age is less than or equal to 65, $\widehat{OR} = 10/2 = 5.0$, and for those whose age is greater than 65, $\widehat{OR} = 8/3 = 2.7$. Confidence intervals can then be computed for each of these age-group specific Odds Ratios if desired. We see some slight evidence that the impact of a history of spontaneous abortion is greater for the younger age group. But the numbers underlying these estimates of the Odds Ratio are necessarily quite small now. To avoid being deceived by small numbers, we want to compare the Odds Ratios allowing for sampling variation. Rather than directly examining changes in the Odds Ratios, we can more easily and equivalently compare the underlying P for each age-group. Note that $\hat{P} = 10/12 = 0.833$ for the younger group, and $\hat{P} = 8/11 = 0.727$ for those over 65 years old. Statistical comparison of these two independent proportion estimates can be achieved using the χ^2 test or the Fisher exact test, if the numbers are small. Table 16.8 lays out the data in a manner that allows easy computation of either test.

Here, the χ^2 test statistic is 0.38, with a p-value of 0.54. The exact test yields a p-value of 0.64. As we might suspect, the numbers are much too small for us to consider the observed differences in the Odds Ratios as definitive evidence of an interactive effect.

16.4.2 Possible confounding and interactive effects due to nonmatching variables

We have now discussed simple techniques that allow study of the exposure–disease relationship, allowing for both the potential confounding and interactive effects of the matching factors. However, there may be other important variables, measured as

Table 16.9 *Matched pair case-control data on history of spontaneous abortion and CHD, stratified on smoking*

Nonsmokers					Smokers				
		Control						Control	
		≥1 SA	No SA					≥1 SA	No SA
Case	≥1 SA	3	6			Case	≥1 SA	1	5
	No SA	2	10				No SA	0	3
				21					9

part of the study design, that we would like to examine to see if they may have a confounding role or be effect modifiers. The most direct way to do this is to further stratify the data into strata defined by constant levels of the new variable. The data are already very finely stratified by the matching factors, but carefully, so that there is balance on the case-control marginal. Unfortunately, with any additional stratification, this benefit of the matched design may be quickly lost since there is no guarantee that the case and control will share a common value of the new confounder and so may be "separated" by the additional stratification. Such separated pairs then contribute no information on exposure effects, as there is now only one individual in the stratum. This seriously affects the precision of this kind of adjusted analysis.

Using our example again, we introduce a new variable that is a binary measure of smoking history. Table 16.9 gives the original matched pair data, now stratified by smoking history *only for those pairs who happened to be concordant for smoking*. Matched pairs where the case and control have different smoking histories are split by stratification on smoking and provide no information on the relationship of spontaneous abortion to CHD, controlling for smoking. Here, we can see that 30 of the matched pairs were also concordant on smoking while 20 were not. Of these 30 pairs, both case and control were nonsmokers 21 times, and both were smokers 9 times.

If we assume that smoking is not an effect modifier, then both tables in Table 16.4 provide estimates of the same fixed Odds Ratio for a history of spontaneous abortions, controlling for smoking, and so the discordant pairs can be combined to give a summary estimate (and confidence interval) for this common Odds Ratio. Essentially, by retaining only those pairs who happen to be concordant for smoking history, this variable looks like one of the matching factors (although with far fewer pairs since it was not *preselected* as a matching variable). From Table 16.9, we see that $\widehat{OR} = 11/2 = 5.5$, this now adjusted for smoking. Qualitatively, this is somewhat higher than the unadjusted estimate, $\widehat{OR} = 3.6$, computed in Section 16.3.

The data in Table 16.9 cannot be used to estimate the Odds Ratio for CHD associated with smoking since they only include pairs concordant on smoking. For this estimate, we reverse the roles of smoking and spontaneous abortion history in Table 16.9, now examining the pairs that are concordant on the latter and discordant on the former.

Table 16.10 *Matched pair case-control data on smoking and CHD, stratified on history of spontaneous abortion*

No SA		Control			≥1 SA		Control	
		Smoker	Nonsmoker				Smoker	Nonsmoker
Case	Smoker	3	3		Case	Smoker	1	1
	Nonsmoker	4	10			Nonsmoker	2	3
				20				7

This yields Table 16.10. With the identical assumption of no interaction, we can combine the discordant pairs in the two tables in Table 16.10 to yield an estimate $\widehat{OR} = 4/6 = 0.7$, indicating a slight protective effect of smoking. However, both the McNemar test statistic and the confidence interval for this Odds Ratio show that this could easily be due to random variation.

With regard to the possible interactive effects of smoking, we can compare the two Odds Ratios in Table 16.9 from the separate smoking strata, using the same techniques that we used in Section 16.4.1. Here, the Odds Ratio in the smoking stratum is not immediately estimable because there are no discordant pairs with an exposed control (but see Section 16.2.2 for a small-sample Odds Ratio estimate); however, the P estimates are $\hat{P} = 6/8 = 0.75$ and $\hat{P} = 5/5 = 1.0$ for nonsmokers and smokers, respectively. Rather than using the χ^2 test to compare these two estimates to assess equality, with such small numbers we use the exact test, which yields a p-value of 0.49. However, Table 16.10 also provides additional information on interaction, now using the concordant pairs on spontaneous abortion history that are discordant on smoking. The exact test on this data compares the P estimates 3/7 and 1/3 to yield a p-value of 0.67. These two independent sources of data on interaction can, of course, be combined using the Cochran–Mantel–Haenszel approach of Chapter 9.1.1 or its exact equivalent (Chapter 9.1.2) to produce a summary p-value. In our example, this produces an even larger p-value since Table 16.9 shows a qualitative synergistic interaction between the two risk factors (being a smoker increases the effect of spontaneous abortions), whereas Table 16.10 displays qualitative antagonism (a spontaneous abortion history makes smoking more protective); these two qualitative effects cancel each other out somewhat when combined. Thus, allowing for little data to analyze, there is no indication that smoking influences the effect of a history of spontaneous abortions on the risk for CHD.

The analyses of Sections 16.4.1 and 16.4.2 show that matched data give extremely little room to maneuver when adjusting for unmatched potential confounding variables or examining interaction effects. If either of these goals is an important objective of the analysis, then it is almost compulsory that we turn to regression models in order to maintain a reasonable level of precision.

16.5 The logistic regression model for matched data

Now we apply the logistic regression model to the analysis of matched data. Continuing our theme of treating matched pair studies as simply yielding stratified data, albeit with only two observations per stratum, the direct way to construct a logistic regression model is to include stratification effects using indicator variables (as described in Chapter 12.6.1) in addition to exposure variables of interest. If there are N matched pairs reflecting presumably N distinct levels of the matching factors, $N - 1$ indicator variables are needed to allow variation of risk over the strata. Thus, in the simplest case with one risk factor X, a possible logistic regression model that incorporates the matched design is given by:

$$\log\left(\frac{p_x}{1 - p_x}\right)_i = \log(\text{odds for } D|X = x, \text{ } i\text{th level of matching factors})$$
$$= a + a_1 I_1 + \cdots + a_{N-1} I_{N-1} + bx$$
$$= a_i^* + bx,$$

assuming that, for the ith level, $I_i = 1$, with all other indicator variables zero. The notation $a_i^* = a + a_i$ is a simple way of summarizing this model. Note the interpretation here that a_i^* is the log odds of D in the ith level of the matching factor when $X = 0$; b represents the log Odds Ratio associated with a unit increase in X, assuming that the level of the matching factors is held constant. This simple model does not yet permit interactive effects between X and the matching variables.

We can easily extend this model to allow multiple risk variables, including terms that describe possible interactions between risk factors and between a risk factor and one or more of the matching variables. Specifically, a multiple logistic regression model for matched data with k explanatory variables, $X_1, \ldots, X_k$, is described by:

$$\log\left(\frac{p_x}{1 - p_x}\right)_i = \log(\text{odds for } D|X_1 = x_1, \ldots, X_k = x_k,$$
$$i\text{th level of matching factors}) \tag{16.5}$$
$$= a_i^* + b_1 x_1 + \cdots + b_k x_k.$$

Unfortunately, we have seen that maximum likelihood is not an effective method when the data are this finely stratified or, in other words, when there are so many unknown parameters. Note that here the set of a_i^* contains N unknown parameters where N is the number of matched pairs. Fortunately, there is a modification to the likelihood function that allows us to proceed. For matched case-control studies, this modification involves conditioning on the total number of exposures (for a binary exposure) in each matched set before we calculate the likelihood function; that is, we assume that the number of exposures is fixed at the observed value in each matched pair. Recall that this is exactly how we set about computing the Odds Ratio for a simple binary exposure in Section 16.2. In general, for a more complex exposure, or for more than one exposure variable, we condition on the pattern of overall exposures observed in each matched pair.

For a concrete example, suppose we wish to examine the effect of the *number* of prior spontaneous abortions on the subsequent risk of CHD rather than the simple dichotomous exposure of Section 16.3. A possible logistic regression model to achieve this aim is given by

$$\log \left(\frac{p_x}{1 - p_x} \right)_i = \log(\text{odds for } D|SA = x, \ i^{\text{th}} \text{ level of matching factors})$$

$$= a_i^* + bx, \tag{16.6}$$

where SA counts the number of prior spontaneous abortions. Here, b represents the log Odds Ratio associated with an increase of one spontaneous abortion. The results of fitting this specific model are described in Section 16.5.1. Before computing the contribution to the likelihood for the ith pair, we condition on the number of prior spontaneous abortions observed for each woman in the pair. For example, in one pair the case reported two prior spontaneous abortions and the control, one. We thus condition on observing the two responses, $SA = 2$ and $SA = 1$, without indicating which response arose from the case and which from the control.

With this conditioning, the only random phenomenon left to assess is how the fixed pattern of exposures is distributed to the case and control. That is, with two possible exposure patterns, we calculate the probability that the case (and the control) is assigned its observed exposure, given (or conditional on) the fact that we know these two exposure patterns belong to this particular matched pair. For the pair we looked at in the last paragraph, we compute the probability that the case was the woman who reported $SA = 2$ and the control $SA = 1$, given that the two responses in the pair were $SA = 2$ and $SA = 1$. In general, the probability that the case reported $SA = x_1$ is just $P(SA = x_1|D)$; similarly, the probability that the control reported $SA = x_2$ is $P(SA = x_2|\bar{D})$. Thus, the conditional probability that $SA = x_1$ for the case and $SA = x_2$ for the control, *given that* $SA = x_1$ and $SA = x_2$ were observed in the pair, is

$$\frac{P(SA = x_1|D)P(SA = x_2|\bar{D})}{P(SA = x_1|D)P(SA = x_2|\bar{D}) + P(SA = x_2|D)P(SA = x_1|\bar{D})}$$

$$= \frac{P(D|SA = x_1)P(\bar{D}|SA = x_2)}{P(D|SA = x_1)P(\bar{D}|SA = x_2) + P(D|SA = x_2)P(\bar{D}|SA = x_1)}$$

$$= \frac{P(D|SA = x_1)/P(\bar{D}|SA = x_1)}{(P(D|SA = x_1)/P(\bar{D}|SA = x_1)) + (P(D|SA = x_2)/P(\bar{D}|SA = x_2))}$$

$$= \frac{e^{a_i^* + bx_1}}{e^{a_i^* + bx_1} + e^{a_i^* + bx_2}}$$

$$= \frac{1}{1 + e^{b(x_2 - x_1)}}, \tag{16.7}$$

the first step using Bayes' formula of Chapter 3.4.1 and the last steps following from the model (Equation 16.6). Note that this conditional probability for concordant pairs, where $x_1 = x_2$, does not depend on b and thereby provides no information on the effect of SA on CHD. For the specific pair, with the case reporting two prior spontaneous abortions and the control one, this conditional probability is simply

$$\frac{1}{1 + e^{-b}}.$$

Computing these conditional probabilities and multiplying them across the independent matched pairs leads to what is known as the *conditional likelihood*. The conditional likelihood can then be used in exactly the same way as the likelihood function for unmatched data, as discussed in Chapter 13.1. The advantage of this is immediate, in that the conditional likelihood does not depend on the matched pair specific parameters a_i^*, but only on the remaining parameters in the model; see Equation 16.7. The by-now familiar maximum likelihood estimates, associated confidence intervals, Wald, score, and likelihood ratio tests are all now available to us based on this conditional likelihood. This technique is known as the *conditional maximum likelihood* method to distinguish it from the maximum likelihood methods used for unmatched data. As noted in Section 16.2, the Odds Ratio estimate, $\widehat{OR} = B/C$, for matched pairs with a binary exposure, results from conditional maximum likelihood.

The conditioning is much simpler for matched cohort studies where the exposure patterns are fixed in each matched pair. In this case we condition on the number of D outcomes in each matched pair to produce the relevant conditional likelihood. Further, for case-control designs, the ideas of conditional likelihood are easily extended to matched designs that allow a small number of cases or controls in each matched set, with (again) a similar modification to cohort studies with more than one exposed or unexposed in each matched group. In sum, conditional maximum likelihood is an appealing alternative to the maximum likelihood approach of Chapter 13.1 in that it avoids the problems of stratified data with few observations in each stratum. On the other hand, it is more difficult computationally when there are many observations per stratum, so that in such cases we usually rely on the simpler unconditional maximum likelihood.

One immediate implication of the use of conditional likelihood is that it does not permit estimation of any parameters in the set $\{a_i^* : i = 1, \ldots, N\}$. Thus, as noted earlier, conditional likelihood analysis of matched data sacrifices the ability to estimate the effects of the matching variables on D in exchange for improved precision in estimating the effects of the main risk factors of interest. With case-control designs— due to the nature of this form of sampling (Chapter 13.3)—these parameters cannot be interpreted anyway, as they represent baseline (i.e., $X_1 = \cdots = X_k = 0$) log odds of disease at the various levels of the matching factors. We are still able, however, to assess the interactive role of matching variables on the relationship between unmatched risk factors and D.

16.5.1 Example—pregnancy and spontaneous abortion in relation to coronary heart disease in women: part 2

We now apply conditional maximum likelihood to estimation of various logistic regression models for incidence of CHD based on a woman's history of spontaneous abortions. Table 16.11 provides definitions of variables that appear in the estimated logistic models summarized in Table 16.12. The maxima of the log likelihoods in Table 16.12 refer to the conditional likelihood as discussed in Section 16.5.

Table 16.11 *Coding for variables in matched case-control study of pregnancy history and CHD*

SA = Number of spontaneous abortions

$$X = \begin{cases} 1 & \text{any history of spontaneous abortions } (SA \geq 1) \\ 0 & \text{no history of spontaneous abortions } (SA = 0) \end{cases}$$

$$X_1 = \begin{cases} 1 & SA = 1 \\ 0 & \text{otherwise} \end{cases}$$

$$X_2 = \begin{cases} 1 & SA = 2 \\ 0 & \text{otherwise} \end{cases}$$

$$X_3 = \begin{cases} 1 & SA \geq 3 \\ 0 & \text{otherwise} \end{cases}$$

$$Xord = \begin{cases} 0 & SA = 0 \\ 1 & SA = 1 \\ 2 & SA = 2 \\ 3 & SA \geq 3 \end{cases}$$

$$Y = \begin{cases} 1 & \text{average age in pair} > 65 \\ 0 & \text{average age in pair} \leq 65 \end{cases}$$

$$Z = \begin{cases} 1 & \text{smoker} \\ 0 & \text{nonsmoker} \end{cases}$$

Table 16.12 *Conditional logistic regression models relating history of spontaneous abortions to incidence of coronary heart disease*

Model (No.)	Parameter	Estimate	SD	OR	p-Value	Max. Log Likelihood
(1) $\log\left(\frac{p}{1-p}\right) = a_i + bx$	b	1.281	0.506	3.600	0.011	-30.76
(2) $\log\left(\frac{p}{1-p}\right)$	b	1.609	0.775	5.000	0.038	
$= a_i + bx + c(x \times y)$	c	-0.629	1.029	0.533	0.541	-30.57
(3) $\log\left(\frac{p}{1-p}\right)$	b	1.338	0.521	3.813	0.010	
$= a_i + bx + cz$	c	0.279	0.501	1.322	0.577	-30.60
(4) $\log\left(\frac{p}{1-p}\right) = a_i + bx$	b	1.039	0.627	2.825	0.097	
$+cz + d(x \times z)$	c	-0.002	0.609	0.998	0.998	
	d	0.819	1.027	2.267	0.426	-30.27
(5) $\log\left(\frac{p}{1-p}\right) = a_i + b_1 x_1$	b_1	1.252	0.654	3.496	0.056	
$+b_2 x_2 + b_3 x_3$	b_2	0.648	0.734	1.912	0.377	
	b_3	2.173	1.099	8.786	0.048	-29.96
(6) $\log\left(\frac{p}{1-p}\right)$	b	0.589	0.251	1.802	0.019	-31.14
$= a_i + b(xord)$						
(7) $\log\left(\frac{p}{1-p}\right) = a_i + b(SA)$	b	0.473	0.215	1.605	0.028	-30.89

Model (1) examines the simple summary of history of spontaneous abortions discussed in Section 16.3 (see Table 16.6). Since x is a binary risk factor, the regression analysis provides an identical estimate of the Odds Ratio, namely, $e^{1.281} = 3.6 = 18/5$. The associated 95% confidence interval for the log Odds Ratio is just $1.281 \pm (1.96 \times 0.506) = (0.289, 2.273)$ or, for the Odds Ratio, $(1.34, 9.71)$. This differs slightly from $(1.39, 9.35)$, described in Section 16.3, since the latter is based on a confidence interval for P (before transforming to the Odds Ratio) rather than on the log scale. The Wald test statistic is 2.53 with a p-value of 0.01; the square of the Wald statistic is 6.42, close to the McNemar test statistic of 7.35 in Section 16.3. Although not reported in Table 16.11, the maximized conditional likelihood in the model with no exposure variables, $\log[p/(1-p)] = a_i^*$, is $34.66 [= 50 \times \log(1/2)]$, as this model assumes no dependence on x. (The conditional probability of the observed case and control exposure, given the exposure pattern in the pair, is then just $1/2$; see Equation 16.7 with $b \equiv 0$), yielding a log likelihood ratio test statistic of 7.80 when compared to Model (1), even more similar to the McNemar statistic. Each of these three tests indicates that the data provide strong evidence of an association between a history of spontaneous abortions and incidence of CHD, controlling for the effects of age and place of residence.

Model (1) assumes no (multiplicative) interaction between age and place of residence and a history of spontaneous abortions. Model (2) now includes the possibility of variation in the Odds Ratio across two simple age groups. Again, since both variables X and Y are binary, Model (2) exactly parallels our consideration of interaction in Section 16.4.1, yielding an Odds Ratio associated with the occurrence of one or more spontaneous abortions of $e^{1.609} = 5.0$ for the younger-age group, and $e^{1.609-0.629} = 2.7$ for the older group. A test of the null hypothesis $H_0 : c = 0$ in Model (2) yields a p-value of 0.54 using either the Wald or likelihood ratio test statistics, just as we saw in Section 16.4.1.

Model (3) introduces another risk factor, smoking, that is not a matching factor. The Odds Ratio associated with smoking is 1.3, which does not yield a significant p-value. The Odds Ratio for a history of spontaneous abortion rises slightly to 3.8, reflecting only a small confounding effect for smoking. Although this analysis is similar to the investigation of Section 16.4.2, the qualitative results for smoking differ since smoking now appears as risky rather than protective. These results cannot be viewed as contradictory in light of large standard errors surrounding the estimates by both strategies. However, the Odds Ratio estimate from Model (3) is more precise, since the regression model, unlike the earlier stratification approach, uses information on the matched pairs that are discordant on smoking history. Model (4) shows qualitatively that the Odds Ratio associated with a history of spontaneous abortions is greater for smokers than nonsmokers ($e^{\hat{b}+\hat{d}} = e^{1.858} = 6.41$ as compared with $e^{\hat{b}} = e^{1.039} = 2.83$), as we saw before from Table 16.9. Of course, the information is insufficient to determine whether this is an interactive effect present in the population, as indicated by the p-value from either the Wald or likelihood ratio tests. These results again differ slightly from those in Section 16.4.2, even though both risk factors are binary, because the conditional likelihood approach uses information from 10 pairs that are discordant on both smoking and spontaneous abortion history.

Finally, Models (5), (6), and (7) consider different approaches to relating number of spontaneous abortions to the risk of CHD. In the 100 women, 7 had prior experience of more than 3 spontaneous abortions (4 had 4, 2 had 6, and 1 had 7). Both Models (6) and (7) show evidence of a trend in CHD risk as the numbers of previously experienced spontaneous abortions increase. Comparing Model (6) to Model (5) gives a likelihood ratio test statistic of 2.36, yielding a p-value of 0.31 when compared to a χ^2 distribution with 2 degrees of freedom. Thus, the linear model in either *Xord* or *SA* appears to reasonably fit the variation in CHD risk over different numbers of spontaneous abortions, despite the apparent dip in risk when *Xord* = 2 compared to *Xord* = 1; note that only 9 of the 100 women reported *SA* = 2.

16.6 Example—the effect of birth order on respiratory distress syndrome in twins

We use a simple example to illustrate the application of the ideas of Section 16.2 to matched cohort designs. Arnold et al. (1987) examined the risk of birth order on respiratory distress syndrome (RDS) in twins. While it is known that there is a higher risk of RDS for second-born twins, the study was intended to investigate whether this relationship could be explained by other factors associated with birth. A series of 221 preterm twin births was collected for study. Considering birth order as a risk factor, such twin pairs then represent a matched cohort study (always one firstborn and one secondborn) with matching factors including variables such as gestational age, method of delivery, secular trends, and various maternal risk factors.

In analogy to Tables 16.2 and 16.6, Table 16.13 classifies these matched pairs according to the observed occurrence of RDS at birth in one, neither, or both twins. The estimate of the Odds Ratio for RDS associated with birth order is then $31/8 = 3.9$, reflecting a sizeable increase in risk associated with being secondborn. The McNemar test statistic is $(31-8)^2/(31+8) = 13.56$, with a p-value of 0.0002, displaying strong evidence of the expected association between birth order and RDS.

Table 16.13 *Matched pair cohort data relating birth order to respiratory distress syndrome in twins*

		First Born	
		RDS	No RDS
Second Born	RDS	24	31
	No RDS	8	158
			221

Table 16.14 *Examination of interactive effect of mode of delivery on the association between birth order and RDS*

		Vaginal	Abdominal
Discordant pairs	Second born has RDS	24	7
	First born has RDS	3	5

Table 16.15 *Conditional logistic regression models relating birth order and mode of delivery to respiratory distress syndrome*

Model (No.)	Parameter	Estimate	SD	OR	p-Value	Max. Log Likelihood
(1) $\log\left(\frac{p}{1-p}\right) = a_i + bx$	b	1.355	0.397	3.875	0.001	-19.79
(2) $\log\left(\frac{p}{1-p}\right) = a_i + bx + c(x \times y)$	b	0.336	0.586	1.400	0.57	
	c	1.743	0.847	5.714	0.04	-17.57

For the 39 discordant pairs, further stratification on the mode of delivery, a matching factor, yielded the data of Table 16.14, the analog of Table 16.8. This table reveals that the estimated Odds Ratio for RDS associated with birth order is 8.0 (= 24/3) for vaginal deliveries and 1.4 (= 7/5) for abdominal deliveries. This indicates the possibility of a strong interactive effect with the conclusion that birth order may only be a risk factor in vaginal deliveries. The χ^2 test applied to Table 16.14 is 4.76 with a p-value of 0.03; the Fisher exact test gives a p-value of 0.08. Thus, even with these small numbers, the data suggest a strong interactive effect.

Table 16.15 gives the results of fitting two simple logistic regression models to this matched data that confirm this interaction. Here the binary variable X is coded as 1 for second-born twins, and 0 for firstborn; similarly, Y is coded 0 and 1 for abdominal and vaginal deliveries, respectively. Note the significant interaction effect in Model (2); this model predicts an Odds Ratio of $e^{0.336} = 1.4$ for RDS, associated with being second born in abdominal deliveries. For vaginal deliveries, the estimated Odds Ratio is $e^{0.336+1.743} = 8.0$. These estimates exactly replicate the simple estimates above because of the binary nature of both birth order and mode of delivery. Note that Model (2) yields an insignificant p-value (0.57) associated with the birth order effect in abdominal deliveries; not shown in the table is the Wald statistic p-value for the same relationship in vaginal deliveries, which is 0.001.

It is worth noting that in this example the twins are naturally occurring matched pairs, unlike the typical epidemiological setting with matched individuals. This raises a possible complication to the analysis due to the issue of independence of the two-pair members. All of our analyses have assumed that, conditional on relevant quantities (such as matching factors, disease outcome, and overall exposure patterns in a case-control study), the two observations are statistically independent. This is questionable in the case of twins unless one assumes that it is possible to find, hypothetically, an appropriate list of common (matched) attributes that twins share, so that when such factors are assumed to be fixed (i.e., conditioned upon), the random "responses" of each twin are independent. For example, in this matched cohort study, we must assume that there is a list of (unknown) matching factors for the twins so that the RDS response of one twin is independent of the other, once we have accounted for these common features. Alternative analysis methods that do not make this assumption are available; see the comments in Chapter 17.2.

16.7 Comments and further reading

Matched designs were introduced as a way of improving precision in estimates of risk relationships when they must be adjusted for possible confounding effects of a set of factors that have many distinct levels. Extensive simulations have been carried out to investigate the necessary conditions for precision gains and to see just how much is gained over standard unmatched designs. See, for example, Kupper et al. (1981) and Karon and Kupper (1982). Gains in precision are most pronounced when the matching factors are strongly associated with both D, the outcome of interest, and with the relevant exposure variable; that is, when the matching variables are expected to be strong confounders. On the other hand, precision may actually be lost through matching, particularly if the matching factors are unrelated to the disease (that is, are not risk factors). This occurs because although the balance on one marginal is favorable by design (the disease marginal in a matched case-control study), we have no control on the other balance (the exposure marginal in a matched case-control study); this balance can be made worse by matching, particularly if the matching factors and exposure are strongly associated. Such a scenario arises when there are a substantial number of matching factors so that the cases and controls are so similar in all regards that they also tend to be similar with regard to the exposure. This leads to a great number of concordant pairs, so that there is little information available on the exposure–disease relationship of interest. This situation is one form of what is commonly referred to as *overmatching*.

The techniques to accommodate matched case-control data, including conditional maximum likelihood for logistic regression models, apply directly to the analysis of the risk-set sampling designs of Chapter 5.4.1. In this case, the data arise from matching on the time at risk (during the risk interval) whether or not any additional matching on other factors was implemented in the design. Subsequent estimates of Odds Ratios are interpreted as Relative Hazards in light of conditioning on time at risk. A slight variation on the logistic regression model for such data is described in Chapter 17, Sections 17.3 and 17.4.

An alternative form of risk-set sampling in nested case-control studies, known as *counter-matching*, seeks not to make cases and controls as alike as possible in terms of potential confounders, but as distinct as possible in terms of the exposure variables of interest (Langholz and Borgan, 1995). For example, in the simplest situation of a binary exposure factor, each randomly sampled case is paired with a control with the *opposite* exposure status, thereby forcing the pair to be discordant. That is, a sampled exposed case is paired with a randomly selected unexposed control, and vice versa. The intent of countermatching is the same as regular matching, that is, increased precision in measuring an exposure effect as compared to standard sampling procedures. This kind of sampling can be accommodated in the analysis with appropriate weighting and therefore can be implemented through conditional maximum likelihood methods with only minor adjustment. Langholz and Clayton (1994) discuss various scenarios where countermatching is an attractive option, in particular situations where exposure is rare or where countermatching can be performed on a proxy of an exposure for which accurate measurement is expensive. Andrieu et al. (2001) consider the use of countermatching to improve efficiency in studies designed to elucidate interaction effects, especially gene–environment interactions. Countermatching on proxies for both genetic variables and environmental variables appears to be most efficient.

16.7.1 When can we break the match?

Many matched studies are small in terms of the total number of matched sets, in part because matching is often costly and difficult to implement. Further, after matching in pairs we may be left with a substantial number of concordant pairs, as in Table 16.6 where 27 of the original 50 pairs are concordant and play no further role in the simple analysis of spontaneous abortion history. For both these reasons, it may be tempting to "break the match" and see what happens if we analyze the data using methods for unmatched data. Is this appropriate? Does it gain us any precision?

In cohort studies, matching on exposure results in the absence of an association between exposure and the matching factors, with the consequence that the sample data cannot show confounding (Chapter 8.1.2). In this case, the pooled data created after breaking matches and combining yields a valid estimate. However, variance estimates for the measures of association, derived from unmatched sampling, are incorrect and cannot be used. Accounting for the matching factors is therefore usually necessary to produce appropriate assessment of variability. Further, if there is differential misclassification of the outcome variable, then we still need to account for matching factors in order to obtain valid effect measure estimates.

The answer to the question of breaking the match is clearer for matched case-control studies in which, by design, matching removes the association between disease and the matching factors. However, this is not quite what is required to purge confounding, since there needs to be no association *conditional on the exposure variable* (Chapter 8.1.2). Thus, pooling the sample data will still yield a biased estimate of the Odds Ratio, except in special circumstances when the population Odds Ratio is exactly one, or when exposure probabilities are constant for all cases and for all controls. Therefore, for matched case-control data it is generally inappropriate to break the match. We must control for the matching factors in the analysis.

These remarks must not be construed to mean that all forms of pooling are inappropriate. In particular, if pair matching is implemented on a factor that only assumes a few distinct values, then it is not only valid to combine pairs that have identical values of the matching factor, but also beneficial for reasons of precision. If there are sufficient number of pairs at each of the common levels of the matching factor, the data can now be analyzed as frequency-matched data. For example, if case-control matched pair data are matched solely on sex, the pairs should be combined into two categories, male and female, and analyzed using stratified techniques for the two sex strata.

Further, in some situations the bias induced by breaking the match may be small relative to the gain in precision that arises from using all the data (including concordant pairs) in the pooled analysis. Under this scenario, it may be preferable to use the pooled estimator if the size of the bias is not of great concern. Liang and Zeger (1988) and Kalish (1990) suggest two ways of averaging the pooled and matched estimators to take advantage of the desirable properties of both. In practice, one can always obtain a sense of the bias and variance gain associated with the pooled estimator by comparing these quantities with the relevant matched estimators. For example, from Table 16.6, the pooled estimator is easily seen to be 3.17, with an associated 95% confidence interval of (1.35, 7.44), using the techniques of Chapter 7.1. The comparison to the matched estimate of 3.6, with 95% confidence interval (1.39, 9.35) of Section 16.3, clearly displays for the pooled estimator a small amount of bias toward the null, with only a slight gain in precision. In this case, there appears to be only a slight precision advantage to the pooled estimator, which probably is not worth the increased bias.

16.7.2 Final thoughts on matching

Gains in precision are less pronounced in case-control than in cohort designs; losses in precision are more pronounced in matched case-control studies. This phenomenon is related to the comparison of variability across these two designs in an unmatched environment, discussed in Chapter 9.5.1.

For many interval-scaled matching factors, exact matches are usually impossible. For example, to match on age by finding a case and a control with identical birth dates would make matching impractical. In such instances, *caliper matching* is usually implemented by finding individuals "close enough" on the matching factor scale. For age this might entail selecting a matched control within 5 years of age of the case. A preferable solution, though, is to simply widen the categories for age that define a match, thus using 5-year age groups to define matching levels. This approach avoids the possibility that controls tend to be systematically younger than their matched case, for example. With very broad categories, it is possible that some confounding will remain due to matching factor variation within category. This is particularly insidious, as matching tends to suggest entire removal of confounding bias. Although, in principle, the exact level of the matching variable can still be controlled in the analysis as an unmatched factor, this is likely to reduce the gains in precision that motivated matching in the first place.

Measurement error remains a major concern with matched data, particularly for unmatched factors. Techniques briefly introduced in Chapter 7.5.1, like the SIMEX method, can be used to investigate the impact of such random errors if additional information is available on the properties of measurement error.

In many situations, a matched design may be appealing because of the immediate availability of control information at the time case data are collected; for example, when sampling from medical records from a variety of sources, or in the case of neighborhood or family matching. On the other hand, if there are several matching factors, it can often be difficult and expensive to locate a control match for all sampled cases. Occasionally a suitable match cannot be located and so the investigator might discard the case information; in such cases, the inadvertent decrease in overall sample size can easily dilute or eliminate any precision gains from matching. Similarly, if implementation costs associated with matching are considerably higher than unmatched sampling, anticipated precision benefits may be lessened or even eliminated by reducing the overall sample size to keep the cost the same as for an unmatched study.

Given these considerations, the most advantageous situation for matching is when there is one or more strong confounders that are extremely hard to measure quantitatively. This is likely when the confounders represent geographic location (as in the example of CHD and women in Sections 16.3 and 16.5.1), or when there is a need to control for family traits or environment. Matching on sibship status, for example, may be appealing, though subject to the caution noted at the end of Section 16.6. For both place of residence or employment and family characteristics, it is usually extremely difficult to define simple quantitative scales that fully capture the necessary variables, so that matching can then be an effective strategy for confounding control.

16.8 Problems

Question 16.1

Johnson and Johnson (1972) investigated 175 cases of Hodgkin's disease. As controls they used siblings of the Hodgkin's patients, choosing the closest sibling of the same gender and within 5 years of age to form a matched pair. The matching reduced the data to 85 patient–sibling pairs. The paper was designed to refute an earlier claim that having a tonsillectomy increased the chances of contracting Hodgkin's disease. Breaking the match, the 85 matched pairs provided information on prior tonsillectomy (T) experience as shown in Table 16.16.

Johnson and Johnson analyzed Table 16.16, thereby ignoring the matching. Repeat their analysis by performing a test and giving an associated p-value, and by estimating the Odds Ratio for Hodgkin's disease associated with a prior tonsillectomy, providing a corresponding 95% confidence interval.

Table 16.16 *Case-control data on tonsillectomy history (T) and Hodgkin's disease, with match broken*

		Hodgkin's Disease		
		D	$\bar{D}$	
	T	41	33	74
Tonsillectomy status	$\bar{T}$	44	52	96
		85	85	170

Table 16.17 *Matched pair case-control data on tonsillectomy history (T) and Hodgkin's disease*

		Control		
		T	$\bar{T}$	
Case	T	26	15	
	$\bar{T}$	7	37	
				85

Table 16.18 *Frequency of exposure patterns for N 1:3 matched case-control sets with binary exposure*

Exposure Pattern	Number of Matched Sets
Case exposed, all three controls exposed	A
Case exposed, two controls exposed	B
Case exposed, one control exposed	C
Case exposed, all three controls unexposed	D
Case unexposed, all three controls unexposed	E
Case unexposed, two controls unexposed	F
Case unexposed, one control unexposed	G
Case unexposed, all three controls exposed	H
Total	N

The correct way of looking at the data takes account of the pairing, as in Table 16.17. Perform the appropriate matched pair analysis by testing the null hypothesis of no association, giving a p-value. Also estimate the Odds Ratio, supplemented by an associated confidence interval. Compare your results with the previous analysis.

Question 16.2

Consider a 1:3 matched case-control study with a dichotomous exposure, where every case is matched to three controls on a set of matching factors. For each matched set of four subjects, there are eight possible outcomes with regard to the observed exposure pattern. Suppose there are a total of N matched sets of four. Each possible exposure pattern and the frequency with which it is observed are is given in Table 16.18. For example, all individuals are exposed in A of the N matched sets. Using the Mantel–Haenszel approach, show that an appropriate estimator of the Odds Ratio linking exposure to disease is given by $\widehat{OR} = (\frac{B}{4} + \frac{2C}{4} + \frac{3D}{4})/(\frac{F}{4} + \frac{2G}{4} + \frac{3H}{4})$.

Question 16.3

Redelmeier and Tibshirani (1997a,b,c) investigated the role of cell phone use on the risk of automobile accidents. They used data available from a collision-reporting

Table 16.19 *Matched pair case-crossover data on cell phone use (CP) and automobile accidents*

		Day before Collision	
		CP	$\bar{C}P$
Day of Collision	CP	13	157
	$\bar{C}P$	24	505
			699

center in Toronto and information from cell phone logs to determine whether a cell phone was in use just (up to 10 min) before the accident in question. For control information, they used the drivers involved in the accident as their own controls with a risk period defined by the exact same 10 min time window from the day previous to the accident. This study design, known as a *case-crossover design*, thus uses each driver as his own match. Data on 699 accidents, in particular, cell phone use on the day of the accident and the prior day, are given in Table 16.19. Using matched data techniques, estimate the Odds Ratio associating cell phone use with the risk of accidents. Provide a 95% confidence interval to supplement the point estimate. Critique the assumptions underlying the statistical methodology in light of comments regarding twin studies in Section 16.6.

The data were unable to elucidate whether drivers were in their car when using a cell phone on the day prior to the accident. Assume a certain fraction of drivers were out of their cars the previous day; how would this bias the estimate of the Odds Ratio? Another concern is that some cell phone calls on the day of the accident may have occurred immediately after the accident but be misclassified as "before accident" if the timing of the accident was even slightly misreported. How would this misclassification distort an estimate of the Odds Ratio?

Question 16.4

Herman et al. (1983) discuss a matched case-control study investigating the relationship between various factors and the risk for stroke in a Dutch population. The data include 132 cases. For each case, one or more controls were selected matching the case on age and gender. After much analysis, the authors reported the (conditional) logistic regression model described in Table 16.20 using the codings for variables of Table 16.21. Assuming that the fitted model provides a reasonable description of the population, (1) describe carefully the effect education has on the risk for stroke. Similarly, describe the effects of (2) previous history of acute myocardial infarction, (3) previous history of high blood pressure, (4) positive Rhesus factor, and (5) gender. What assumptions do the authors invoke by not including the single variables (1) age and (2) high blood pressure in the model described in Table 16.20?

Question 16.5

The data set *infertility*, found by going to http://www.crcpress.com/e_products/downloads/, provides matched case-control data (Trichopoulos et al., 1976) that

Table 16.20 *Conditional logistic regression model for data from Tilberg, the Netherlands, October 1978–July 1981*

	Logistic Coefficient	Standard Error	Wald Statistic
Education	−0.604	0.321	−1.882
Education × gender	0.741	0.393	1.885
Physical activity, leisure time	−0.716	0.230	−3.113
Acute myocardial infarction	2.999	1.374	2.183
(Acute myocardial infarction) × age	−1.320	0.664	−1.988
Cardiac arrhythmias	5.856	3.103	1.887
(Cardiac arrhythmias) × age	−1.926	1.165	−1.653
(High blood pressure) × gender	1.507	0.546	2.760
(High blood pressure) × age	−0.408	0.222	−1.838
Diabetes mellitus	0.796	0.497	1.602
Obesity × age	0.394	0.159	2.478
Transient cerebral ischemic attack	1.991	0.454	4.385
Rhesus factor	−1.598	0.762	−2.097
(Rhesus factor) × age	1.385	0.401	3.454

Table 16.21 *Variable codes for use in logistic model*

Sex	0 = female, 1 = male
Age	0 = 40–49 years, 1 = 50–59 years,
	2 = 60–69 years, 3 = 70–74 years
Education	0 = 6–7 years. 1 = 8–9 years, 2 = 10^+ years
Physical activity, leisure time	0 = little, 1 = regular light, 2 = regular heavy
Acute myocardial infarction	0 = no, 1 = yes
Cardiac arrhythmias	0 = no, 1 = yes
High blood pressure	0 = no, 1 = yes
Diabetes mellitus	0 = no, 1 = yes
Obesity	0 = no, 1 = yes
Transient cerebral ischemic attack	0 = no, 1 = yes
Rhesus factor	0 = negative, 1 = positive

Note: For medical variables, the answer "yes" refers to a previous medical history of the condition.

relates a history of induced or spontaneous abortions to the risk of secondary infertility. In this data set, two controls are selected for each of 83 cases of secondary infertility, matched on age, education, and parity. For one case, only one control was retained. Use conditional logistic regression techniques to investigate the relationship between binary measures of a past history of either spontaneous or induced abortions on the risk for secondary infertility. Now use the full detail in the scale of both these risk factors that gives the exact number of prior spontaneous or induced abortions, with particular attention as to whether including these ordered variables linearly in the model provides an adequate fit.

Question 16.6

Referring to the analysis of Question 16.5 on the data set *infertility*, now examine the interactive effects of the matching variable, parity, on either a prior history of spontaneous or induced abortions.

CHAPTER 17

Alternatives and Extensions to the Logistic Regression Model

There are many variations on the logistic regression model beyond the applications to unmatched and matched binary outcome data considered in Chapters 12 to 16. These include (1) variations in the basic linear form assumed for risk variables in the model, (2) more complex outcome data, and (3) more structured forms of data sampling. We briefly discuss each of these in turn. In Sections 17.3 to 17.5, we turn in a different direction to consider a detailed look at how risk changes dynamically over the risk period via a regression model for the hazard function.

17.1 Flexible regression model

So far, we have assumed that the scale of exposure variables is known before data analysis begins, although we considered methods of letting the data guide this choice in Chapter 15.1. The *generalized additive model* of Hastie and Tibshirani (1990) maintains the additive structure of the logistic regression model, but allows the data to fit the manner in which each exposure variable influences the log odds of disease. For example, with two exposure variables, X and Z, we can fit the model

$$\log\left(\frac{p_x}{1 - p_x}\right) = \log(\text{odds for } D|X = x) = a + f(x) + g(z),$$

where the two functions f and g are unspecified. This model replaces the linear terms (bx and cz in the usual formulation of logistic regression) with arbitrary, presumably nonlinear functions, f and g; instead of estimating the coefficients b and c, we now use the data to estimate functions that describe how unit changes in X and Z modify the risk of D. If f and g are reasonably smooth, their values have a natural interpretation: with Z held fixed, the slope of the function f at x is approximately the log Odds Ratio associated with a unit increase in X, near $X = x$, with an equivalent interpretation for the function g. The fact that the functions are estimated from the data and not prespecified allows very flexible dependence of the risk on changes in X and Z. The model is easily extended to include more than two factors, and it is possible to mix linear terms with the unspecified functions.

Figure 17.1 illustrates the fit of the following generalized additive model

$$\log(\text{odds for } D|x, wt, chol) = a + bx + f(wt) + g(chol).$$

to data from the Western Collaborative Group Study, using the variable names of Table 15.1. Figure 17.1 displays the estimates of f [s(bodyweight)] and g [s(cholesterol)], where for plotting esthetics we have omitted the individual with serum cholesterol of

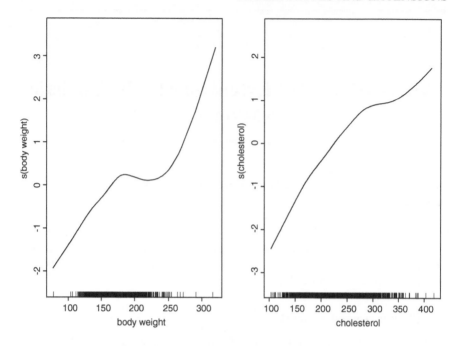

Figure 17.1 *Generalized additive model for the effects of body weight and serum cholesterol, at baseline, on incidence of CHD in the Western Collaborative Group Study, adjusting for behavior type.*

645 mm%, noted in Chapter 15.4. The shape of f is similar to what we previously observed in a univariate analysis in Figure 15.1. The marks on the X-axis in both plots indicate the location of the data values of both body weight and serum cholesterol. It is helpful to plot the two functions on the same Y-axis scale, since then the shapes of the curves can be compared with regard to their influence on CHD risk; for example, since the rough "slopes" of the two curves are similar, an increase of 50 mg/100 ml of serum cholesterol raises the risk of CHD more than does an increase of 50 lb in body weight.

Both the estimates of the functions f and g are reasonably linear, confirming earlier analyses, although as in Figure 15.1 there is an interesting "flat" part of the curve estimating f for weights ranging from about 180 to 230 lb; here the data suggest that increases or decreases in weight within that range make no difference to the risk of CHD. A problem with these flexible curves is that they can be overly influenced by small deviations; adding pointwise 95% confidence intervals to the curves as in Figure 17.2 helps identify the parts of the curves that are estimated with the most accuracy. Figure 17.2 dramatically displays where the shapes are less well identified by the data, regions—at both ends—where the data are sparse. Finally, the estimated value of b the log Odds Ratio, associated with behavior type, controlling for body weight and cholesterol in this manner, is 0.803, giving an Odds Ratio of 2.23, similar to previous analyses that only adjust for a few confounders.

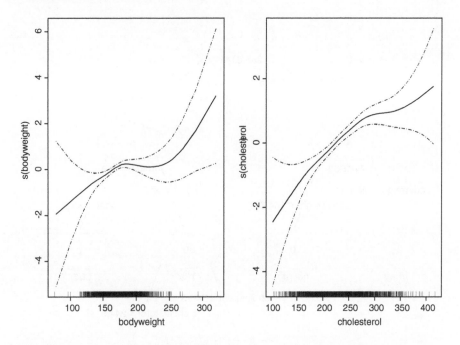

Figure 17.2 *Pointwise 95% confidence intervals for the estimated functions in a generalized additive model for the effects of body weight and serum cholesterol, at baseline, on incidence of CHD in the Western Collaborative Group Study, adjusting for behavior type.*

The generalized additive model maintains the "additive" structure that is at the core of logistic regression and the other regression models of Chapter 12. Such models are convenient and remarkably flexible. Nevertheless, there is some discomfort philosophically with the idea that changes in risk associated with one exposure should necessarily "add" with changes from a completely different exposure, particularly when exposures are measured on different scales. For example, why should the additional risk associated with being a type A individual be added to the extra risk that arises from being 50 lb overweight? *Classification trees* provide a very different kind of regression model that abandon additivity in favor of very simple scales for all the exposures. For an introduction, see Zhang and Singer (1999) and Zhang et al. (1996). Long et al. (1993) compare the application of tree methods and logistic regression models in medical problems. Zhang and Bracken (1996) apply tree methods to the study of risk factors for spontaneous abortions.

The simplest version of a classification tree divides the population into partitions defined by each exposure variable being in some contiguous interval (e.g., weight between 150 and 163 lb, height between 5 ft 10 in. and 6 ft, and behavior type A) such that the risk in each partition is assumed to be constant. Using enough partitions allows us to model changes in risk over the entire range of all risk factors. The data are used to select the "best" partition according to some criteria (here, we use the likelihood function). For the Western Collaborative Group Study, consider the effects on CHD

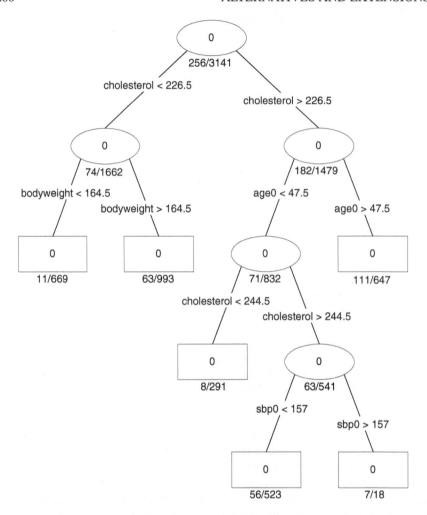

Figure 17.3 *Part of a classification tree for incidence of CHD in the Western Collaborative Group Study, based on baseline measurements of age (age0), body weight, height, serum cholesterol, systolic (sbp0) and diastolic blood pressure, and behavior type. Numbers below each node give the number of individuals (denominator) and the number of CHD cases (numerator) classified to that node.*

risk of baseline measurements on age, body weight, height, serum cholesterol, systolic and diastolic blood pressure, and behavior type. The scales used for each variable are described in Table 15.1 (again omitting one individual with a serum cholesterol of 645 mm%. Figure 17.3 displays part of a classification tree derived from the data.

A classification tree is constructed by (1) systematically splitting a variable at each level (i.e., cholesterol <200 mg/100 ml and cholesterol >200 mg/100 ml), (2) finding the split that "best" fits the data according to a selected criterion (here the likelihood function), (3) repeating this separately for all explanatory variables under consideration, and finally (4) selecting the "best-of-the-best" split across variables. This process yields the first partition of the sample; in Figure 17.3, the best split corresponds to cholesterol being greater than or less than 226.5 mg/100 ml. This entire process is now repeated separately on both subgroups of the population defined for the first split. In Figure 17.3, the best split among those individuals with cholesterol >226.5 mg/100 ml is between age at recruitment of greater than vs. less than 47.5 years old; on the other side, the best split among those individuals with cholesterol <226.5 mg/100 ml is based on body weight being greater than or less than 164.5 lb. Note that it is possible that this second split, on either side, could use serum cholesterol again. Again the process is repeated on the four new partitions and so on. Repeated splits on the same variable in one region of the tree indicates a form of dose-response. Splitting on different variables in different parts of the tree reflects a form of effect modification; for example, age is important among those with high cholesterol but not in the low cholesterol group. The fraction of CHD cases at the different nodes indicates that the algorithm successfully looks for partitions where the incidence proportions differ most across a split. In particular, at the first split, the Odds Ratio comparing the high and low cholesterol group split at 226.5 mg/100 ml is $OR = (182 \times 1588)/(74 \times 1297) = 3.01$. Be aware that the confidence interval techniques of Chapter 7.1.2 are inappropriate for these Odds Ratios because the split itself was selected by the data (to maximize the resulting Odds Ratio in some sense) and not prespecified.

Classification trees are most often used for prediction rather than regression modeling, but they illustrate that highly nonlinear models can be easy to interpret and yield different results from logistic regression. It is interesting that even though Figure 17.3 only shows a part of a tree, there is no splitting on either height or diastolic blood pressure. These variables were also considered unimportant in the model selecting process of Chapter 15.2; in addition, the multivariate logistic regression model also retained systolic blood pressure at the expense of diastolic blood pressure. In this top part of the tree, behavior type has yet to make an appearance.

Both generalized additive models and classification trees use a high number of degrees of freedom to achieve their extreme flexibility. For example, the two functions of cholesterol and body weight estimated in Figures 17.1 and 17.2 required close to 6 degrees of freedom between them, just for these two variables. As such, both methods are subject to overfitting where the characteristics of the final estimates may be determined more by the data than by actual structure in the population. It is therefore important to use various tools of model selection to avoid data-driven anomalies. Considerable effort has been given in both technologies to modify the basic estimation strategies to avoid overfitting.

17.2 Beyond binary outcomes and independent observations

While pointing out the value of more refined disease assessment, we have throughout focused on problems where the only measure of the outcome is binary. In many studies, a more refined scale may be available that, at the very least, classifies disease status into several categories. For example, rather than using merely a diagnosis of AIDS in a study of HIV disease, it is possible to define outcome categories in terms of CD4 counts or other immunological variables. As with categorical risk factors, we must first distinguish between outcome categories that possess a natural order, *ordinal responses*, even if only a nominal scale is available, and those that possess no natural ordering, or *polytomous responses*. HIV patients with CD4 counts exhibit ordering, whereas a classification of AIDS outcomes into reason for diagnosis (e.g., Kaposi's sarcoma, pneumocystis carinii pneumonia (PCP), etc.) may not. Extensions of the logistic regression model are available for either case and are discussed in Hosmer and Lemeshow (2000). Greenland (1994) considers a variety of logistic regression models for ordinal response data.

Independence of individual observations is another key assumption that we have depended on extensively. While it holds for most population-based epidemiological studies, it is unlikely when data are collected on small structured groups as part of the study design. For example, cohort data may be collected on all individuals in a variety of occupational workgroups, with the result that individuals may be more alike when they share a group and thus a particular occupational setting, than individuals from different groups even after taking account of all measured exposures. In family studies, common to genetic epidemiological investigations, exposure and outcomes may be collected on all family members or all siblings, where it is difficult to support the independence assumption. This is exactly the issue raised in Chapter 16.6 in our discussion of matched twin studies.

Longitudinal studies, or repeated measures designs, provide an alternative source of correlated disease outcome data. In such studies, there may be, for example, repeated observations of a binary measure of a child's respiratory health over time, measured to assess whether exogenous variables (such as air pollution levels) and endogenous variables (including parents' smoking habits) may be risk factors for the selected outcome. Clearly, longitudinal observations of the same subject are likely to be correlated as compared with observations from different subjects.

Fortunately, the topic of correlated binary outcome data has received enormous attention over the past 20 years and there are a number of extensions to the logistic regression model that are suitable for these data structures. Zeger and Liang (1986) provide estimation procedures for the logistic regression model with correlated binary outcomes, with a more detailed discussion given in Diggle et al. (2002). Logistic regression models become more difficult to interpret, let alone fit, with longitudinal data. First, the availability of multiple measurements allows us to consider the effects of a risk factor both *for a single person* and *for the population as a whole*. Odds Ratios associated with these two approaches differ, requiring care in both model fitting and interpretation. Second, many approaches to longitudinal outcome data ignore the issue of time-dependent confounding, a topic we touch on briefly in Section 17.6. Nevertheless, longitudinal investigations are particularly attractive because of their potential for additional precision and their ability to elucidate causal effects.

17.3 Introducing general risk factors into formulation of the relative hazard—the Cox model

In Chapter 4.5 we introduced the Relative Hazard, $RH(t)$, at time t associated with a binary exposure, when comparing risks at t within an interval $[0, T]$. Specifically, we showed that if the cumulative risk is small over $[0, T]$ and proportional hazards hold $(RH(t) = RH$, for t in $[0, T])$, then $OR(T) \approx RH(T) = RH$ so that the Odds Ratio at the end of the interval is approximately the same as the constant Relative Hazard (see Equation 4.6). We now consider extending these ideas to allow for more complex exposures.

Suppose that a risk factor X is measured on a continuous scale. For a moment, consider two subpopulations, the first of which has exposure at the level $X = x_1$ and the second at level $X = x_0$. With the logistic regression model of Chapters 12 and 13, we might relate cumulative (cumulative) incidence at these two levels through the model $\log[\frac{p_x}{(1-p_x)}] = a + bx$, so that the log Odds Ratio comparing the two groups is just $b(x_1 - x_0)$. Here, of course, the Odds Ratio refers to cumulative risks over the entire interval $[0, T]$. To apply this approach to the Relative Hazard, assumed constant over time, we use $\log RH \equiv \log RH(t) = c(x_1 - x_0)$. Here we have a different slope coefficient, c, to reflect that we are now modeling the Relative Hazard rather than the Odds Ratio, although for rare diseases we would expect the coefficients and models to be very similar due to Equation 4.6. Restating this expression for the Relative Hazard in terms of the hazard function then gives

$$h(t|X = x) = h(t|X = 0)e^{cx} \equiv h_0(t)e^{cx},$$

or, equivalently,

$$\log[h(t|X = x)] = \log h_0(t) + cx.$$

Here $h(t|X = x)$ denotes the hazard function at time t for the subpopulation whose exposure level is $X = x$. This model is often referred to as the *Cox model* (Cox, 1972). The function $h_0(t)$ is known as the *baseline hazard* function because it describes the hazard function for the "baseline" level of exposure $X = 0$. The coefficient c is formally interpreted as the log Relative Hazard associated with a unit increase in the level of X. For example, if $c > 0$, then e^c measures the relative increase in hazard, *at all times* t, when comparing two levels of exposure, X, that differ by one unit on the X scale. On the other hand, if $c = 0$, then all exposure levels have identical hazard functions over the interval of risk. Often the Cox model is described as the *proportional hazards model*, since the hazard functions for different exposure groups are necessarily proportional. However, this assumption can easily be relaxed in the Cox model, as we note in Section 17.5.1.

Just as in logistic regression, we can extend the Cox model to simultaneously allow for the effects of multiple risk factors as follows:

$$\log[h(t|X_1 = x_1, \ldots, X_k = x_k)] = \log h_0(t) + c_1 x_1 + \cdots + c_k x_k. \qquad (17.1)$$

Now the baseline hazard function $h_0(t)$ is the hazard function when $X_1 = \cdots = X_k = 0$, and the coefficient c_j is the log Relative Hazard associated with a unit increase in X_j, holding the other risk factors, $X_i : i \neq j$, in the model fixed. The issues of confounding, interactive effects and ordered and unordered categorical exposures are all addressed in the same way as with logistic regression. Estimates of the coefficients $c_1, \ldots, c_k$ can be obtained by maximizing a modified kind of likelihood function (the so-called *partial likelihood*) that avoids estimation of the arbitrary baseline hazard

Table 17.1 *Coding for variables used in logistic and Cox regression models for the Western Collaborative Group Study*

$$X_1 = \begin{cases} 1 \text{ age is between 50 and 59 years} \\ 0 \text{ age is between 39 and 49 years} \end{cases}$$

$$X_2 = \begin{cases} 1 \text{ systolic blood pressure} \geq 126 \text{ mmHg} \\ 0 \text{ systolic blood pressure} < 126 \text{ mmHg} \end{cases}$$

$$X_3 = \begin{cases} 1 \text{ behavior type A} \\ 0 \text{ behavior type B} \end{cases}$$

$$X_4 = \begin{cases} 1 \text{ blood cholesterol} \geq 223 \text{ mg/100 ml} \\ 0 \text{ blood cholesterol} < 223 \text{ mg/100 ml} \end{cases}$$

$$X_5 = \begin{cases} 1 \text{ smoker} \\ 0 \text{ nonsmoker} \end{cases}$$

function $h_0(t)$ in Equation 17.1; this technique yields all the various tools associated with maximum likelihood we learned for logistic regression, including standard deviations of the coefficient estimates and Wald, score, and likelihood ratio tests. The approach used here is very closely related to the conditional likelihood strategy for matched data in Chapter 16. In fact, it is helpful to look at incidence time data as a form of stratified or matched data, where the matching variable is "time at risk" (see Section 17.4). Further, the modified likelihood can be shown to be appropriate under various forms of case-control sampling appropriate for data collected in time over the risk interval (see, for example, Chapter 5.4.1).

As already noted, if the outcome D is rare, we would expect little difference in the regression coefficients between a logistic regression model based on certain risk factors and the corresponding Cox model with the same factors, assuming proportional hazards. We illustrate this by comparing the logistic regression and Cox models for a set of simple covariates, applied to data from the Western Collaborative Group Study. Codings for the variables are given in Table 17.1. The fitted models for the two approaches are given in Table 17.2.

Note the close similarity between the estimated Odds Ratios and Relative Hazards associated with each variable in the model. The estimated standard deviations of the estimated coefficients are also so similar that the Wald test statistics for the association of any specific risk factor with CHD incidence, in the presence of the other variables, yield essentially the same p-values. Finally, we note that the likelihood ratio test statistic associated with fitting all five variables as opposed to none (the constant risk model) is 161.3 for the logistic regression model and 165.6 for the Cox model. Both are comparable to a χ^2 distribution with 5 degrees of freedom, under the null hypothesis that none of the five putative risk factors is associated with incidence of CHD. Again, the two approaches give essentially identical results.

Will the logistic regression and Cox models ever yield different results? That is, under what conditions will an incidence time analysis, assuming proportional hazards, present a different picture of the effects of risk factors than analysis of cumulative

Table 17.2 *Logistic regression and Cox models for the Western Collaborative Group Study*

Variable	Logistic Regression Model					
	Parameter	Estimate	SD	OR	Wald Statistic	p-Value
Intercept	a	−4.402	0.206			
Age	b	0.539	0.137	1.714	3.934	0.0001
Systolic blood pressure	c	0.730	0.147	2.075	4.966	<0.0001
Behavior type	d	0.760	0.143	2.138	5.315	<0.0001
Cholesterol	e	0.952	0.150	2.591	6.347	<0.0001
Smoking	f	0.555	0.137	1.742	4.051	0.0001

Note: Logistic regression model: $\log\left(\frac{p}{1-p}\right) = a + bX_1 + cX_2 + dX_3 + eX_4 + fX_5$.

Variable	Cox Model					
	Parameter	Estimate	SD	RH	Wald Statistic	p-Value
Age	g	0.529	0.127	1.697	4.165	<0.0001
Systolic blood pressure	h	0.677	0.139	1.968	4.871	<0.0001
Behavior type	i	0.735	0.136	2.085	5.404	<0.0001
Cholesterol	j	0.915	0.143	2.497	6.399	<0.0001
Smoking	k	0.532	0.129	1.702	4.124	<0.0001

Note: Cox regression model: $\log(h(t)) = \log(h_0(t)) + gX_1 + hX_2 + iX_3 + jX_4 + kX_5$.

incidence data? After all, accumulation of the exact time of incident events—the times of CHD events in the Western Collaborative Group Study—tends to be substantially more costly than collection of cumulative incidence at the end of a study. Leaving aside the issue of whether continuous follow-up information on events is less likely to suffer from misclassification of outcomes, one advantage of the Cox model is that it allows estimation of the baseline hazard function, $h_0(t)$, in addition to Relative Hazard coefficients, thereby providing insight into how the hazard evolves over time for any exposure group. However, even this estimate is not available for case-control sampling and the extra information hardly seems worth the additional cost. With this point of view, the Cox model does not seem worth the bother. Nevertheless, there are scenarios where allowing for time in the analysis makes all the difference, and in the next section we discuss when and why the two models might yield different results.

17.4 Fitting the Cox regression model

As already indicated, the Cox regression model can be fit to data via a modification of the maximum likelihood technique. Without describing this procedure in full technical detail, we shall see how the approach differs from logistic regression for the simple case of a binary exposure. We illustrate the ideas using data from the Western Collaborative Group Study.

Suppose we choose the binary exposure variable, smoking (see Table 17.1), to investigate its relationship to incidence of CHD. For each observed time of a CHD

Table 17.3 *Coronary heart disease and smoking, stratified by time at risk at observed CHD events*

Time of CHD Event (Days)			CHD Event Yes	CHD Event No
18	Smoking	Yes	1	1501
		No	0	1652
21	Smoking	Yes	1	1500
		No	0	1652
22	Smoking	Yes	0	1500
		No	1	1651
...	...	...	...	...
3122	Smoking	Yes	1	125
		No	0	136
3229	Smoking	Yes	0	20
		No	1	26

event, we can construct a 2 × 2 table for individuals based on their smoking status with outcome variable being whether or not they experienced a CHD event *at that particular time*. For example, Table 17.3 lists a few of these tables; in the data set, the earliest time from enrollment to a CHD event was 18 days. Table 17.3 shows that a single individual, a smoker, experienced a CHD event at that particular time since enrollment, and a further 3153 individuals (= 1501 smokers +1652 nonsmokers), at risk on day 18, did not experience such an event. This accounts for all 3154 individuals in the original sample. The next smallest time was at 21 days, when again a smoker suffered a CHD event, while 3152 other individuals at risk did not. Note that the sample size for this 2 × 2 table is now 3153, since the individual who experienced the event at 18 days has been removed from the "at risk" population entering day 21. Table 17.3 also displays the 2 × 2 tables for the longest event times: at day 3122 there were 262 individuals still at risk, of whom 1 smoker experienced a CHD event. All individuals from the original sample who had either experienced a CHD event earlier or who had ceased follow-up prior to day 3122 are now excluded from this 2 × 2 table; only 47 individuals remain at risk entering day 3229, at which time 1 nonsmoker experienced a CHD event. Note the drop of 215 in sample sizes between these two "final" 2 × 2 tables, from 262 at day 3122 to 47 at day 3229; one of these 215 was no longer at risk at day 3229 because they had the CHD event at day 3122, but the other 214 individuals ceased follow-up at some time between 3122 and 3229 days from enrollment.

The complete version of Table 17.3 lists a series of 248 2 × 2 tables, each of which provides a piece of information, albeit small, regarding the association of smoking status and the risk of a CHD event (of the 257 observed CHD event times, 9 are days on which exactly 2 events occurred). To combine these 2 × 2 tables for assessing this association, we use the Cochran–Mantel–Haenszel test statistic of Chapter 9.1.1.

Although it appears at first glance that the data in these tables may not be independent, since most individuals appear in many tables at different risk times, the absence of any assumed structure in the baseline hazard function of the proportional hazards model (Equation 17.1) allows for use of the Cochran–Mantel–Haenszel procedure. Further, the proportional hazards assumption shows that the relative hazard, and thus approximately the Odds Ratio, stays constant over the 2×2 tables defined by time at risk, thus providing the "no interaction" assumption necessary for effective use of the Cochran–Mantel–Haenszel test.

The Cochran–Mantel–Haenszel procedure, applied to time-to-event data in the manner described, is known as the *log rank* test and is widely used in the analysis of clinical trials in addition to epidemiologic studies. The method accommodates the possibility of differing follow-up periods: those with short follow-up only contribute information to the "early" 2×2 tables, whereas individuals with long follow-up will appear in most of the 2×2 tables until the time they drop out or experience a CHD event. This approach, however, assumes that factors that determine when follow-up ends (i.e., dropping out) do not affect the risk of suffering CHD. In particular, the log rank test is inappropriate if some individuals tend to be lost to follow-up because they begin to experience CHD disease and thereby have a higher risk of a subsequent CHD event than others who have been followed for a similar length of time, but are not lost to follow-up.

In the Western Collaborative Group Study, the log rank test for the data outlined in Table 17.3 yields a test statistic of 23.76. As for the Cochran–Mantel–Haenszel test, comparison of this value to tables of the χ^2 distribution with 1 degree of freedom provides evaluation of the null hypothesis that smoking is unrelated to the hazard or risk of CHD events. In this case, the p-value is approximately 10^{-6}. For comparison, the square of the Wald statistic derived from fitting a Cox model with only this measure of smoking is 23.02; the likelihood ratio test statistic comparing this to a model with no risk factors is 23.81. Both test statistics yield very similar results to the log rank test. On the other hand, the χ^2 test statistic of Chapter 6, which ignores the time of CHD events and the issue of loss to follow-up, is 22.76.

17.5 When does time at risk confound an exposure–disease relationship?

In the log rank test, stratification by time at risk illustrates the essential difference between the approaches of the Cox model and the logistic regression model of Chapters 13 to 15. Namely, the proportional hazards model controls for the effect of time at risk, prior to consideration of the association between the risk factors and the outcome, assuming no interaction between time at risk and these factors (the proportional hazards assumption). Loosely speaking, the proportional hazards model allows for the potential confounding effects of time at risk whereas the logistic regression model does not. If there is no such confounding, the two approaches can be expected to yield similar results, as illustrated in Table 17.2 for the Western Collaborative Group Study with a simple set of covariates.

By the same token, we anticipate different results when time at risk does confound an exposure of interest. Thus, to appreciate situations where logistic regression and the Cox model provide differing fits, we merely need to understand when time at risk is a confounding variable. In the simplest case, the conditions of Chapter 8.1.2 show that in order for confounding to occur, it is necessary that (1) time at risk be causally associated with outcome risk, and that (2) time at risk be associated with exposure. In almost all epidemiological settings, we expect the first of these conditions to hold. In short, how long an individual has been at risk usually affects the probability that the outcome will soon occur; in fact, the outcome risk most often, although not always, increases with time of risk. In fact, the only case where this situation does not hold is when time at risk is unrelated to the hazard (that is, the hazard function is constant). Thus, the presence of confounding by time at risk hinges on the second condition, association with exposure.

17.5.1 Time-dependent exposures

With exposures that are measured at enrollment and remain constant in time, it appears as though there can be no association between subsequent time at risk and exposure, so that time at risk confounding cannot occur. On the other hand, if exposure levels change throughout the risk period, then by definition there will likely be association between time at risk and exposure, and time at risk confounding will occur. With such time-dependent risk factors, we thus expect to see different results from logistic regression and proportional hazards models. In fact, there is no immediate way that the logistic regression model can accommodate time-varying exposures, whereas it is straightforward to allow this phenomenon when fitting the Cox model. To see this, consider the stratification by time at risk described in the previous section; there is no requirement that individuals stay in the same exposure group from one 2×2 table to another. In sum, a time at risk model, such as the Cox model, is required when exposure levels change over time. Further, incorporation of time into the covariates of the Cox model allows us to relax the assumption of proportional hazards considerably. For example, consider the simple model

$$\log[h(t|X = x)] = \log h_0(t) + cx + d(x \times t),$$

which extends Equation 17.1 to allow for time-dependent explanatory variables, here a simple constructed variable, $x \times t$, capturing exposure effect modification by time. In this model, the log Relative Hazard associated with a unit increase in X is given by $c + dt$, and thus can either decrease ($d < 0$) or increase ($d > 0$) as time evolves. For this version of the model, strict proportional hazards across two exposure groups no longer holds. For an introduction to the use of time-dependent risk factors in the Cox model, see Fisher and Lin (1999).

17.5.2 Differential loss to follow-up

Even when exposure levels remain fixed over time, as in our previous analyses of the Western Collaborative Group Study where we only examine baseline measures, it is possible that an association with time at risk can be induced indirectly. One such

Table 17.4 *Differential loss to follow-up*

		First Risk Period	Second Risk Period
Without loss to follow-up	E	100	100
	$\bar{E}$	100	100
With loss to follow-up	E	100	75
	$\bar{E}$	100	100

scenario arises from *differential loss to follow-up*. This occurs when the probability of being lost to follow-up over time varies by exposure level (when logistic regression models are used, this appears as differential misclassification of the outcome).

We illustrate this schematically by considering a hypothetical example where the outcome is CHD and the risk factor, E, is smoking status. To avoid changes in the risk set sizes due to occurrence of CHD, we allow for individuals who experience a CHD event to be replaced, at that time, by a newly sampled individual with an identical exposure level. With no loss to follow-up, the exposure groups stay the same size over time. For example, Table 17.4 describes this phenomenon when there are two major risk periods; in the first "risk period" there are 100 at risk with E and 100 at risk without E. With no loss to follow-up, these numbers remain the same in the second, later risk period. On the other hand, we now consider the possibility of loss to follow-up; simplistically, suppose as before that at the beginning of the first "risk period" there are 100 at risk with E and 100 at risk without E. However, by the beginning of the second risk period, while there are still 100 at risk without E, there are now only 75 at risk with E, because 25 individuals in this group have died from smoking-related disease other than CHD (and hence are lost to follow-up). Table 17.4 clearly shows that while there is no association between E and time at risk with no loss to follow-up, an association is created by differential loss to follow-up.

17.6 Comments and further reading

The original paper that introduced the Cox model (Cox, 1972) is one of the most widely cited articles in the scientific literature, reflecting the many areas of application where event time investigations are important. However, the Cox model is but one possibility in studying the relationship between the hazard function and risk factors, and other choices can be found in many introductions to the broad topic of *survival analysis*; see, for example, Kalbfleisch and Prentice (2002), Hosmer and Lemeshow (1999), and Collett (1994). In particular, both generalized additive models and tree-based methods can be applied to follow-up data with event times known (Hastie and Tibshirani, 1990; LeBlanc and Crowley, 1995; Segal, 1995). Carmelli et al. (1991; 1997) illustrate application of classification trees to survival data arising from further follow-up of the Western Collaborative Group Study. Note that the Cox model is well suited to handle case-control studies with risk-set sampling (Chapter 5.4.1), since the data are already "stratified" on time in the analysis, as discussed earlier in this chapter. It thus provides an alternative to the use of a logistic regression model for such data, previously discussed in Chapter 16.7; the two approaches tend to give very similar results. Prentice (1986) considers application of the Cox model to case-cohort data.

A principal advantage of time-based models is their ability to address exposures that themselves change over time (Section 17.5.1). All but a few exposures in epidemiological studies have the potential for variation over time, and our treatment of them as fixed must, at best, be considered a proxy for more subtle behavior. Further, longitudinal data that capture such time variation in key risk factors and their confounders have far greater potential of unraveling causal effects than studies with only a single measurement of these variables. However, when both risk factors and confounders are time-dependent, the issues of confounding in Chapter 8 become significantly more delicate. This is particularly true when such confounders are *endogeneous* variables measured on an individual that have the property that they can be affected by other risk variables (in contrast, an *exogeneous* time-dependent variable, like air pollution counts, presumably cannot be changed by other individual factors). Causal graphs of longitudinal variables now require their consideration at different points in time, as in the simple example illustrated in Figure 8.3(b). As another example, in the Western Collaborative Group Study, serum cholesterol could have been measured over time, rather than just at baseline. We have already considered the possibility that this variable might confound the role of behavior type, perhaps due to a common (unmeasured) source variable that causes both factors, suggesting the need for adjustment in estimation of the effect of behavior type. On the other hand, over time, behavior type may directly affect serum cholesterol levels; in particular, Type A individuals may aggressively seek treatment for high cholesterol and take advantage of cholesterol-reducing medication. This "aspect" of serum cholesterol is therefore on the pathway between behavior type and disease, indicating that it should not be controlled in the analysis. This contradiction—adjust and do not adjust for cholesterol—is an indication of the failure of stratification to accommodate confounding that itself is time-varying (Robins, 1989; Jewell and Hubbard, to appear). Fortunately, there has been substantial recent progress on alternative analysis techniques that, with the appropriate *longitudinal* data, appropriately control for time-dependent confounding; see Robins (1997), van der Laan and Robins (2002), and Jewell and Hubbard (to appear).

17.7 Problems

Question 17.1

The data set *wcgs*, found by going to http://www.crcpress.com/e_products/downloads/, contains information on the length of time until CHD incidence or the end of follow-up for each individual. Use this information and the log rank test to investigate the association between behavior type and the hazard for CHD, accounting for the time at risk.

Question 17.2

Table 17.2 gives the results of fitting a Cox model to the Western Collaborative Group Study data, using binary versions of five risk factors: age, systolic blood pressure, behavior type, cholesterol, and smoking. Fit a similar Cox model using the continuous versions of these variables, where appropriate, as recorded in the data set *wcgs*. Interpret your results and compare the findings to those reported in Table 17.2.

Question 17.3

Still using the data set *wcgs*, consider a time-dependent risk factor defined by multiplying behavior type by time at risk. Fit a Cox model that includes this variable along with the original behavior type to examine whether the Relative Hazard for CHD, associated with behavior type, changes monotonically over time. Carry out a similar analysis using baseline smoking as a risk factor instead of behavior type. Interpret the results from both analyses.

CHAPTER 18

Epilogue: The Examples

In all examples discussed in the book, we have focused on statistical estimation of a variety of measures of association and regression models. It is crucial to interpret these results in the context of the details of the study and current epidemiological understanding of the disease and exposures. For two of the main case studies, the Western Collaborative Group Study and the study of coffee drinking and pancreatic cancer, we take these last few words to draw attention to further findings.

As previously indicated when we introduced the Western Collaborative Group Study, the original CHD incidence data were based on an average of about 9.5 years of follow-up after recruitment. Enrolled individuals were subsequently followed well beyond the original time frame of the study. Ragland and Brand (1988) discuss data on heart disease *mortality* after about 22 years of follow-up, finding little association between behavior type and heart disease mortality. This anomalous result, as compared with the observed association with CHD incidence, may be due in part to the possibility that Type A behavior type is associated with a better prognosis after a CHD event as compared with Type B individuals. In other words, the very characteristic that might increase the risk of a CHD event may, in turn, be linked with a greater chance of a more successful recovery! Carmelli et al. (1991, 1997) study even longer follow-up information on both heart disease and cancer mortality using classification trees.

The findings of MacMahon et al. (1981) on coffee drinking and incidence of pancreatic cancer were controversial almost from the moment they appeared. To say that reaction was intense would be an understatement, and the report warranted editorial comment from *The New York Times*, in part because of the fact that coffee drinking is so ubiquitous. Cases were defined to be all incident pancreatic cancers, with minor restrictions, that occurred in Boston and Rhode Island hospitals over a 5-year period. Controls were sampled from the patient populations of the physicians treating the cases, excluding any patients who suffered from smoking and alcohol-related diseases. There was substantial criticism of the choice of controls, in that if an individual who smokes and drinks heavily also tends to drink coffee, the controls would be less likely to be coffee drinkers than individuals in the Target Population from which cases were drawn, whether or not there is a relation between coffee consumption and pancreatic cancer. Selection bias might then underly the apparent association between coffee and pancreatic cancer incidence, and perhaps explain the lack of a strong dose-response effect, noted in Chapters 11 and 13. The authors argued against such selection bias in that the restrictions merely excluded individuals who would have been overrepresented otherwise. Additional concern was raised by the inclusion of individuals with gastroenterologic conditions in the controls, people who might drink less coffee because of their medical condition. The study attempted to avoid this phenomenon in both cases and controls by asking about coffee consumption habits prior to their disease, but differential recall remained a possibility. Other selection issues focused on the differential level of nonresponse and possible error due to interviewer bias. This debate was carried out in a series of letters in *The New England Journal of Medicine* ("Coffee and Cancer of the Pancreas," 1981, Vol. 304, 1604–1606; "More on Coffee and Pancreatic Cancer," 1987, Vol. 316, 483–484). An interesting aside is that all the publicity that the putative link received in the media did not appear to make any appreciable difference in the public's coffee consumption (Samet et al., 1982), at least in the short term.

The 1981 study motivated a number of subsequent investigations that tried to reproduce the original finding. Although a few investigations reported a weak association, most were unsuccessful; in fact, the same authors (with C. C. Hsieh) described their own negative attempt at confirmation (Hsieh et al., 1986). Some other studies did display a weak association in a variety of circumstances, suggesting that it is impossible to "completely exonerate coffee" (see second reference in the last paragraph). Overall, there now appears to be little convincing evidence that coffee consumption is related to the risk of pancreatic cancer (Tavani and La Vecchia, 2000).

There has been remarkably little follow-up to the study of Winkelstein et al. (1958) on the link between hormonal or pregnancy factors and the incidence of CHD in women. A confirmatory study was soon implemented (Winkelstein and Rekate, 1964) and several investigations have established that women with early bilateral oophorectomy have greater risk of CHD (Stampfer et al., 1990). Given the relative frequency of spontaneous abortions, Winkelstein (1995) continues to recommend further examination of the role of this risk factor in heart disease.

Perhaps these case studies illustrate the obvious, that with observational studies, "it ain't over 'til it's over." The recent controversy surrounding results from the Women's Health Initiative, a randomized trial that gives insight into the role of hormone replacement therapy in incidence of heart disease and breast cancer, has renewed the debate about the value and interpretation of observational studies vis-à-vis randomized trials. Several thoughtful commentaries on this topic are in the January 2003 issue of *Epidemiology*. What is certain is that while no amount of creative statistical arguments can rescue either a seriously flawed study or highly inaccurate data, careful application of the ideas covered in this book provides substantial insight from epidemiological studies and helps avoid both glaring and subtle dangers that face all of us who are engaged in unraveling the mysteries of human diseases.

References

Andrieu, N., Goldstein, A.M., Thomas, D.C., and Langholz, B. (2001). Counter-matching in studies of gene-environment interaction: Efficiency and feasibility. *American Journal of Epidemiology* 153, 265–274.

Armitage, P. (1955). Tests for linear trends in proportions and frequencies. *Biometrics* 11, 375–386.

Armstrong, B.K., White, E., and Saracci, R. (1994). *Principles of Exposure Measurement in Epidemiology*. New York: Oxford University Press.

Arnold, C., McLean, F.H., Kramer, M.S., and Usher, R.H. (1987). Respiratory distress syndrome in second-born versus first-born twins. *New England Journal of Medicine* 317, 1121–1125.

Ascher, M.S., Sheppard, H.W., Winkelstein, W., Jr., and Vittinghoff, E. (1993). Does drug use cause AIDS? *Nature* 362, 103–104.

Begg, C. (2001). The search for cancer risk factors: When can we stop looking? *American Journal of Public Health* 91, 360–364.

Berger, J. and Sellke, T. (1987). Testing a point null hypothesis: The irreconcilability of P-values and evidence. *Journal of the American Statistical Association* 82, 112–139.

Berkson, J. (1946). Limitation of the application of fourfold tables to hospital data. *Biometrics Bulletin* 2, 47–53.

Breslow, N.E. and Day, N.E. (1980). *Statistical Methods in Cancer Research. 1: The Analysis of Case-control Studies*. Lyon: I.A.R.C.

Breslow, N.E. and Day, N.E. (1987). *Statistical Methods in Cancer Research. 2: The Design and Analysis of Cohort Studies*. Lyon: I.A.R.C.

Carmelli, D., Halpern, J., Swan, G.E., Dame, A., McElroy, M., Gelb, A.B., and Rosenman, R.H. (1991). 27-year mortality in the Western Collaborative Group Study: Construction of risk groups by recursive partitioning. *Journal of Clinical Epidemiology* 44, 1341–1351.

Carmelli, D., Zhang, H., and Swan, G.E. (1997). Obesity and 33-year follow-up for coronary heart disease and cancer mortality. *Epidemiology* 8, 378–383.

Carroll, R.J. (1998). Measurement error in epidemiologic studies. In *Encyclopedia of Biostatistics*. Editors-in-Chief: Armitage, P. and Colton, T. New York: John Wiley & Sons.

Carroll, R.J., Kuchenhoff, H., Lombard, F., and Stefanski, L.A. (1996). Asymptotics for the SIMEX method in structural measurement error models. *Journal of the American Statistical Association* 91, 242–250.

Carroll, R.J., Ruppert, D., and Stefanski, L.A. (1995). *Measurement Error in Nonlinear Models*. London: Chapman & Hall.

Clayton, D. and Hills, M. (1993). *Statistical Models in Epidemiology*. New York: Oxford University Press.

Cochran, W.G. (1954). Some methods for strengthening the common χ^2 tests. *Biometrics* 10, 417–451.

Colditz, G.A., Rosner, B.A., and Speizer, F.E. (1996). Risk factors for breast cancer according to family history of breast cancer. *Journal of the National Cancer Institute* 88, 365–371.

Cole, S. and Hernán, M.Á. (2002). Fallibility in estimating direct effects. *International Journal of Epidemiology* 31, 163–165.

Collett, D. (1994). *Modelling Survival Data in Medical Research*. London: Chapman & Hall.

Collett, D. (2002). *Modelling Binary Data*. Second Edition. London: Chapman & Hall.

Collings, B.J., Margolin, B.H., and Oehlert, G.W. (1981). Analyses for binomial data, with application to the fluctuation test for mutagenicity. *Biometrics* 37, 775–794.

Cook, J. and Stefanski, L.A. (1995). A simulation extrapolation method for parametric measurement error models. *Journal of the American Statistical Association* 89, 1314–1328.

Cornfield, J. (1951). A method of estimating comparative rates from clinical data. Applications to cancer of the lung, breast and cervix. *Journal of the National Cancer Institute* 11, 1269–1275.

Cox, D.R. (1972). Regression models and life tables (with discussion). *Journal of the Royal Statistical Society B* 34, 187–220.

D'Agostino, R.B., Chase, W., and Belanger, A. (1988). The appropriateness of some common procedures for testing the equality of two independent binomial populations. *American Statistician* 42, 198–202.

Diggle, P., Heagerty, P., Liang, K.-Y., and Zeger, S. (2002). *Analysis of Longitudinal Data*. Second Edition. New York: Oxford University Press.

Dobson, A.J. (2001). *An Introduction to Generalized Linear Models*. Second Edition. London: Chapman & Hall.

Dodge, Y. (1985). *Analysis of Experiments with Missing Data*. New York: John Wiley & Sons.

Dole, N., Savitz, D.A., Hertz-Picciotto, I., Siega-Riz, A.M., McMahon, M.J., and Buekens, P. (2003). Maternal stress and preterm birth. *American Journal of Epidemiology* 157, 14–24.

Dosemeci, M., Wacholder, S., and Lubin, J.H. (1990). Does non-differential misclassification of exposure always bias a true effect towards the null value? *American Journal of Epidemiology* 132, 746–748.

Dupont, W.D. and Page, D.L. (1985). Risk factors for breast cancer in women with proliferative breast disease. *New England Journal of Medicine* 312, 146–151.

Easton, D.F., Peto, J., and Babiker, A.G. (1991). Floating absolute risk: An alternative to relative risk in survival and case-control analysis avoiding an arbitrary reference group. *Statistics in Medicine* 10, 1025–1035.

Edson, M. (1999). *W;t: a Play*. New York: Farrar, Straus & Giroux.

Efron, B. and Tibshirani, R.J. (1993). *An Introduction to the Bootstrap*. London: Chapman & Hall.

Feychting, M., Forssen, U., and Floderus, B. (1997). Occupational and residential magnetic field exposure and leukemia and central nervous system tumors. *Epidemiology* 8, 384–389.

Fisher, L.D. and Lin, D.Y. (1999). Time-dependent covariates in the Cox proportional hazards model. *Annual Review in Public Health* 20, 145–157.

Fisher, R.A. (1932). *Statistical Methods for Research Workers*. Edinburgh: Oliver & Boyd (13th, 1958).

Fleiss, J.L. (1981). *Statistical Methods for Rates and Proportions*. Second Edition. New York: John Wiley & Sons.

Forastiere, F., Goldsmith, D.F., Sperati, A., Rapiti, E., Miceli, M., Cavariani, F., and Perucci, C.A. (2002). Silicosis and lung function decrements among female ceramic workers in Italy. *American Journal of Epidemiology* 156, 851–856.

Friedman, G.D., Kannel, W.B., Dawber, T.R., and McNamara, P.M. (1966). Comparison of prevalence, case history, and incidence data in assessing the potency of risk factors in coronary heart disease. *American Journal of Epidemiology* 83, 366–377.

Gart, J.J. (1976). Letter: Contingency tables. *The American Statistician* 30, 204.

Goodman, S.N. (1993). P-values, hypothesis tests and likelihood: Implications for epidemiology of a neglected historical debate (with commentary and response). *American Journal of Epidemiology* 137, 485–496.

Goodman, S.N. and Royall, R. (1988). Evidence and scientific research. *American Journal of Public Health* 78, 1568–1574.

Greenland, S. (1986). Adjustment of risk ratios in case-base studies (hybrid epidemiologic designs). *Statistics in Medicine* 5, 579–584.

Greenland, S. (1988). On sample-size and power calculations for studies using confidence intervals. *American Journal of Epidemiology* 128, 231–237.

Greenland, S. (1994). Alternative models for ordinal logistic regression. *Statistics in Medicine* 13, 1665–1677.

Greenland, S. (1995). Avoiding power loss associated with categorization and ordinal scores in dose-response and trend analysis. *Epidemiology* 6, 450–454.

Greenland, S. (2000). An introduction to instrumental variables for epidemiologists. *International Journal of Epidemiology* 29, 722–729.

Greenland, S. and Brumback, B. (2002). An overview of relations among causal modelling methods. *International Journal of Epidemiology* 31, 1030–1037.

Greenland, S. and Finkle, W.D. (1995). A critical look at methods for handling missing covariates in epidemiologic regression analysis. *American Journal of Epidemiology* 142, 1255–1264.

Greenland, S. and Kleinbaum, D.G. (1983). Correcting for misclassification in two-way tables and matched-pair studies. *International Journal of Epidemiology* 12, 93–97.

Greenland, S. and Morgenstern, H. (2001). Confounding in health research. *Annual Review of Public Health* 22, 189–212.

Greenland, S., Pearl, J., and Robins, J.M. (1999). Causal diagrams for epidemiologic research. *Epidemiology* 10, 37–48.

Greenland, S. and Thomas, D.C. (1982). On the need for the rare disease assumption in case-control studies. *American Journal of Epidemiology* 116, 547–553.

Halloran, M.E. and Struchiner, C.J. (1995). Causal inference for infectious diseases. *Epidemiology* 6, 145–151.

Hastie, T. and Tibshirani, R. (1990). *Generalized Additive Models*. New York: Chapman & Hall.

Helms, M., Vastrup, P., Gerner-Smidt, P., and Mølbak, K. (2003). Short and long term mortality associated with foodborne gastrointestinal infections: Registry based study. *British Medical Journal* 326, 357–360.

Herman, B., Schmitz, P.I.M., Leyten, A.C.M., van Luijk, J.H., Frenken, C.W.G.M., op de Coul, A.A.W, and Schulte, B.P.M. (2003). Multivariate logistic analysis of risk factors for stroke in Tilburg, the Netherlands. *American Journal of Epidemiology* 118, 514–525.

Hirji, K.F., Mehta, C.R., and Patel, N.R. (1987) Computing distributions for exact logistic regression. *Journal of the American Statistical Association* 82, 1110–1117.

Hosmer, D.W., Hosmer, T., Lee Cessie, S., and Lemeshow, S. (1997). A comparison of goodness-of-fit tests for the logistic regression model. *Statistics in Medicine* 16, 965–980.

Hosmer, D.W. and Lemeshow, S. (1999). *Applied Survival Analysis: Regression Modeling of Time to Event Data*. New York: John Wiley & Sons.

Hosmer, D.W. and Lemeshow, S. (2000). *Applied Logistic Regression*. Second Edition. New York: John Wiley & Sons.

Hsieh, C.C., MacMahon, B., Yen, S., Trichopoulos, D., Warren, K., and Nardi, G. (1986). Coffee and pancreatic cancer (chapter 2). *New England Journal of Medicine* 315, 587–589.

Jewell, N.P. (1984). Small sample bias of point estimators of the odds ratio from matched sets. *Biometrics* 40, 421–435.

Jewell, N.P. (1986). On the bias of commonly used measures of association for 2 × 2 tables. *Biometrics* 42, 351–358.

Jewell, N.P. and Hubbard, A. *Analysis of Longitudinal Studies in Epidemiology*. To appear.

Jewell, N.P. and Shiboski, S. (1990). Statistical analysis of HIV infectivity based on partner studies. *Biometrics* 46, 1133–1150.

Johnson, S.K. and Johnson, R.E. (1972). Tonsillectomy history in Hodgkin's disease. *New England Journal of Medicine* 287, 1122–1125.

Kalbfleisch, J.D. and Prentice, R.L. (2002). *The Statistical Analysis of Failure Time Data*. Second Edition. New York: John Wiley & Sons.

Kalish, L.A. (1990). Reducing mean squared error in the analysis of pair-matched case-control studies. *Biometrics* 46, 493–499.

Karon, J.M. and Kupper, L.L. (1982). In defense of matching. *American Journal of Epidemiology* 116, 852–866.

Kleinbaum, D.G., Kupper, L.L., and Morgenstern, H. (1982). *Epidemiologic Research*. New York: Van Nostrand Reinhold.

Kupper, L.L., Karon, J.M., Kleinbaum, D.G., Morgenstern, H., and Lewis, D.K. (1981). Matching in epidemiologic studies: Validity and efficiency considerations. *Biometrics* 37, 293–302.

Lagakos, S.W. (1988). Effects of mismodeling and mismeasuring explanatory variables on tests of their association with a response variable. *Statistics in Medicine* 7, 257–274.

Lane-Claypon, J.E. (1926). A Further Report on Cancer of the Breast. Reports on Public Health and Medical Subjects 32. London: Her Majesty's Stationery Office.

Langholz, B. and Borgan, Ø. (1995). Counter-matching: A stratified nested case-control sampling method. *Biometrika* 82, 69–79.

Langholz, B. and Clayton, D. (1994). Sampling strategies in nested case-control studies. *Environmental Health Perspectives—Supplement* 102, 47–51.

Langholz, B. and Goldstein, L. (1996). Risk set sampling in epidemiologic cohort studies. *Statistical Science* 11, 35–53.

Larntz, K. (1978). Small-sample comparisons of exact levels for chi-squared goodness-of-fit statistics. *Journal of the American Statistical Association* 73, 253–263.

LeBlanc, M. and Crowley, J. (1995). A review of tree-based prognostic models. In *Recent Advances in Clinical Trial Design and Analysis*. Editor: Thall, P.F. New York: Kluwer, 113–124.

Lehtinen, M., Koskela, P., Jellum, E., Bloigu, A., Anttila, T., Hallmans, G., Luukkaala, T., Thoresen, S. Youngman, L., Dillner, J., and Hakama, M. (2002). Herpes simplex virus and risk of cervical cancer: A longitudinal, nested case-control study in the Nordic countries. *American Journal of Epidemiology* 156, 687–692.

Levy, P.S. and Lemeshow, S. (1999). *Sampling of Populations: Methods and Applications*. Third Edition. New York: John Wiley & Sons.

Liang, K.-Y. and Zeger, S. (1988). On the use of concordant pairs in matched case-control studies. *Biometrics* 44, 1145–1156.

Liu, G. (2000). Sample size for epidemiologic studies. In *Encyclopedia of Epidemiologic Methods*. Editors: Gail, M.H. and Benichou, J. New York: John Wiley & Sons.

Long, W.L., Griffith, J.L., Selker, H.P., and D'Agostino, R.B. (1993). A comparison of logistic regression to decision tree induction in medical domain. *Computers and Biomedical Research* 26, 74–97.

Lotufo, P.A., Chae, C.U., Ajani, U.A., Hennekens, C.H., and Manson, J.E. (2000). Male pattern baldness and coronary heart disease. The Physicians' Health Study. *Archives of Internal Medicine* 160, 165–171.

MacMahon, B., Yen, S., Trichopoulos, D., Warren, K., and Nardi, G. (1981). Coffee and cancer of the pancreas. *New England Journal of Medicine* 304, 630–633 and 1604–1606.

MacMahon, S., Peto, R., Cutler, J., Collins, R., Sorlie, P., Neaton, J., Abbott, R., Godwin, J., Dyer, A., and Stamler, J. (1990). Blood pressure, stroke and coronary heart disease: Part 1, prolonged differences in blood pressure: Prospective observational studies corrected for the regression dilution bias. *Lancet* 335, 765–774.

Magliozzi, T., Magliozzi, R., and Berman, D. (1999). *A Haircut in Horse Town: And Other Great Car Talk Puzzlers*. New York: Perigee Books.

Mantel, N. (1977). Letter: Contingency tables—a reply. *The American Statistician* 31, 135.

Mantel, N. and Haenszel, W. (1959). Statistical aspects of the analysis of data from retrospective studies of disease. *Journal of the National Cancer Institute* 22, 719–748.

McKnight, B. (1998). Effect modification. In *Encyclopedia of Biostatistics*. Editors-in-Chief: Armitage, P. and Colton, T. New York: John Wiley & Sons.

Mehta, C.R. and Patel, N.R. (1998). Exact inference for categorical data. In *Encyclopedia of Biostatistics*. Editors-in-Chief: Armitage, P. and Colton, T. New York: John Wiley & Sons.

Mehta, C.R., Patel, N.R., and Gray, R. (1985). On computing an exact confidence interval for the common odds ratio in several 2×2 contingency tables. *Journal of the American Statistical Association* 80, 969–973.

Moore, D.S. and McCabe, G.P. (2002). *Introduction to the Practice of Statistics*. Fourth Edition. New York: W.H. Freeman & Company.

National Research Council (1986). *Environmental Tobacco Smoke. Measuring Exposures and Assessing Health Effects*. Washington, D.C.: National Academy Press.

Neuhaus, J. (1999). Bias and efficiency loss due to misclassified responses in binary regression. *Biometrika* 86, 843–855.

Newman, S.C. (2001). *Biostatistical Methods in Epidemiology*. New York: John Wiley & Sons.

Olshan, A.F., Smith, J.C., Bondy, M.L., Neglia, J.P., and Pollock, B.H. (2002). Maternal vitamin use and neuroblastoma. *Epidemiology* 13, 575–580.

Pearl, J. (1995). Causal diagrams for empirical research (with discussion). *Biometrika* 82, 669–710.

Pearl, J. (2000). *Causality*. New York: Cambridge University Press.

Perez-Padilla, R., Perez-Guzman, C., Baez-Saldana, R., and Torres-Cruz, A. (2001). Cooking with biomass stoves and tuberculosis: a case control study. *International Journal of Tuberculosis and Lung Disease* 5, 441–447.

Prentice, R.L. (1986). A case-cohort design for epidemiologic cohort studies and disease prevention trials. *Biometrika* 73, 1–11.

Prentice, R.L. and Pyke, R. (1979). Logistic disease incidence models and case-control studies. *Biometrika* 66, 403–411.

Ragland, D.R. and Brand, R.J. (1988). Coronary heart disease mortality in the WCGS: Follow-up experience of 22 years. *American Journal of Epidemiology* 127, 462–475.

Redelmeier, D. and Tibshirani, R. (1997a). The association between cellular telephone calls and motor vehicle collisions. *New England Journal of Medicine* 336, 453–458.

Redelmeier, D. and Tibshirani, R. (1997b). Interpretation and bias in case-crossover studies. *Journal of Clinical Epidemiology* 50, 1281–1287.

Redelmeier, D. and Tibshirani, R. (1997c). Is using a car phone like driving drunk? *Chance* 10, 5–9.

Roberts, R.S., Spitzer, W.O., Delmore, T., and Sackett, D.L. (1978). An empirical demonstration of Berkson's bias. *Journal of Chronic Diseases* 31, 119–128.

Robins, J.M. (1989). The control of confounding by intermediate variables. *Statistics in Medicine* 8, 679–701.

Robins, J.M. (1997). Causal inference from complex longitudinal data. In *Latent Variable Modelling with Applications to Causality.* Editor: Berkane, M. New York: Springer-Verlag, 69–117.

Robins, J.M. (2001). Data, design, and background knowledge in etiologic inference. *Epidemiology* 11, 313–320.

Robins, J.M., Breslow, N., and Greenland, S. (1986). Estimators of the Mantel–Haenszel variance consistent in both sparse data and large strata limiting models. *Biometrics* 42, 311–324.

Robins, J.M. and Greenland, S. (1992). Identifiability and exchangeability for direct and indirect effects. *Epidemiology* 3, 143–155.

Robins, J.M., Hernán, M.Á., and Brumback, B. (2000). Marginal structural models and causal inference in epidemiology. *Epidemiology* 11, 550–560.

Robins, J.M. and Rotnitzky, A. (1995). Semiparametric efficiency in multivariate regression models with missing data. *Journal of the American Statistical Association* 90, 122–129.

Robins, J.M., Rotnitzky, A., and Zhao, L.P. (1994). Estimation of regression coefficients when some regressors are not always observed. *Journal of the American Statistical Association* 89, 846–866.

Robinson, L.D. (1991). The Effects of Covariate Adjustment upon Precision for Some Common Generalized Linear Models. Ph.D. dissertation. University of California, Berkeley.

Robinson, L.D. and Jewell, N.P. (1990). Some surprising results about covariate adjustment in logistic regression models. *International Statistical Review* 58, 227–240.

Rodrigues, L. and Kirkwood, B.R. (1990). Case-control designs in the study of common diseases: Updates on the demise of the rare disease assumption and the choice of sampling scheme for controls. *International Journal of Epidemiology* 19, 205–213.

Rosenman, R.H., Brand, R.J., Jenkins, C.D., Friedman, M., Straus, R., and Wurm, M. (1975). Coronary heart disease in the Western Collaborative Group Study: Final follow-up experience of $8^1/_2$ years. *Journal of the American Medical Association* 223, 872–877.

Rosenman, R.H., Friedman, M., Straus, R., Wurm, M., Kositchek, R., and Werthessen, N.T. (1964). A predictive study of coronary heart disease: The Western Collaborative Group Study. *Journal of the American Medical Association* 189, 15–22.

Rosner, B., Spiegelman, D., and Willett, W.C. (1990). Correction of logistic regression relative risk estimates and confidence intervals for measurement error: The case of multiple covariates measured with error. *American Journal of Epidemiology* 132, 734–745.

Rosner, B., Willett, W.C., and Spiegelman, D. (1989). Correction of logistic regression relative risk estimates and confidence intervals for systematic within-person measurement error. *Statistics in Medicine* 8, 1051–1070.

Rothman, K.J. (1976). Causes. *American Journal of Epidemiology* 104, 587–593.

Rothman, K.J. and Greenland, S. (1998). *Modern Epidemiology.* Second Edition. Philadelphia: Lippincott-Raven.

Rotnitzky, A. and Robins, J. (1997). Analysis of semiparametric regression models with non-ignorable nonresponse. *Statistics in Medicine* 16, 81–102.

Royston, P. and Altman, D.G. (1994). Regression using fractional polynomials of continuous covariates: Parsimonious parametric modelling (with discussion). *Applied Statistics* 43, 429–467.

Rubin, D.B. and Schenker, N. (1991). Multiple imputation in health-care databases: An overview and some applications. *Statistics in Medicine* 10, 585–598.

Samet, J.M., Kutvirt, D.M., and Christensen, L.M. (1982). Media coverage of coffee study has little impact on coffee consumption. *New England Journal of Medicine* 307, 129.

Sato, T. (1992a). Maximum likelihood estimation of the risk ratio in case-cohort studies. *Biometrics* 48, 1215–1221.

Sato, T. (1992b). Estimation of a common risk ratio in stratified case-cohort studies. *Statistics in Medicine* 11, 1599–1605.

Schlesselman, J.J. (1982). *Case-control Studies: Design, Conduct, Analysis.* New York: Oxford University Press.

Schulman, K.A., Berlin, J.A., Harless, W., et al. (1999). The effects of race and sex on physicians' recommendations for cardiac catheterization. *New England Journal of Medicine* 340, 618–626.

Scott, A.J. and Wild, C.J. (1997). Fitting regression models to case-control data by maximum likelihood. *Biometrika* 84, 57–71.

Segal, M.R. (1995). Extending the elements of tree-structured regression. *Statistical Methods in Medical Research* 4, 219–236.

Self, S., Prentice, R., Iverson, D., Henderson, M., Thompson, D., Byar, D., Insull, W., Gorbach, S.L., Clifford, C., Goldman, S., Urban, N., Sheppard, L., and Greenwald, P. (1988). Statistical design of the women's health trial. *Controlled Clinical Trials* 9, 119–136.

Selvin, S. (1996). *Statistical Analysis of Epidemiologic Data.* Second Edition. New York: Oxford University Press.

Shekelle, R.B., Shryock, A.M., Paul, O., Lepper, M., Stamler, J., Liu, S., and Raynor, W.J. (1981). Diet, serum cholesterol, and death from coronary heart disease. The Western Electric Study. *New England Journal of Medicine* 304, 65–70.

Siemiatycki, J. and Thomas, D.C. (1981). Biological models and statistical interactions: An example from multistage carcinogenesis. *International Journal of Epidemiology* 10, 383–387.

Sommer, A., Tarwotjo, I., Djunaedi, E., West, K.P., Loedin, A.A., Tilden, R., Mele, L., and the Aceh Study Group (1986). Impact of vitamin A supplementation on childhood mortality: A randomized controlled community trial. *Lancet* 1, 1169–1173.

Stafford, R. Unpublished work.

Stampfer, M.J., Colditz, G.A., and Willett, W.C. (1990). Menopause and heart disease. A review. *Annals of the New York Academy of Sciences* 592, 193–203.

Tavani, A. and La Vecchia, C. (2000). Coffee and cancer: a review of epidemiological studies, 1990–1999. *European Journal of Cancer Prevention* 9, 241–256.

Thompson, W.D. (1991). Effect modification and the limits of biological inference from epidemiologic data. *Journal of Clinical Epidemiology* 44, 221–232.

Trichopoulos, D., Handanos, N., Danezis, J., Kalandidi, A., and Kalapothaki, V. (1976). Induced abortions and secondary infertility. *British Journal of Obstetrics and Gynaecology* 83, 645–650.

Tuyns, A.J., Péquignot, G., and Jensen, O.M. (1977). Le cancer de l'oesophage en Ille-et-Vilaine en fonction des niveaux de consommation d'alcool at de tabac. *Bulletin du Cancer* 64, 45–60.

Vach, W. (1994). *Logistic Regression with Missing Values in the Covariates.* Lecture Notes in Statistics 86. New York: Springer-Verlag.

Vach, W. (1998). Missing data in epidemiologic studies. In *Encyclopedia of Biostatistics.* Editors-in-Chief: Armitage, P. and Colton, T. New York: John Wiley & Sons.

Vach, W. and Blettner, M. (1991). Biased estimation of the odds ratio in case-control studies due to the use of ad-hoc methods of correcting for missing values for confounding variables. *American Journal of Epidemiology* 134, 895–907.

Vach, W. and Schumacher, M. (1993). Logistic regression with incompletely observed categorical covariates—a comparison of three approaches. *Biometrika* 80, 353–362.

van Belle, G. (2002). *Statistical Rules of Thumb.* New York: John Wiley & Sons.

van der Laan, M. and Robins, J. (2002). *Unified Methods for Censored Longitudinal Data and Causality.* New York: Springer-Verlag.

Wacholder, S. (1991). Practical considerations in choosing between the case-cohort and nested case-control design. *Epidemiology* 2, 155–158.

Wacholder, S., McLaughlin, J.K., Silverman, D.T., and Mandel, J.S. (1992a). Selection of controls in case-control studies, I. Principles. *American Journal of Epidemiology* 135, 1019–1028.

Wacholder, S., McLaughlin, J.K., Silverman, D.T., and Mandel, J.S. (1992b). Selection of controls in case-control studies, II. Types of controls. *American Journal of Epidemiology* 135, 1029–1041.

Wacholder, S., McLaughlin, J.K., Silverman, D.T., and Mandel, J.S. (1992c). Selection of controls in case-control studies, III. Design options. *American Journal of Epidemiology* 135, 1042–1051.

Waksberg, J. (1978). Sampling methods for random digit dialing. *Journal of the American Statistical Association* 73, 40–46.

Weinberg, C.R., Umbach, D.M., and Greenland, S. (1994). When will nondifferential misclassification preserve the direction of a trend? *American Journal of Epidemiology* 140, 565–571.

Weitoft, G.R., Hjern, A., Haglund, B., and Rosén, M. (2003). Mortality, severe morbidity, and injury in children living with single parents in Sweden: A population-based study. *Lancet* 361, 289–295.

Willett, W. (1998) *Nutritional Epidemiology.* 2nd Edition. New York: Oxford University Press.

Winkelstein, W., Jr. (1995). Spontaneous abortion and coronary heart disease. *Journal of Clinical Epidemiology* 48, 500.

Winkelstein, W., Jr. and Rekate, A.C. (1964). Age trend of mortality from coronary heart disease in women and observations on the reproductive patterns of those affected. *American Heart Journal* 67, 481–488.

Winkelstein, W., Jr., Stenchever, M.A., and Lilienfeld, A.M. (1958). Occurrence of pregnancy, abortion, and artificial menopause among women with coronary artery disease: A preliminary study. *Journal of Chronic Diseases* 7, 273–286.

Woodward, M. (1999). *Epidemiology Study Design and Data Analysis.* New York: Chapman & Hall.

Zeger, S. and Liang, K.-Y. (1986). Longitudinal data analysis for discrete and continuous outcomes. *Biometrics* 42, 121–130.

Zelen, M. (1971). The analysis of several 2×2 contingency tables. *Biometrika* 58, 129–137.

Zhang, H. and Bracken, M.B. (1996). Tree-based, two-stage risk factor analysis for spontaneous abortion. *American Journal of Epidemiology* 144, 989–996.

Zhang, H., Holford, T., and Bracken, M.B. (1996). A tree-based method of analysis for prospective studies. *Statistics in Medicine* 15, 37–49.

Zhang, H. and Singer, B. (1999). *Recursive Partitioning in the Health Sciences.* New York: Springer-Verlag.

Glossary of Common Terms and Abbreviations

Acyclic Graph Causal graph where no directed path forms a closed loop, so that no variable can cause itself in a feedback loop

Additive Interaction Scenario where Excess Risks for two exposures taken singly do not merely add to obtain the Excess Risk for combined exposure to both factors together; equivalent to homogeneity of the Excess Risk for one factor over levels of the other

Ancestor of A Node, B, in a causal graph where there is a directed path beginning at B and leading to A

AR Attributable risk

Attributable Risk Fraction of cases in population that would be eliminated if eradication of exposure leaves all individuals with observed risk for the unexposed

Backdoor Path from A to B A path in a causal graph that leaves the variable A along an edge pointing into A, and then proceeds to B

Berkson's Bias Selection bias that arises from using samples of hospitalized individuals to estimate association of characteristics in the population

Binary Outcome Data Data for which the outcome variable can assume only two values

C Extraneous factor, potential confounding variable

Case-Cohort Study Study based on a random sample of cases and a random sample of the entire study population

Case-Control Study Study based on random samples of populations with differing disease characteristics

Causal Graph Graph that displays causal and other relationships between variables of interest

Centering Practice of normalizing a variable by measuring from a central value in meaningful increments; used to minimize collinearity when fitting interaction or quadratic terms in a regression model

CHD Coronary heart disease

χ^2 **Test** Test for independence of exposure and disease

χ^2_{gof} **Test** Test statistic used to examine adequacy of a model relating exposure variables to disease, often used to examine whether some form of linear trend is appropriate

χ^2_H **Test** Test statistic used to examine homogeneity of measure of association relating exposure and disease, across levels of other extraneous factors, usually constructed using either the Woolf or Breslow–Day methods

$\chi^2_{overall}$ **Test** Test statistic used to examine independence of exposure and disease when there are several exposure categories

χ^2_{trend} **Test** Test statistic used to examine monotonic trend in risk of disease over increasing levels of an ordered exposure variable

Child of A Node, B, in a causal graph where there is a directed edge pointing from A to B

Classification Tree Flexible regression model for associating many risk factors to the risk of disease, that does not assume additivity of effects from different risk factors

Cochran–Mantel–Haenszel Test Summary test of independence of exposure and disease, controlling for the potential confounding effects of variables, C, and assuming there is no interaction between these variables, C, and the exposure and disease relationship

Cohort Study Study based on random samples of populations with differing exposure characteristics

Collapsibility Situation where tables yielding exposure and disease distribution, stratified by other variables, can be pooled into a summary table without altering the level of observed association between the exposure and disease as given by a specific measure of association

Collider Variable, or node, A, on a path in a causal graph where the edges of the path entering and leaving A both have arrows pointing into A

Collinearity High correlation between risk factors in a regression model, often caused where one factor is an interaction or quadratic term including the other factor

Conditional Maximum Likelihood Variant of maximum likelihood procedure used to estimate regression models with matched, or finely stratified, data

Confounding Distortion of a causal effect induced by the association of variables with both exposure and disease

Counterfactuals Putative disease outcomes for individuals under alternative exposure conditions than those actually experienced

Cox Model Regression model that associates risk factors with the hazard of a disease; used to model data on incidence times and varying lengths of follow-up time in a study; accommodates time-varying exposures and differential loss to follow-up

D Disease or outcome variable

Degrees of Freedom Comparative measure of flexibility between two competing models or hypotheses; often used to specify a particular χ^2 null distribution for comparison of the two models, associated with the likelihood ratio test

Descendant of A Node, B, in a causal graph where there is a directed path beginning at A and leading to B

Differential Measurement Error Measurement errors in individual's exposure that vary depending on their disease status

Directed Graph Causal graph where every edge has a directed arrow reflecting cause and effect

Directed Path Series of edges in a causal graph that follows a single direction from node to node

E Exposure variable

$E(a)$ Expectation of a random variable a

Edge Link between two variables, or nodes, in a causal graph

ER Excess Risk

Excess Risk Absolute difference in incidence proportions, or risks of disease outcome in exposed and unexposed subpopulations

Fractional Polynomial Polynomials of a risk factor that include simple and fractional powers of the risk factor; used to provide flexible model that allows risk of disease to change smoothly with the risk factor without making rigid assumptions such as linearity

Frequency Matching Practice of choosing groups of individuals that share the distribution of matching factors that have few large categories, used when selecting exposed and unexposed groups in a cohort study, or cases and controls in a case-control study

Generalized Additive Model Flexible regression model for associating many risk factors to the risk of disease, that maintains additivity of effects from different risk factors without necessarily assuming a linear model for any specific factor

$h(t)$ Hazard function at time t

$h_E(t)$ Hazard function for exposed individuals at time t; analogous definition for $h_{\bar{E}}(t)$

Hazard Function Instantaneous incidence rate at specific point in time

Hosmer–Lemeshow Test Global or overall test of the goodness of fit, or adequacy, of a regression model for disease risk; may detect gross inadequacies of a specified model

$I(t)$ Incidence Proportion over the risk interval from 0 until time t, using appropriate time scale

Incidence Proportion Proportion of defined population, at risk at beginning of time interval, that become incident cases of disease by end of the interval

Likelihood Function Probability of data given a certain model that relates risk of disease to risk factors; used to provide estimates and confidence intervals for model parameters

Likelihood Ratio Test Test that examines hypotheses regarding parameters of a model that relates risk of disease to risk factors; based on comparison of values of the maximized log likelihood function at differing assumptions specified by nested null and alternative hypotheses

Linear Regression Model for Risk Model that assumes risk of disease changes linearly with changes in each risk factor

log$x$ The logarithm of a number x; used here to refer to the natural logarithm of x, $\log_e x$, or $\ln x$

Logistic Regression Model for Risk Model that assumes that the log odds of disease changes linearly with changes in each risk factor

Log Linear Regression Model for Risk Model that assumes that the logarithm of the risk of disease changes linearly with changes in each risk factor

Log Rank Test Test of independence of risk factor and incidence of disease that uses exact times of disease incidence and accounts for varying times of follow-up

Low Birthweight Infant birthweight less than 2500 g

Lowess Algorithm to produce estimates of risk, or log odds, of disease that change smoothly with changes in a risk factor without making rigid assumptions such as linearity

Mantel–Haenszel Estimate Summary estimate of a measure of association based on a weighted average of stratum-specific measures

Maximum Likelihood Estimate Estimate of a parameter of a model that relates risk of disease to risk factors

McNemar Test Test of independence of exposure and disease based on matched data

Measurement Error Errors in measurement of exposure or disease

Misclassification Measurement errors in binary factors including exposure or disease

Multiplicative Interaction Scenario where Relative Risks, or Odds Ratios, for two exposures taken singly do not merely multiply to obtain the Relative Risk (or Odds

Ratio) for combined exposure to both factors together; equivalent to homogeneity of the Relative Risk (or Odds Ratio) for one factor over levels of the other

n Total sample size

n_A Number of sampled individuals with characteristic A

$N_E(t)$ Number of exposed individuals at risk of disease at time t; analogous definition for $N_{\bar{E}}(t)$

Nested Case-Control Study Case-control study based on sampling cases and controls from a larger subpopulation or cohort

Nested Models Two models for which one of the models is a special case of the more general second model

Node Symbol for a variable in a causal graph

Observational Study Study based on sampling populations without control over exposure variables

OR Odds Ratio

$\widehat{OR}$ Sample estimate of population Odds Ratio; analogous definition for $\widehat{RR}$, $\widehat{ER}$, $\widehat{AR}$, etc.

Odds Ratio Ratio of odds of disease outcome in exposed and unexposed sub-populations

Pair Matching Practice of choosing two individuals that share the same value of specified matching factors, used when selecting exposed and unexposed individuals in a cohort study, or a case and control in a case-control study

Partial Likelihood Variant of maximum likelihood used to estimate regression models with exact times to either incidence or end of follow-up

π_{case} Sampling fraction, or probability, for cases in a case-control study

$\pi_{control}$ Sampling fraction, or probability, for controls in a case-control study

$P(A)$ Probability of event A, or probability that a randomly sampled individual from a population has characteristic A

$P(A|B)$ Conditional probability of event A, given B, or probability that a randomly sampled individual from a population has characteristic A, given that they have characteristic B

Point Prevalence Proportion of defined at risk population that are affected by disease at specified point in time

Population-Based Study Study based on random sample of population with sampling not based on individuals' exposure or disease characteristics

Probit Regression Model for Risk Model that assumes that the inverse cumulative function of the standard Normal distribution, applied to the risk of disease, changes linearly with changes in each risk factor

Proportional Hazards Assumption that the Relative Hazard associated with exposure comparisons remains constant over time

Randomization Assumption Key assumption that which exposure condition is observed for an individual does not depend on the outcomes of any counterfactual for that individual

Randomized Study Study based on randomizing exposure or intervention variables to participants

Relative Hazard Ratio of hazard functions in exposed and unexposed subpopulations

Relative Risk Ratio of incidence proportions, or risks of disease outcome, in exposed and unexposed subpopulations

RH Relative Hazard

RR Relative Risk

$S(t)$ Survival function, equals $1 - I(t)$, proportion of defined population, at risk at beginning of time interval, that is disease free (has not experienced the outcome) by time t

SIMEX Simulation-Extrapolation method for adjusting sample estimators to allow for measurement error by adding additional error through simulation, and then extrapolating back to the scenario of no measurement error

Study Population Population from which we are able to sample in performing an epidemiological study

Target Population Population to which we wish to apply information gained from epidemiological study

Type B Behavior type characterized by aggressiveness and competitiveness

Type A Behavior type characterized by relaxedness and noncompetitiveness

V Variance of a random variable

Wald Test Test that examines hypotheses regarding parameters of a model that relates risk of disease to risk factors; based on maximum likelihood estimate and its associated variability

Woolf's Estimate Summary estimate of a measure of association based on a weighted average of stratum-specific measures

$z_{1-\frac{\alpha}{2}}$ The $\left(1 - \frac{\alpha}{2}\right)$th percentile of the standard Normal distribution

Index

Note: Italicized pages refer to notes, illustrations, and tables.

2 × 2 tables, 59
  calculating expectations in, *155*
  Cochran-Mantel-Haenszel test, 126
  generic form of, *45*
  Mantel-Haenszel method, 130
  simple notation for, 155
  summary of test of association in, 123–125
  symbols for entries in, *60, 166*

A

Abortion, 260
  and incidence of coronary heart disease, 265–266, 271–274
  and pregnancy, 6
  and smoking, 267–268
Accident fatalities, 3
Acyclic directed causal graphs, 103–105
  and confounding, 107–108
  instrumental variables in, 117
Additive interaction, 149–150, 161
Additive models, generalized, 285–289
Age, 1
  baseline measurement of, *288*
  as confounding variable, 123
  in Cox model, *293*
  as exposure variable, 170
  as factor in treatment of diseases, 3
  in logistic regression models, *293*
  as risk factor for coronary heart disease, 247–250
  time as, 9
AIDS, 1, 289
Air pollution, 290
Alcohol consumption, 15–16
  binge drinking in, 16
  and pancreatic cancer, 78

as specific risk exposure, 1
Analysis of covariance, 139
Analysis of variance, 139
Ancestor nodes, 105
Antagonism, 147, 161
Antibodies, 52
Antilogarithm, 78
A priori method, 5
Asbestos exposure, 149, 152
Association
  overall test of, 165–166
  relative risk as primary source of, 184
  summary test of, 123–124
Association, measures of
  attributable risk, 38–40
  errors in, 86–87
  excess risk, 37–38
  odds ratio, 32–33
  plot of, *36*
  relative hazard, 35–37
  relative risk, 31–32
Assumptions, in causal graphs, 105–106
Attributable risk, 38–40
  See also Risks
  in case-control studies, 50
  estimation of, 84–85
Austria, 3
Autism, 102

B

Backdoor paths, in causal graphs, 107–109
Backward stepwise regression method, 246
Barrier contraceptives, 169
Baseline groups, 148
Baseline hazard function, 291

Bayesian methods, 62, 270

Behavioral indicators, 1

Behavior type and coronary heart disease
  counterfactual patterns in, *151*
  in Cox model, *293*
  homogeneity tests in, *159*
  in logistic regression models, *293*
  measurement errors, *88*
  stratified by body weight, *124*, 157
  x_2 test statistic for, 82–83

Berkson's bias, 26–28

Bias, 75

Binary exposure, 188–190
  in coffee drinking and pancreatic cancer, 227
  in Western Collaborative Group Study (WCGS), 207–209

Binary outcome data, 4, 289–290

Binary risk factor, 31

Binary variables, 82

Binomial distribution, 262

Biological agents, 16

Biomarkers, 16, 237

Birth order, 274–276

Birthweight, 4
  and attributable risk for infant mortality, 39–40
  in cohort studies, 48
  and excess risk for infant mortality, 37–38
  and infant mortality, 20, 32
  linear regression analysis of, 182–183
  and marital status of mother, 20–21, *60*
  in population-based studies, 46
  and relative risk for infant mortality, 32

Blood banks, 51–52, 55

Blood pressure, 2
  See also Coronary heart disease
  baseline measurement of, *288*
  confounding effects of, 180
  in Cox model, *293*
  in logistic regression models, *293*
  as risk factor for coronary heart disease, 82, 247–250

BMDP® (statistical software), 8

Body weight and coronary heart disease
  baseline measurement of, *288*
  centering variables in, 233
  counterfactual patterns in, 150–151
  degrees of freedom, 224
  estimated standard errors in, 224
  goodness of fit test for, 171–173
  indicator variables for discrete exposures in, 191–196
  likelihood function in, 202–204
  Mantel-Haenszel test statistics for, 131–133
  quadratic models, 233–235
  regression coefficients in, 206–207
  relative risks for, 135–136

Bonferroni corrected level, 126

Bootstrap method, 90, 239

Boston, Massachusetts, 78, 301

Box plots, 255

Breast cancer
  and childbearing, 162
  family history of, 161
  and hormone placement therapy, 302
  incidence of, 12
  and level of serum cholesterol, 117
  risk of, 53–54

Breslow-Day method, 158, 230

C

Caffeine, 95

Calendar time, 9

California, mortality data for Caucasian males in, *14*

Caliper matching, 278

Cancer registries, 51

Carcinogenesis, 161

Cardiac catheterization, 41

Case-cohort studies, 53–55
  estimation of relative risk in, 86
  odds ratio in, 86, 218

Case-control studies, 48–50
  See also Cohort studies;
    Population-based studies; Study designs
  on coffee drinking and pancreatic cancer, 78–79
  confounding in, 119
  disadvantages of, 55

estimation of attributable risk in, 85
frequency matching in, 257–258
key variants of, 50–55
for large samples, 67–68
logistic regression models in,
    212–215, 218
matching in, 180
nested, 51
pair matching in, 258–262
risk-set sampling of controls in, 51–53
sampling distribution in, 77
sampling fractions in, 213
Categorical data, 5
Catheterization, 41
Causal effects
of coffee drinking, 95–96
computation of, 96
of intervention assignment, 118
of vaccination, 102
Causal graphs, 102–105
assumptions in, 105–106
backdoor paths in, 107–109
of childhood vaccinations and health
    conditions, 106–107
in choosing crucial confounders,
    111–112
controlling confounding in, 109–112
vs. counterfactuals, 116
in goodness of fit procedures, 254
in inferring presence of confounding,
    107–109
nodes of, 103–105
Causal inference, 94
confounding variables, 99–100
counterfactuals, 94–99
Causality, 5
Causal relative risk, 97–99
Causal risk, 152
Causation, 116
Centering variables, 233
Centers for Disease Control, 8
Cervical cancer, 51
Childhood mortality, 118
Child nodes, 104
Cholecystitis, 26–28
Cholesterol, 11
baseline level, 255, *288*
and breast cancer, 117

confounding effects of, 180
and coronary heart disease, 82
in Cox model, *293*
in logistic regression models, *293*
measurement over time, 298
missing data, 238
predictors of, 239
as risk factor for coronary heart
    disease, 247–250
Chronic diseases, 147
Chronic exposures, 16
Chronological time, 9
Cigarette lighters, 93
Classification trees, 287–289
Clinical records, 26–27
Clinical treatment, 2
Clinical trials, 3
Closed populations, incidence
    proportions in, 15
Cluster sampling, 28
CMV (cytomegalovirus), 160–161
Cochran-Mantel-Haenszel test,
    125–128
in confounding effects of extraneous
    variables, 175–176
in homogeneity tests, 159
in logistic regression models, 224
log rank test, 295
in pair matching, 259, 262–264
in Western Collaborative Group
    Study (WCGS), 132–133
Coffee drinking, 3
abstainers, 167
causal effect of, 95
odds ratio in, 86–87
population data on, *97–98*
Coffee drinking and pancreatic cancer, 6
counterfactuals in, *95*
eliminating confounding effects in,
    100–103, 138–139
logistic regression models, 215–218,
    227–230
odds ratio in, 78–79
ordered categories in, 244
overview of, 301
sex as variable in, *124*
trend in risk, 173–175
x_2 test statistic for, 167

Cohort studies, 47–48
  See also Case-control studies;
    Population-based studies; Study
    designs
  assessment of significance in, 62–64
  disadvantages of, 55
  estimation of attributable risk in, 85
  estimation of excess risk in, 83–84
  excess risk in, 77
  for large samples, 67–68
  relative risk in, 77
  variance in, 77–78
Collapsibility, 112–115, 222
Collection of data, 2
Colliders, 104
  controlling for, 110–111
  medical care access as, 109
Collinearity, 232
  in explanatory variables, 235
  and risk factors, 140
Colon cancer, 108
Colon polyps, 108
Concordant pairs, 260, 278
Conditional likelihood method, 143, 271
Conditional maximum likelihood, 236,
  271
Conditional probabilities, 24–26
  Berkson's bias, 26–28
  in case-control studies, 49
  in cohort studies, 48
  independence of two events in, 26
  in odds ratio, 71
  in population-based studies, 45, 46
  in relative risk, 33, 81–82
Confidence intervals, 5
  for excess risk, 136–138
  for logarithmic relative risk, 134–135
  for log odds ratio, 130
  for odds ratio, 77–78, 80, 128–134,
    215
  for relative risk, 134–136
  for unknown population proportion,
    22–24
Confidence limits, 24
  for attributable risk, 84
  in likelihood function, 205
Confounding, 93
  adjustments for, 175–176

assessment with logistic regression
    models, 221–223
  control by stratification, 100–102
  controlling, 109–112
  definition of, 98
  eliminating effects of, 101
  empirical approach to, 142–143
  inferring presence of, 107–109
  and interaction effects, 265–268
  necessary conditions for, 118
  with nonmatching variables, 266–268
  and precision, 138–142
  quantitative measures of, 116
  schematic of, *99*
  and statistical interaction, *113*
Confounding factors, 93, 181
Confounding variables, 99–100
  in frequency matching, 257–258
  and stratification, 118–119
Consistency of association, 152–159
Consumption of coffee. *See* Coffee
    drinking
Consumption of tobacco. *See* Smoking
Contraceptives, 169
Controls, risk-set sampling of, 51–53
Control sampling, 51–53, 55
Coronary heart disease, 10
  and abortion, 260, 265–266, 271–274
  and behavior type. *See* Behavior type
    and coronary heart disease
  and body weight. *See* Body weight
    and coronary heart disease
  excess risk estimation of, 37, 136–138
  and hormone placement therapy, 302
  incidence rate of, 37
  lifestyle variables, 82
  mortality in, 301
  and pregnancy, 264–265
  prevalence and incidence data on, *11*
  relative risk for, 37, 135–136
  risk factors, 2, 3, 6
  and smoking, 267–268, *294*, 297
  and spontaneous abortion, 264–265
Counterfactuals, 94–99
  vs. causal graphs, 116
  and interaction, 150–152, 161–162
  origin of, 116
Countermatching, 276–277

Covariance, analysis of, 139
Covariates, 2, 251
Cox model, 290–293
Cox regression model, 293–295
Cross-validation, 255
Cumulative incidence proportion, 10, 35
Cytomegalovirus (CMV), 160–161

D

Data collection, 2
Degrees of freedom, 166, 224
Delayed entry, 16
Delivery (childbirth), 274–276
Density sampling, 51, 52, 55
Descendant nodes, 105
Deviance, 206
Deviations, sum of, 127
Diabetes, 26–28
Diagnosis, *4*, 9
Diastolic blood pressure, *288*
Dietary factors, 2
Dietary fat, 117
Dietary fiber, 108
Diet sugar, *110*
Differential errors, 87
Differential loss to follow-up, 296–297
Directed causal graphs, 103–108
Discordant pairs, 261
Discrete exposures, 165
    See also Exposures
    coffee drinking and pancreatic
        cancer, 167, 173–175
    confounding in, 175–176
    exact tests, 175–176
    goodness of fit, 170–171
    indicator variables for, 191–196
    interaction in, 175–176
    nonlinear trends in risk in, 170–171
    overall test of association, 165–166
    qualitative variables in, 169–170
    test for trend in risk in, 167–171
    Western Collaborative Group Study
        (WCGS), 171–173
Disease-based sampling, 48–50
Disease-exposure association, measures
    of
    attributable risk, 38–40
    errors in, 86–87

    excess risk, 37–38
    odd ratio, 32–35
    population in, 44
    relative hazard, 35–37
    relative risk, 31–32
Disease occurrence, measures of
    disease rates, 12–15
    hazard function, 12–14
    incidence, 9–11
    prevalence, 9–11
Diseases, 1–2
    incidence of, 9–11
    incidence rate of, 12–13
    occurrence of. *See* Occurrence of
        diseases
    prevalence of, 9–11
    rates, 12–13
    risk of, 1
Diuretics, 95
Dose-response effect, 185, 191–193
Dummy variables, 191–193

E

Ecologic studies, 3, 16
Educational status, 1
Effect modification, 128
Employment records, 16
Endogeneous variables, 298
Epidemiological studies, 1–2
    statistical approaches to, 2–4
    statistical packages for, 8
Epi Info 2000 (statistical software),
    8
Estimators, 5
    for attributable risk, 84–85
    for excess risk, 83–84
    inverse probability weighted, 144
    for odds ratio, 73–81
    for relative risk, 81–83
Ethnicity, 4
Etiology of diseases, 10
Events, 19
    independence of, 26
    probability of, 25
    reversing roles of, 25
Evolution of diseases, *2*
Exact tests, 71, 175–176
Excess fraction, 40

Excess risk, 37–38
  See also Attributable risk; Odds
      ratio; Relative risk; Risks
  in additive interaction, 150
  in case-control studies, 49–50
  in cohort studies, 77
  confidence interval for, 136–138
  effect of stratification on, 141
  estimation of, 83–84
  homogeneity of, 157–158
  for infant mortality, 37–38
  and linear regression models, 182–183
  in slope parameters, 182
  summary estimates for, 136–138
Exogeneous variables, 298
Expectation, 5
Experimental studies, 3
Explanatory variables, 1
  collinearity in, 232, 235
  measures of, 4
  missing data in, 239
Exponential function, 77
Exposed population, 35
Exposure-based sampling, 47–48
Exposures
  assessment of, 16, 45
  binary, 188–190
  binary outcome data in, 4
  data collection, 4
  discrete, 191–193
  groups, 47
  and incidence, 35–36
  indicator variables, 191–193
  under laboratory conditions, 94
  measurement of, 9
  natural order in levels of, 168
  overall test of association, 165–166
  probabilities, 62
  qualitatively ordered variables of,
      169–170
  randomization of, 99
  reference level of, 160
  and roles of disease, 34–35
  time-dependent, 296
Exposure variables, 2
  in assessment of confounding, 222
  replicates of, 237
  scale of, 243–246

sensitivity and specificity of, 89
Expression, 1–2
Extraneous factors, 93
  summary estimates and confidence
      intervals for excess risk, 136–138
  summary estimates and confidence
      intervals for odds ratio, 128–134
  summary estimates and confidence
      intervals for relative risk, 134–136
  summary test of association, 123–128
Extreme interaction, 160–161
Eye color, 5

F

Family history, 108–109
Family income, *4*
Family size, *4*
Fetal alcohol syndrome, 16
Fibers, intake of, 108
Finland, serum banks in, 51
First-born children, 274
Fisher exact test, 71
Flexible regression model, 285–289
Fluoridation, 110–111
Forward stepwise regression method,
  246
Fractional polynomials, 245–246
Frequency histograms, *75*, *76*
Frequency matching, 119, 257–258
  See also Matched studies; Pair
      matching

G

Gall bladder, inflammation of, 26–28
Gambling, 32
Generalized additive models, 285–289
Generalized linear model, 196
Gestational age, 274–276
GLIM® (statistical software), 8
Gold standard method, 87, 237
Goodness of fit, 170–171, 250–252

H

Hair color, 5
Hazard functions, 13–14, 35
Hazard rate, 52
Health insurance, *4*, 74, 93

Height
    baseline measurement of, *288*
    as risk factor for coronary heart
        disease, 247–250
Herpes simple virus type 2 (HSV-2), 51
Heterogeneity tests, 230
High blood pressure, 2
Higher order interaction, 226
High-sugar diet, 110–111
HIV (human immunodeficiency virus)
    infection, 1
    and AIDS studies, 289–290
    risk of, 196
    and use of barrier contraceptives, 169
Homogeneity tests, 155–156
    Breslow-Day method, 158
    for excess risk, 157–158
    for odds ratio, 158
    power of, 158–159
    for relative risk, 157–158
Hormone placement therapy, 302
Hosmer-Lemeshow test, 252–254
Hospitalization rates, 28
Hospital records, 26–27
HSV-2 (herpes simple virus type 2), 51
Human cytomegalovirus (CMV),
    160–161
Hume, David, 116
Hypergeometric distribution, 70, 169
Hypothesis tests, 5, 61–62, 215

I

Immunosuppression, 160
Incidence, 9–11
    age-sex variation in, 118
    and exposure, 35–36
Incidence proportion, 10, 12
    in closed populations, 15–16
    and hazard function, 35
    and probability, 21–22
Incidence rate, 12
    of coronary heart disease, 37
    measurement with hazard function,
        35
Independence, 59–61
    of events, 26
    x_2 test for, 69–70

Independent observations, 289–290
Independent variables, 2
Indicator variables, 191–193, 226
Indonesia, childhood mortality in, 118
Induction, 1–2
Infant birthweight. *See* Birthweight
Infant mortality
    attributable risk for, 39–40
    by birthweight, *21*
    conditional probabilities of, 24–26
    excess risk for, 37–38, 182
    linear regression analysis of, 182–183
    by mother's marital status, *21*,
        39–40, 188–190
    probability of, 20
    regression models, *189*
    relative risk for, 32
    risk factors for, 40
Infection, 9, 160
Infectious agents, 22
Instrumental variables, 117
Intent-to-treat analysis, 118
Interaction, 94
    additive, 149–150
    adjustments for, 175–176
    and confounding, 101, *113*
    and counterfactuals, 150–152,
        161–162
    extreme, 160–161
    higher-order, 226
    in logistic regression models, 225–227
    with matching variables, 265–266
    multiplicative, 148–149
    with nonmatching variables, 266–268
Intercept coefficient, 192, 225
Intercept parameters, 182
    interpretation of, 187–188
    in logistic regression models, *293*
    and outcome-dependent sampling,
        214
Interval prevalence, 10
Intervention, 2
    additive interaction in, 161
    and attributable risk, 39
    causal effect of, 118
    randomized, 117
Inverse probability weighted estimators,
        144

Inverse weighting, 116
Item nonresponse, 238

J

Job records, 16
Joint probabilities, 45
  in case-control studies, 49
  in cohort studies, 48
  in population-based studies, 46

K

Kaposi's sarcoma, 290
Kundera, Milan, 95

L

Latency period, 1
Left truncation, 16
Levels of exposures, 165
  coffee drinking and pancreatic
    cancer, 167, 173–175
  confounding in, 175–176
  and dose-response effect, 185
  exact tests, 175–176
  goodness of fit in risk, 170–171
  indicator variables, 191–196
  interactions in, 175–176
  nonlinear trends in risk, 170–171
  overall test of association, 165–166
  qualitatively ordered variables in,
    169–170
  regression models, 179
  sampling fractions in, 213
  trend of risks in, 167–171
  Western Collaborative Group Study
    (WCGS), 171–173
Lifestyle variables, 82
Likelihood function, 199–201
  based on logistic regression models,
    200–201
  steepness of, 204
Likelihood intervals, 62
Likelihood ratio method, 205–206
  as alternative to x_2 test, 209
  and goodness of fit test, 251–252
  and partial likelihood function, 292
Linear regression models, 181–183
  for body weight and coronary heart
    disease, *195*

and estimating trend in risk, 169
for infant mortality and mother's
  marital status, *189*
Links, 196
Logarithmic relative risk, 134–135
Logarithmic transformation, 75–76
Log_e (natural logarithm), 76
Logistic regression models, 186–187
  See also Regression models
  in assessment of confounding,
    221–223
  binary outcomes in, 289–290
  in case-control studies, 212–215, 218
  centering variables in, 233
  of coffee drinking and pancreatic
    cancer, 215–218, 227–230
  collinearity in, 233
  of coronary heart disease and body
    weight, *195*
  for coronary heart disease and
    spontaneous abortions, *272*
  with correlated binary outcomes, 290
  Cox model, 291–295
  differential loss to follow-up, 296–297
  flexible, 285–289
  goodness of fit, 250–252
  for incidence of coronary heart
    disease in women, 271–274
  independent observations, 289–290
  for infant mortality and mother's
    marital status, *189*
  interaction in, 225–227
  likelihood function, 200–201, 219
  log likelihood function, 204–206
  for matched data, 269–271
  maximum likelihood estimate,
    204–206
  measurement errors in, 237
  missing data in, 237–240
  multiple, 190–196
  null hypotheses, 206–207
  parameters in, 187–188
  quadratic models in, 233–235
  restrictions on use of maximum
    likelihood method in, 235–236
  risk factors in, 250
  and time-dependent exposures, 296
  Western Collaborative Group Study

(WCGS), 208–212, 223–225, 230, *231*

Log likelihood function, 204–206

Log linear regression model, 183–184
  for body weight and coronary heart disease, *195*
  for infant mortality and mother's marital status, *189*

Log odds, 186, 196

Log odds ratio, 129–130
  in interaction in multiple logistic regression model, 225–227
  in interpretation of logistic regression parameters, 187–188

Log rank test, 295

Log risk, 196

Longitudinal studies, 290
  causal graphs in, 298
  causality in, 5
  data collection in, 4

Low birthweights of infants
  marginal frequency of, 62
  and marital status of mother, *64*
  and use of vitamin supplements, 72–73

Lung cancer, 147
  lifetime risk of, 32
  risk factors, 149, 152

M

Malnutrition, 2

Mantel-Haenszel method, 130–131
  in estimating excess risk, 136–138
  in estimating relative risk, 135–136
  in logistic regression models, 223
  and pair matching, 259
  in pair matching, 262–264
  in Western Collaborative Group Study (WCGS), 132–133

Marginal probabilities, 45
  in case-control studies, 49
  in cohort studies, 48
  in population-based studies, 46

Marginals, in stratification, 179–180

Marital status of mother
  and attributable risk for infant mortality, 39–40

in cohort studies, 48
  and excess risk for infant mortality, 38
  and infant birthweight, 20–21, *60*, *64*
  likelihood function, 199–201
  in population-based studies, 46

Matched studies
  breaking the match in, 277–278
  confounding and interaction effects, 265–268
  coronary heart disease in women, 264–265
  effect of birth order on respiratory distress syndrome in twins, 274–276
  frequency matching, 119, 257–258
  logistic regression models for, 269–274
  pair matching, 258–262

Matching, 180
  frequency, 257–258
  pair, 258–262

Matching variables
  interaction effects of, 265–266
  and risk factors, 269

Maximum likelihood method, 200–201
  in analysis of stratified data, 143
  estimated standard errors of, 222
  in estimating parameters in regression models, 218
  and log likelihood function, 204–206
  restrictions on use of, 235–236

McNemar's test, 262, 263

Measurement errors, 86–90, 237

Measures of association
  attributable risk, 38–40
  errors in, 86–87
  excess risk, 37–38
  odds ratio, 32–33
  plot of, *36*
  relative hazard, 35–37
  relative risk, 31–32

Medical records, 26–27

Medical treatment, 2

Mental health services, *4*

Misclassification, 86–90, 176

Missing data, 116, 237–240

Model building, 246–250

Model parameters, 182
Model selection methods, 255
Monotonic dose-response effect, 191–193
Mortality, 13–15
  in coronary heart disease, 301
  hazard function based on, *14*
Multiple imputation, 239
Multiple logistic regression model,
  190–191
  indicator variables for discrete
    exposures in, 191–196
  interaction in, 225–227
  for Western Collaborative Group
    Study (WCGS), *249–250*
Multiplicative interaction, 148–149
  in logistic regression models, 225
  null hypothesis in test for, *153*

N

Natural logarithm ($\log_e$), 76
Negative risks, 184
Nested case-control studies, 51
New England Journal of Medicine, The,
  302
New York Times, 301
Nightline, 41
Noncentral hypergeometric distribution,
  70, 156
Nondifferential errors, 87, 237
Nondifferential misclassification, 176
Nonmatching variables, 266–268
Nonresponse, 237
Nonsmokers, 149, 267–268
Normal density, plot for, *184*
Normal distribution, 22–24, 262
Norway, serum banks in, 51
Null hypothesis, 62
  of homogeneity, 159
  of independence, 61, 172, 174
  likelihood based methods, 205–206
  and regression coefficient, 206–207
  typical set of risks under, 168

O

Observable risks, 152
Observational studies, 3
  conditional probabilities in, 24–26

inference based on estimated
  probability in, 22–24
probability and incidence proportion
  in, 21–22
simple random samples in, 20–21
Occupational conditions, 16
Occurrence of diseases, 9
  incidence, 9–11
  prevalence, 9–11
  and probability, 22
  rates of, 12–15
Odds ratio, 32–33
  See also Attributable risk; Excess
    risk; Relative risk
  as approximation to relative risk,
    33–34
  associated with smoking, 273
  average estimates across strata for,
    130–131
  in case-cohort studies, 54, 218
  in case-control studies, 49–50, 54
  coffee drinking and pancreatic
    cancer, 227–228
  conditional maximum likelihood
    estimate of, 261–262
  confidence interval for, 77–78,
    128–134
  of coronary heart disease and body
    weight, 194–195
  of discordant pairs, 261
  estimation of, 73–81
  for expected data table, 52–53
  frequency histograms, *75, 76*
  and frequency matching, 259
  homogeneity of, 157–158
  individual stratum estimates of,
    129–130
  log, 129–130, 187–188, 225–227
  as measure of association of interest,
    153–154
  as measure of effect, 149
  modified estimator of, 86
  and multiple logistic regression
    model, 190–191
  in multiplicative interaction, 149
  in pair matching, 261–262
  pooled, 115
  vs. relative hazard, 291–293
  vs. relative risk, *34*, 41

roles of disease and exposure in, 34–35
sampling distribution of, 74–77
small sample adjustments, 79–81, 264
stratum-specific, 115, 125–127
summary estimates for, 128–134
Ordered categories, 244
Ordered discrete variables, 4
Ordinal responses, 290
Organ donor testing, 160
Organ rejection, 160
Outcomes, 19
conditional probability of, 24
potential, 116
Outcome variables, 4, 9
Outliers, 254
Overfitting of models, 255
Overmatching, 276

P

Pair matching, 258–264
See also Frequency matching; Matched studies
Pancreatic cancer, 3
case-control study of, *79*
and coffee drinking. *See* Coffee drinking and pancreatic cancer
population data on, *97–98*
population risks of, 96
risk factors, 225–226
and sex of individual, 99
sex strata, 257–258
and tea drinking, 95
Parent nodes, 104
Parents' smoking habits, 290
Partial likelihood, 291
PCP (pneumocystis carinii pneumonia), 290
Pearson x_2 test, 251–252
Period prevalence, 10
Pipelines, 99–100
Pneumocystis carinii pneumonia (PCP), 290
Point estimation, 215
Point prevalence, 10, 12
Poisson regression models, 16
Polyps, 108
Polytomous responses, 290

Pooled analysis, 278
Pooled odds ratio, 115
Population, 5, 43–44
association, 105
attributable risk, 40
estimated probability in, 22
incidence proportion in, 9, 35
period prevalence in, 9
random sampling of, 20, 28–29
sampling of, 28–29
study, 43–44, 53, 55
study designs based on, 45–47
subgroups of, 47
target, 43–44, 55
Population-based studies, 45–47
See also Case-control studies; Cohort studies; Study designs
assessment of significance in, 59–61
estimation of attributable risk in, 84
estimation of excess risk in, 83–84
hypothesis tests in, 61–62
interpretation of p-values in, 61–62
sampling distribution in, 77
Population probabilities, 45–46
Posttransplants, 160–161
Potential outcomes, 116
Power, 5
Precision, 180
Predictors, 1
Pregnancy
and incidence of coronary heart disease, 259, 271–274
risk during, 16
and spontaneous abortion, 6, 264–265
Premenarcheal childhood, 12
Prenatal care, 46–47
Prevalence, 9–11
Probability, 19
of composite events, 25
conditional. *See* Conditional probabilities
and incidence proportion, 21–22
inference based on, 22–24
Probit model, 184–185, *189*, *195*
Promotion, 1–2
Proportional hazards, 36
See also Relative hazards
and coufounding effects, 295

Proportional hazards (*Continued*)
  Cox model, 291
  and odds ratio, 52
Proportions, scaled difference in, *67*
Prospective studies, 45
Prostate cancer, 3
Prostate specific antigen (PSA), 3
PSA (prostate specific antigen), 3
Public health, 2
P-values, 5, 61–62

Q

Quadratic models, 233–235
Quasi-experimental studies, 3

R

Random digit dialing, 55
Random error, 87, 90
Random experiments, 19
Random guesses, 239
Randomized assumption, 98, 101
Randomized clinical trials, 3
Random sampling, 20
  advantages and disadvantages of,
    28–29
  in estimating measures of association,
    43
  in population-based studies, 45–46
Random variables, 5, 72
Rare diseases, 33, 41
Reference groups, 27, 148
Refractive errors, 27–28
Regression calibration, 237
Regression coefficient, 206–207
Regression models, 176
  in analysis of exposures at discrete
    levels, 179–181
  with binary exposure, 188–190
  flexible, 285–289
  linear, 181–183
  log linear, 183–184
  multiple logistic, 190–196
  probit, 184–185
  simple logistic, 186–188
Relative hazards, 35–37
  See also Proportional hazards
  risk factors in, 290–293
  and risk-set sampling, 52–53

and time-dependent exposures, 296
Relative risk, 31–32
  See also Attributable risk; Excess
    risk; Odds ratio; Risks
  in case-cohort studies, 86
  in case-control studies, 49–50
  causal, 97–99
  in cohort studies, 77
  and collapsibility over strata, 112–115
  conditional probabilities in, 33, 81–82
  confidence interval for, 134–136
  of coronary heart disease, 37
  effect of stratification on, 141
  estimation of, 81–82, 88–90
  homogeneity of, 157–158
  logarithmic, 134–135
  and log linear regression models,
    183–184
  Mantel-Haenszel estimate of, 135
  as measure of effect, 148, 149–150
  in multiplicative interaction, 148–149
  for CMV (cytomegalovirus) infection,
    160–161
  null hypothesis in, 166
  vs. odds ratio, 33–34, 41
  for posttransplant CMV diseases, 160
  as primary source of association, 184
  summary estimates for, 134–136
Renal transplants, 160
Repeated measures design, 290
Replicates, 237
Residuals, 251
Respiratory distress syndrome (RDS),
  274–276
Restrospective studies, 45
Rhode Island, 78, 301
Risk factors, 1
  adjusting for, 181
  binary, 31
  binary outcome data in, 4
  in confounding effects
    exposure-disease relationship,
    295–296
  interaction, 147
  and matching variables, 269
  and model building, 247
  in relative hazard, 290–293
  vulnerability of studies of, 98
  x_2 test for, *166*

Risks, 1
   attributable, 38–40
   excess, 37–38
   goodness of fit, 170–171
   vs. measures of association, *36*
   negative value for, 184
   nonlinear trends in, 170–171
   observable, 152
   relative, 31–32
   test for trend in, 167–169
   time at, 295–296
Risk-set sampling, 51–53, 218

S

Sample size
   in case-control studies, 67–69
   in cohort studies, 67–69
   and estimators of odds ratio, 79–81
   planning, 86
   and x_2 test, 70–71
Sampling, 5
   advantages and disadvantages of,
     28–29
   disease-based, 48–50
   distribution, 22–24
   exposure-based, 47–48
   fractions, 213, 218
   outcome-dependent, 214
   of population, 43–44
   random, 20
   random error in, 90
   risk-set, 51–53, 218
   statistical tools in, 2
   stratified, 28–29
   variance, 80
Sampling distribution, 74–77
   of attributable risk, 84
   hypergeometric distribution in, 169
   of relative risk, 81
   skewness of, 75
   of small sample estimator, 80
   with zero expectation, 77–78
SAS® (statistical software), 8
Scatterplot, 245–246, 255
Score method, 205
Screening, 3
Seat-belt laws, 3, 39
Second-born children, 274

Second-order interaction, 226
Secural trends, 274–276
Selection bias, 237
Self-reports, 16
Semiparametric theory, 240
Sensitivity, 87–88
Serum banks, 51–52, 55
Serum cholesterol. *See* Cholesterol
Severity of diseases, 3
Sex, 1
   as binary outcome variable, 4
   as confounding variable, 123
   as factor in pancreatic cancer, 99, 101
   as factor in treatment of diseases, 3
Significance, assessment of
   in case-control designs, 64–68
   in cohort designs, 62–64
   in population-based designs, 59–62
SIMEX (simulation exploration)
   method, 88–89, 237
Simple logistic regression models,
   186–188
Simple random samples, 20, 28–29
Single imputation method, 239
Slope coefficient, 192–193, 225, 231
Slope parameters, 182, 187–188
Smoking, 15–16
   and abortion, 267–268
   confounding effects of, 180
   and coronary heart disease, 3, 82,
     267–268, *294*, 297
   in Cox model, *293*
   in logistic regression models, *293*
   pack-years of, 16
   and pancreatic cancer, 78
   and relative risk for lung cancer, 32,
     149
   as risk factor for lung cancer, 152
   as specific risk exposure, 1
Smoothing, 245
Social support, 243
Socioeconomic status (SES), 1
   and access to medical care, 102, 106
   and childhood vaccination, 102, 106
   and family history, 109
   and medical access, 111–112
Specificity, 88
S-Plus®(statistical software), 8

Spontaneous abortion, 260
  and incidence of coronary heart
    disease, 264–266, 271–274
  logistic regression models, 270
  odds ratio for, 273
  and pregnancy, 6
SPSS® (statistical software), 8
Standard normal density, plot for, *184*
STATA® (statistical software), 8, 24
Statistical interaction. *See* Interaction
Statistical software, 2, 8
Strata, 123–125
  collapsibility over, 112–115
  consistency of association, 152–159
Stratification, 100–102
  and collapsibility, 112–115
  by confounding factors, 119
  in controlling confounding, 109
  interaction between variables and
    exposure of interests in, 175–176
  logistic regression effect in, 219
  marginals in, 179–180
  and precision, 224–225
  symbols for entries in, *124*
Stratified sampling, 28–29
Stratum-specific odds ratio, 115,
  125–127
Stress, 243
Structural equation models, 106
Study designs, 3–4
  case-control, 48–50
  cohort, 47–48
  comparison of, 65–68
  population-based, 45–47
Study population, 43–44
  control sampling in, 55
  frequency matching, 257–258
  nonresponse in, 237
  subcohorts of, 53
Summary test of association, 123–125
  Cochran-Mantel-Haenszel test,
    125–128
  samples sizes in, 128
Survival analysis, 297
Survival functions, 14, *15*
Sweden, serum banks in, 51
Symptoms of diseases, 1
Synergism, 147, 161
Systolic blood pressure, *288*, *293*

T

Target population, 43–44
  causal relative risk in, 98
  control sampling in, 55
  missing data in, 238
  slope coefficient, 214
Tea drinking, 78, 95
Time, 9
Time at risk, 295–296
Time-dependent exposures, 296
Tirol, Austria, 3
Tobacco consumption. *See* Smoking
Tooth decay, 110–111
Transformation, 75–76
Treatment of diseases, 2
T-tests, 5
Tubercle bacilli, 2
Tuberculosis, 2
Twins, 274–276
Type I errors, 5
Type II errors, 5

U

Unexposed population, 35
Unmarried mother, 199–201
  confidence intervals for population
    proportion of, 23
  and infant births, 23
  and infant birthweight, *60*, *64*
  and infant mortality, 46–47
  marginal frequency of, 62
  nutrition, 46–47
  prenatal care of, 46–47
  relative risk for infant mortality, 32
Unordered discrete variables, 4
Urination, frequency of, 95
USA Today, 41

V

Vaccination
  causal effect of, 102
  causal graphs of, 106–107
  and health condition, 108–109
Validation information, 16
Variables, 4
  absence of variation in, 109
  instrumental, 117
  lifestyle, 82
  matching, 258–262, 265–266

nonmatching, 266–268
outcome, 9
Variance, 5
    analysis of, 139
    in cohort studies, 77–78
Vitamin A, 118
Vitamins, use of, 74

W

Wald method, 205
    as alternative to x_2 test, 209
    in logistic regression models,
        223–224
Washington Post, The, 41
Water fluoridation, 110–111
Western Collaborative Group Study
    (WCGS), 6
    coding for variables, *208*
    Cox model, *293*
    excess risk estimation of coronary
        heart disease in, 136–138
    exposure scale in, 244
    flexible regression model, 285–287
    goodness of fit test for, 171–173
    homogeneity tests in, *155*, 156–158
    Hosmer-Lemeshow test statistic for,
        252–254
    indicator variables for discrete
        exposures in, 191–193
    interactive effects in, *231*
    item nonresponse in, 238
    likelihood function, 200–201
    logistic regression models, 207–212,
        223–225, 230, *293*
    log rank test, 295

    Mantel-Haenszel method in, 131–133,
        135–137
    missing data in, 238
    model building in, 247–250
    multiple logistic regression model for,
        249–250
    relative risk, 82–83
    scatterplot in, 245–246
    summary of, 301
    Woolf's method in, 135–137
Women's Health Initiative, 302
Women's Health Trial, 53
Woolf's method, 129–130
    in estimating excess risk, 136–138
    in estimating relative risk, 134–136
    in homogeneity tests, 155, *157*
    in logistic regression models, 223
    in pair matching, 262–264
    in test of consistency of association,
        153–155
    in Western Collaborative Group
        Study (WCGS), 132–133, 230

X

X_2 test, 67
    alternative formulations of, 69–70
    for association, 165–166
    for homogeneity, *154*
    for independence, 126–127
    linear trend in, 170–171
    power of, 65–66
    and sample size, 70–71

Z

Zero expectation, 77